OPTIMAL HEALTH

How to Get It, How to Keep It

by

Dr. Randy W. Martin

Medicine Bear Publishing
Blue Hill, Maine
USA

OPTIMAL HEALTH
How to Get It, How to Keep It

Cover Design by Linda Deming

Comic art on pages 11, 76, 106, 180, 202, 215, 235, and 250 by Gerrit Huig

Editing, Text Design and Production by Sara Lyara Estes

This book is not meant to be a substitute for sound medical advice. If you have a chronic or acute health problem, please consult a health practitioner. Neither the author nor the publisher makes any claims about the effectiveness of the procedures, treatments or products described in this book. Health care is a complex and individual matter and no particular approach can be said to apply to all people and all situations.

ISBN 1-891850-16-4
Library of Congress Catalog Card Number 98-83056
Printed in USA on acid-free paper

MEDICINE BEAR PUBLISHING
P.O. BOX 1075
BLUE HILL, MAINE 04614-1075
USA

Contents

Contents

Contents

Contents

Contents

Contents

GRATITUDE

I'd like to express my thanks to:

- ❖ my patients. It is through their faith, trust, honesty, candor, and participation in their own personal healing process that I have come learn what true health in healing really is.

- ❖ Greg Brodsky, who taught my first class in Oriental healing techniques.

- ❖ Steven Rosenblatt, M.D., who had the courage and vision to start the California Acupuncture College.

- ❖ Denise Cavener, my anatomy teacher at Santa Monica College, who taught me it was OK to start a new career and that a part of me was indeed a scientist.

- ❖ Harry Oxenhandler, M.D., for letting me sing during my first acupuncture treatment and for sending me to Demelza.

- ❖ Demelza for showing me my Saturn return, which gave me the permission and freedom to channel my energy into the healing field.

- ❖ Carolyn Goldman, D.L., for giving me Ignatia 30X, my second homeopathic remedy, which helped me to cry, and clearly showed me the credibility of classical homeopathy.

- ❖ Dr. Hu Claybrooke, for being *the* most incredible teacher and healer; you are missed.

- ❖ Sydney Yudin, for having faith in herbal medicine and passing his knowledge and faith on to me.

- ❖ Drs. K. O. and S. George for their untiring faith in God and in homeopathy.

- ❖ Rabbi Ted Falcon, Ph.D., for his spiritual support and for telling me to become a chiropractor (and for my inner rebel and guide who instead did what he wanted).

- ❖ my mother, who taught me how to "feel" and "intuit" other people's pain.

- ❖ my dad, who taught me the importance of being out in the world and showed me it's okay to be a "health nut."

- ❖ Ellen Asher for helping me believe in myself.

- ❖ Shari Rosner for teaching me it is possible to connect consistently and under any condition or circumstance.

- ❖ Gerrit Huig for his fine artwork.

- ❖ Rabbi David Cooper and Vega Rosenberg for reminding me to stay in the light.

- ❖ Sara Estes for her great editing, insights, and graphic presentation.

- ❖ Medicine Bear Publishing and Jonathon Spinney for their incredible perseverance in getting the job done.

INTRODUCTION

Please accept this book as my humble offering to you. It is meant to stimulate your thoughts and feelings—your process of continued awareness and self-growth.

Some sections are very thorough. Others are mere outlines of the subject at hand. Please view this as a working document. After you have read it through, you may have questions or feel the need for more information.

Many of these essays are taken from articles I have written for other publications or as informational handouts for my patients and students. The field of holistic health is so vast it can be overwhelming, even to me—and I devote most of my waking hours to studying health and what it takes to achieve it.

If you have benefited by any part of this book, or if you feel any part in particular should be expanded, I would enjoy hearing from you. Your feedback is most welcome. I will be incorporating your comments, suggestions, and questions into my next book.

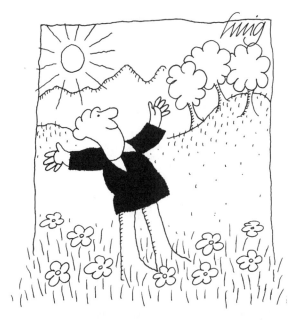

How many a man has dated a new era
in his life from reading a book!
—Henry David Thoreau

I use an eclectic and multidisciplinary approach to the practice of holistic medicine, so much of the material presented in this book will conflict with the theories of classical homeopathy. The suggestions for treatment could potentially antidote your remedies.

If you are taking homeopathic remedies prescribed by a classical homeopath, or are unsure whether you are being seen by a classical homeopath, it is best to check before following any of the herbal or homeopathic suggestions in this book.

MY PERSONAL STORY: HOW I CAME TO BELIEVE IN HOMEOPATHIC AND ORIENTAL MEDICINE

As a child I remember my dad forcing my brother and me to take vitamins. My dad was always into something new and whatever seemed weird. At times we had handfuls of multicolored vitamins to take with our morning orange juice and cereal.

I hated taking vitamins. Besides being a small child who had difficulty swallowing such large pills, I remember thinking it was stupid. But Dad spent a lot of money on them, and if we didn't use them up I knew he would be angry with us. Little did I know that years later I would come to be an expert on such matters. Would I be stretching things to say that he was probably my first influence or mentor in the area of alternative medicine?

Another memory is of my frequent stomach pains and what seemed like weekly visits to Kaiser Permanente of the San Fernando Valley in Los Angeles. I remember the long waits in the waiting room and the constant fear of the doctor and what he might do to me. His cold hands on my stomach, the cold metal instruments on my warm skin, and the secret whispers between the doctor and my mother—it was very frightening for a small child.

I think his name was Dr. Marshall, and my mother considered everything he said to be gospel, but they never did find anything wrong with my stomach and I continued to have stomach and digestive problems.

Now, of course, I know this to be what Oriental medicine calls a Damp Cold Spleen syndrome—nothing a few doses of homeopathic Nux. Vom. 12X or gentian root would have problems curing. My childhood diet was full of cheese, mayonnaise, milk, Cokes, and cold fruit juices and definitely added to my constitutional predisposition to digestive problems.

When I was sixteen and in tenth grade, I was initiated into Transcendental Meditation. Maybe it was that I took after my dad in terms of always wanting to try out things that were on the fringe, but I remember going to a TM lecture and being totally thrilled that I could get high on something natural—meditation. At any rate, my parents split the $35 initiation fee with me and I was off and meditating. At the time I was sure it was something I would continue to do for the rest of my life. But as the game of life progressed and I entered college, I gradually became interested in other things—like drugs.

With the exception of the stomach pain and weak digestion, I never did have any major health problems, thank God. As a college student in northern California at the University of California at Santa Cruz, I remember going to the Kaiser Permanente in San Jose for some type of general checkup. This is where I had a major turn of events. The experience radically changed my life forever.

I went to a medical doctor at Kaiser and begin to ask him some general questions. He said not to worry about any of the physical, health-related problems I was having, but to meditate instead. He was a TM-er himself and he told me that meditation had the power to reduce stress and heal almost any problem I was having.

I remember feeling at the time, "What good is a doctor if he's not gonna tell me what to do differently, or at least run some tests and give me some medications?" A part of me felt disappointed and angry, but another part of me was positively impressed. I remember feeling that he really blew my mind: A doctor telling me to look within! I was shocked and very impressed.

Years passed, and I found myself living and working in a small town in Oregon as an environmental resource planner for the state of Oregon. I had been a child of the Sixties and, as such, I had a major desire to help heal the planet. I decided that I could be most effective by working through, rather than against, the system. So I obtained a master's degree in urban and environmental planning jointly from the University of British Columbia and San Jose State University, and set off to do some serious environmental healing work in Oregon.

The only problem was that *I* needed some healing. I was totally stressed out by the Planning Commission and City Council meetings, and all the citizen groups' constant pressure and antagonism. I found myself responding to the stress by drinking coffee, eating sugar and salt, and getting into a very unhealthy cycle of fasting and bingeing. My blood sugar went crazy and my energy and moods were very unpredictable and unstable. Sadly, I found that in that small coastal Oregon town of only 6,000 people I had nobody to turn to for help.

I tried to get local doctors to give me a glucose tolerance test to check for hypoglycemia, but none of the local doctors believed in this disease. I heard that there was a medical doctor who practiced nothing but acupuncture in Corvallis, a town about an hour away. I secured his phone number and tried to schedule an appointment, but learned he had a three-month waiting list for new patients. I'm sure I made a nuisance of myself by calling so often and sounding so desperate, but I convinced his secretary that I was severely hypoglycemic and she scheduled an appointment for me.

This doctor was like no other doctor I'd ever met. He sat in a little child's chair low to the ground so that I was much larger and taller than him. Whenever I asked a question about my diet he would throw it back at me and force me to answer my own question. In short, he modeled for me what I would later come to term the "mirroring" concept of healing. This technique would eventually become the basis of my own medical practice.

My health, energy, and diet radically and quickly improved due to his care, love, and excellent acupuncture treatments. I used to drive the 2-hour round trip on a weekly basis and looked forward to the acupuncture treatments.

Years later, when I was in acupuncture college myself, I was always amazed that some of my fellow students were studying to become acupuncturists without ever having experienced acupuncture for themselves. For them, it was just a good business venture. In fact, many of them actually took recreational drugs and ate junk foods for the full 4 years of acupuncture college. I found this very strange.

I decided that, as an adjunct to the healing work I was doing with my acupuncturist up in Oregon, I would like to try something else as well. So I made an appointment to see a naturopath at the Portland School of Naturopathy. On some unconscious level, I was probably thinking of changing careers at this point, but on the surface my reason for going to the naturopathic doctor was to deal with my health.

This naturopath gave me my first homeopathic remedy. I will never forget this experience. Not only did the experience of taking the "little sugar pills" feel very rebellious, which I loved, but my acupuncturist told me not to take them because they were poison. The remedy was homeopathic *Merc. Sol. 30X,* composed of minute amounts of mercury. My acupuncturist thought I was taking *poisonous* mercury and that I would harm myself by taking it. Obviously, the acupuncturist knew nothing about homeopathic medicine. I believed the acupuncturist, stopped taking the pills, and never went back to the naturopath. Little did I realize that years later I would be curing strep throats by the dozens with this little jewel of a homeopathic remedy!

It wasn't until many years later that I came in contact with homeopathy again. I moved to Los Angeles for a family crisis and I was seeing a chiropractor and complaining of digestive problems. The chiropractor pulled out a little black book which looked a lot like a bible. She paged through the book and came up with a homeopathic remedy that looked like it precisely matched my symptoms. It was homeopathic *Ignatia*. She gave it to me in a 12X potency, and I had an experience which definitely changed my personal and professional life forever.

The week after my treatment, after having taken the Ignatia two or three times, I found myself feeling very emotional. In fact, I found myself letting out tears. I was able to cry for the first time that I could remember. I was amazed, excited, afraid, confused, and hopeful. "What *was* in those little white pills?" I wanted to know at my next chiropractic visit, and "Where can I get more information about them?"

My chiropractor referred me to her teacher, who quickly became my teacher and my homeopathic doctor, teacher, and mentor. His name was Dr. Hu Claybrooke. He was a master homeopath and an incredible teacher. Unfortunately, after studying with him for only 3 years, he was murdered in a domestic dispute, but I have been fortunate enough to study with the doctor who was *his* mentor and teacher for many years as well.

To make a long story even longer, I subsequently enrolled in acupuncture college while continuing my study of homeopathy. In 1981, while in acupuncture college, I remember being the only acupuncturist I knew to study homeopathy. Everyone else studied Chinese herbs only. As we are now seeing, many doctors in all different fields are beginning to see the value of homeopathy as a specialty or as an adjunct modality.

I could tell many more personal stories of the power of homeopathy and Oriental medicine in my life. I do have many incredible ones to tell, but I'd rather stop here and coach you in how to experience your own stories of awe and wonderment.

So, my friends, shall we begin?

I HAVE ...

by Dr. Randy W. Martin

I have a dream.

I have a dream that instead of yelling and blaming others, I can see and feel what's disturbing in me and focus on understanding and changing it instead.

I dream that instead of going to a doctor to be healed, I can manifest my own inner healer to do the work for me.

That instead of needing to leave L.A. because of the earthquakes, the filth, the poverty, the poison in the air, and the congestion, I can muster the inner strength to create significant political and social and environmental change.

I have a dream that I am surrounded by a nurturing, loving community of friends and a lover who shares my values and sensuality.

I dream that my God cares for me immensely and that I complete her creation with a deep degree of integrity.

In my dream, I am playing with friends, and kids, and dogs, and the cats are lying in the thick green grass purring happily.

My dream is a big part of me. I like it. It moves me.

My dream ... Oh, my God ... My dream ... I dream.

No army can withstand the strength of an idea whose time has come.
—Victor Hugo

OPTIMAL HEALTH: YOUR BIRTHRIGHT?

Why can some people eat candy bars while I can't?

We are all born with certain constitutional imbalances, both weaknesses and strengths. There is nothing we can do to alter this because this predisposition is inherited from our parents and our grandparents. In fact, all people are *not* created equal—at least not physiologically or energetically equal. We are each biologically *individual*. Whatever health weaknesses our parents and grandparents had are generally the ones we will be prone to have ourselves.

That is the bad news. The good news is that by using homeopathic and/or Oriental medical treatments, following a good diet, doing proper exercise geared to one's particular constitution, and working on mental attitude, almost everyone can overcome his or her inherited predisposition to disease and enjoy significantly better health than one would otherwise have expected.

The unfair reality is that some people can get away with eating candy and chocolate and not gain weight or have any health problems, while others have to watch everything they eat to avoid ill effects such as allergic reactions, weight gain, high cholesterol, chronic fatigue, or any number of other health problems.

Let's discuss "health" in a bit more detail. What is it? How can you enjoy it?

What is "health"?

My definition of health is *freedom* on all four levels of life:

- The *physical* level—freedom from the disease of pain, fatigue, or other physical discomfort which limits our ability to act and live life fully

- The *mental* level—openness to think and respond in ways that are not reactive defense mechanisms cultivated from childhood; freedom from irrationality, prejudice, and dogma; the ability to think clearly and to process information in a way that is growth-inducing

- The *emotional* level—the ability to appropriately feel one's emotions and to experience and share with others such feelings as laughter, happiness, grief, sorrow, fear, anger, sympathy, and empathy

- The *spiritual* level—the desire and ability to serve our fellows in the community; compassion and understanding for others, including reverence for the plant and animal kingdoms and our mother earth and father sky; the ability to connect to your spiritual source

How are my symptoms used to bring me closer to optimal health?

Physical symptoms, although they can be very painful to those who suffer them, are valuable to me as a doctor in helping you achieve good health. Your symptoms are like the oil warning light in your car: They point to the deeper imbalance in your body and mind. They speak to me of something bigger. They are the tip of the iceberg. As your doctor, I need to see your physical and emotional symptoms to know what it is you are really suffering from.

In holistic medicine, a diagnosis is not simply the name of your disease. Rather, a diagnosis is based on an in-depth analysis of what is going on with you on all four levels—physical, mental, emotional, and spiritual. Your proper diagnosis and treatment is dependent upon all the signs and symptoms you have.

How does this differ from Western "allopathic" doctors?

Modern allopathic* medicine prescribes the use of suppressive drugs like antibiotics, antihistamines, allergy medicines, or pain relievers, all of which cover up the real cause of a problem by removing the symptoms. Without having access to these symptoms, your holistic doctor may view your entire case analysis as clouded because the information necessary to make an in-depth diagnosis is unavailable.

For example, you might have a headache and take aspirin to cover the pain. Or you may suffer from a bad vaginal infection and use a topical ointment to clear it up. By suppressing the symptoms, you change your entire symptomatic picture. To treat you, I need to know *all the specifics of the case—what your problems are without any alterations or cover-up.*

In addition to covering up the symptoms, allopathic medication changes your Oriental diagnostic "pulse picture" and could alter your tongue diagnosis—both very important factors for a diagnosis in Oriental medicine (see pages 69 and 70). Some allopathic medications—such as antibiotics and muscle relaxants—can change your overall disposition, your emotional attitude, your outlook, and your methods of coping.

What is the treatment objective according to a holistic approach?

My goal as a classical homeopath and doctor of Oriental medicine is to eliminate the need for you to cover up your symptoms with drugs, and to heal the *root* of the problem or imbalance. This is done by uncovering and then treating the cause of your problems using spcific ancient and time-tested modalities based in nature. Later sections in this book discuss the philosophies of Oriental medicine and homeopathy. In some cases, if you eliminated the signs and symptoms by taking allopathic medications or using surgery, *you may have come no closer to good health than if you chose to ignore the problems altogether!*

There are **exceptions** to this rule—times when allopathic drugs and surgery can be lifesaving and life-giving—and it is important to take each case on its merits and evaluate it individually. Often, the holistic and allopathic approaches can be used side by side compatibly. We should be grateful for the lifesaving abilities of allopathic medicine…when used appropriately.

---

* Allopathic—conventional Western medicine. Technically, it treats disease through the use of substances that produce different effects than the disease. There is a focus on treating the *effects* (symptoms) of disease rather than the *cause* of disease. In contrast, homeopathic medicine uses substances that produce the *same* effects of the disease and focuses on treating the *cause* rather than the symptoms (effects).

The object of the holistic* approach to medicine is to redirect the energy patterns that precede physical and emotional symptoms. By balancing the body and mind on an energetic level, your overall health will improve, your immune system will be stronger, you will have more energy, and your mental and emotional outlook will be more positive and balanced.

What can I expect if I choose to use allopathic medications?

If you continue to treat your symptoms with allopathic medications, you will continue to harbor a deeper imbalance. As you grow older, you may begin to develop more serious degenerative diseases. These diseases will often be the same ones your parents or grandparents suffered.

Some allopathic medications can actually weaken your immune system. If used frequently, antibiotics kill not only the unfriendly bacteria in your body but also some of the bacteria your body depends on to help maintain its balance of health and resistance.

It is not uncommon to suffer digestive upsets or for women to get yeast infections soon after taking antibiotics. Antibiotics kill off some of the friendly bacteria which keep the body in a state of positive balance. A better solution is to use herbs, diet, acupuncture, or homeopathic remedies to boost and strengthen your immune system to help it triumph over the unfriendly bacteria.

Allopathic medications and/or surgery can sometimes cause even greater problems than the ones they are meant to cure. They do this by suppressing the body's own, naturally-occurring immune system—what homeopaths call the "vital force." Under natural conditions, without the intervention of allopathic drugs or surgery, the body has its own wisdom. This inner wisdom or vital force actually works to expel any imbalance that you may have by discharging it or "pushing" it onto the surface of your body.

Symptoms such as a skin rash, cold, or yeast infection will be welcomed by a homeopath because they are not bad at all. They are the body's attempt to throw off the inner energy imbalances and to create *homeostasis** within the body. Allopathic drugs and most surgical procedures are meant to remove the symptoms, without regard for their effect on the body's own naturally-occurring homeostatic process. By removing the symptoms they will often suppress the natural discharge process that throws the energy imbalance out to the surface of the body.

Symptoms are defense mechanisms. They are the body's most cost-effective way to eliminate the imbalance and defend you against a deeper or more serious illness. This is best illustrated with an example from psychology. Let us say that a husband has an

---

* Holistic—involves treatment which is aimed at affecting the body, intellect, emotions and spirit. Can include any alternative or traditional modalities, including surgery, prescription medications, acupuncture, massage, chiropractic, etc.

* Homeostasis—a state of balance in the body where all organ systems are working, coordinated with each other and in relative balance

extramarital affair and his wife learns of it, but she decides to overlook her feelings of anger and rage and suppress her feelings. What is likely to happen? Most likely anger and resentment will eventually get the best of her, rise to the surface, and erupt in some form of overpowering emotional outburst or inappropriate action ("acting out"). She may decide to have an affair herself, or she may start acting in apparently odd, irrational ways to get back at him or to get his attention.

It works the same with the body's physiology. If a cyst or mole is cut out, the body will do something else to compensate—to get your attention, to tell you the imbalance that created the growth in the first place still exists and is not being dealt with. The body may choose to create another cyst in the same or in another place. In other words, if a symptom is treated as an enemy and ignored, allopathically medicated, or cut out, the body will create an even more ingenious way to let you know there is something wrong. (See note, page 23)

If a child's skin rash is suppressed by cortisone creams, 5 years later that same child may get asthma, frequent ear infections or colds, or the child may be termed hyperactive and begin to act out in tantrums or violent behavior toward other children. Each person's body is a complex of unknown defense mechanisms, which act out according to genetics and environmental factors. The rule of homeopathy is that when any symptom or discharge is suppressed by an allopathic medication, the underlying imbalance will resurface in another way.

Going back to our psychological example above, if the wife sought the help of a therapist or close friend when she learned of her husband's infidelity, she could have been encouraged to discharge her rage and anger appropriately. Whether the relationship would have been saved is still questionable, but at the very least she would have been able to clear and heal her own emotional state.

What about all the aspirin and other drugs I have already taken?

Most of us have accumulated years and years of physiological and emotional suppression of our natural discharging processes. We have been taught to act as if everything is fine. We take aspirin for a headache, have benign cysts, moles, and warts removed, take decongestants for sinus congestion, have allergy shots for allergies, take antacids for ulcers, etc. Sooner or later, after years and years of this suppression, the body/mind will erupt—with cancer, colitis, tension headaches, anxiety, emotional depression or moodiness, or whatever the particular inherited traits and environmental conditions dictate.

You can change this pattern *today*. It is your choice to refuse to submit to allopathic medication at times when it is not absolutely necessary, to choose to actively improve your health, and to correct your underlying chronic patterns of disease.

What can I do to start on a new wellness program?

If you choose to change the way you look at health and disease; if you see each symptom as an opportunity to tune into your unique imbalances; if you use each new symptom (whether it's emotional depression or constipation) as a barometer to assess your internal unconscious coping mechanisms and vital force—then you are ready to begin the road to optimal health. This path will not only make you feel better emotionally and physically, it is also a philosophy of life—a truly holistic way of seeing the interconnectedness of everything within the body and mind and in the world at large.

I am not telling you that you are responsible for ill health and disease in your body. Much of what happens to us is based on our genetics and environmental influences, which are totally beyond our control. I *am* saying that you can be empowered enough to do something about the portion that you *can* control.

Besides the use of homeopathic medicine and acupuncture, there are other things you can do to actively participate in your wellness process:

- ❁ Notice the patterns of strength and mildness of your symptoms by keeping a personal medical journal (see page 25 on how to keep a journal)

- ❁ Learn to become more aware of and to appreciate the underlying processes that may contribute to and cause your patterns (e.g. stress, diet, smog, dampness, Santa Ana winds, full moon, poor work environment, or other environmental conditions)

- ❁ Gain new behavioral skills to help you to cope with and correct your disease patterns

If you think of yourself as a complex organism burdened by layer upon layer of suppressed disease patterns, the process of regaining your health and re-owning your body and mind can be seen as slowly unpeeling layer upon layer of the skins of an onion. The closer you approach the heart of the onion, the closer you come to optimal health.

What proof can you give me that this philosophy actually works?

What I am proposing is that you have faith—faith in the natural cures that have been given to us, in the interconnectedness of all life, in your own intuition, in your body's own inner healing mechanisms, and in the natural process you must go through if your goal is *real health*. Instead of having a panic attack whenever you don't feel well and taking the first medicine available to numb your current discomfort, you may want to learn to respect your own body-mind process—to feel the pain, "journal" about it, exercise more, and take a natural remedy that will strengthen your system over the long term.

If you really need some kind of proof that homeopathy, acupuncture, diet, and exercise are definitely going to cure you, you may have to undertake a long course of self-study. The data and research are available if you want them. Remember that these forms of medicines have been around a lot longer than the allopathic approach.

I suggest you use yourself as a guinea pig. If my logic seems right to you in your gut, then I invite you to join me. Together we will go for it—***optimal health***. It's your birthright!

Who's Your Doctor and Why?

Increasingly, people come to me for treatment and make comments like, "I came to you because I don't believe in Western medicine." Although it's very exciting that so many people are now looking to acupuncture and homeopathic medicine as an alternative, this kind of comment also concerns me.

Western medicine and alternative medicine both have a place alongside each other—each in its appropriate place. If you need the name of a good physician who *also* values the integrity of homeopathy and acupuncture, please let me know. It's best not to wait for a medical emergency to acquaint yourself with a doctor. You are better prepared if you have already developed an ongoing relationship with a Western-trained physician *and* a homeopath or acupuncturist.

Choosing Your Doctor

Here are some criteria to look for in choosing your holistic or Oriental medical doctor:

How do I know how to choose the right holistic doctor?

The first thing to do is ask your friends to introduce you to their doctor and see how he or she seems to you. If you don't know anyone who sees a holistic doctor, try the phone book. Better yet, try attending lectures to find someone you like.

What should I ask a potential doctor?

The particular questions do not matter as much as *the way in which they are answered*. The doctor should reflect caring, commitment, and nurturing, since these are the qualities you need in a healer.

You may want to ask about his or her education and specialties, but these should not play too much of a role in your selection. Great credentials do not necessarily make a great doctor. In holistic medicine, there really is no such thing as a specialty, because you want a doctor who sees you as a whole person and will treat you as a whole person. If you have endometriosis and cysts, you don't necessarily want a doctor who specializes in these, because each person who has these problems needs to be treated on the basis of her constitution.

Your very best bet is to read up on whatever type of problem you have and ask educated questions. You may want to determine if your doctor uses electrical diagnostic machines, relies on pulse and tongue diagnosis, is a classical homeopath, or just took a few weekend courses in homeopathy.

What else should I pay attention to?

Does the doctor make good eye contact? Do you feel "rushed" with the doctor? Is the office clean? Is the front office staff helpful and congenial? Do you feel "good vibes" in the doctor's office? Are the treatment rooms clean and comfortable?

The length of time spent with you may not be a reliable indication of a doctor's proficiency. A great doctor may be able to take a brief look at you and determine what you need, while a more mediocre doctor may take an hour and a half to do the same thing.

Do not quickly jump to conclusions. Many people want quick results, but this is a flawed way of thinking when it comes to health care. Keep in mind how long you have had your problem. If it is a long-term problem, you can expect treatment to take some time.

Don't wait to see if your friend gets better before starting your own treatment! Your physiology and biology are totally different. Most likely you will heal in different ways and with different timing.

The doctor should return phone calls the day you call. I prefer a doctor who allots time during the day to take and return phone calls. You deserve to work with someone who makes you feel cared about.

If I feel angry at my doctor, should say something?

Yes, most definitely! If you have never had any psychotherapy, you may not be familiar with the concepts of projection and transference. What this means is that if your doctor is a good healer, at some time during the process of your treatment you will undoubtedly project your feelings onto him or her. These are likely to be feelings of anger or pain. Angry feelings are generally anger you feel toward either yourself or the disease, and you won't be able to separate it at the time. Anger can be used productively and should be discussed.

Be open to reading about the psychological concepts of projection and transference and be willing to "own" your anger and take it back from the doctor. Your doctor is not a god. A great doctor will help you see how your attitudes keep you in the process of disease, and will direct you to a therapist or the appropriate books to help you work through emotional stagnation and pain.

Finally, pay close attention to how you feel. Your own inner healer is a part of you. The objective of healing is to empower you in your healing process. Pay attention whether this doctor makes you feel dependent on him/her, or empowers your inner sense of healing. Some degree of dependency is a good thing, but you also want to feel like you are part of a healing team effort.

Surgery and Holistic Health

What do Oriental medicine and homeopathy have to offer someone facing surgery?

Depending on the type of surgery, there are specific herbs and homeopathic remedies that will help prepare body and mind for the invasive trauma. Acupuncture can also relax you and build up your immunity so that your body will not be as adversely affected.

Sometimes surgery is the best health alternative. In these cases, acupuncture can help on an emotional level by giving you the courage to confront the surgery head-on.

People who are balanced, with strong immune systems going into the surgery, are much more likely to come out without complications. They are also more likely to recover more quickly, especially from the effects of anesthesia.

What can you do after surgery?

A patient recently came to me for treatment after breaking his ankle. The ankle was in a cast, and I gave him some specific homeopathic remedies to help the bone heal faster and reduce inflammation in the tendons and ligaments. I did acupuncture around the cast to help heal the wound. His doctor was very surprised at how fast he healed, but this is not an uncommon event!

Homeopathic remedies and acupuncture can also be used after surgery to facilitate the removal of anesthetic from the organs, aid tissue healing so that there will be less scarring, increase one's appetite, detox from pain medications or other remedies, and reduce inflammation and swelling in the area around the surgery. This also applies to dental work. An acupuncture treatment and/or homeopathic remedy will also help you recover from dental work much more quickly.

Acupuncture and homeopathy should also be used after surgery to help correct the underlying problem that led to the need for surgery in the first place. Unless the underlying constitution is treated, the same or a related problem will manifest itself again and again. Surgery is normally only a stopgap measure; it does not eliminate the problem that created the need for surgery in the first place.

Acupuncture is also very effective during a course of chemotherapy and radiation treatments to ease the body back into balance between treatments. It also can be used to help the body eliminate toxic allopathic drugs more quickly.

Can I use acupuncture and homeopathic treatment instead of surgery?

If a surgery is elective and the doctor approves of waiting for a few months, it is worth attempting to heal the problem through a course of acupuncture treatments, herbs, and/or homeopathy before resorting to surgery.

NOTE: I definitely believe in surgery for many types of problems. Each person must be individually analyzed. I am not judging the Western medical profession (which saves many lives) as bad; I am merely presenting the holistic approach, which I try to practice with my patients. To the extent it is possible to keep the surgeon's knife away from your skin, I fully support any and all alternatives!

> *When people are viewed as nothing more than machines, doctors become like mechanics.*
>
> —*K. Lenia Scanlon*

Treatment Philosophy & Approach

My approach to the practice of medicine is a holistic one. I analyze and diagnose problems based on a very broad perspective using Western as well as Oriental medical diagnostic techniques. In many cases, you may be asked questions about the emotional and spiritual aspects of your life as well. Complaints you may have previously been told are "all in your head" may in fact be quite relevant to your total health.

The more you share about yourself, the more peculiar symptoms you are able to divulge, the more effective your treatment will be. This is a team effort, and it is important to this type of treatment that you consider yourself an active participant in your healing process. Any insights or roadblocks you experience along the way should be welcomed and shared, if you feel comfortable in doing so. This is a process-oriented treatment approach rather than the "Band-Aid" approach that most people are familiar with.

Acupuncture treatments usually take place on a once- or twice-weekly basis for three to ten weeks. Constitutional and homeopathic treatments (see page 32) occur once every three to eight weeks for periods of up to a year or more.

After your initial pains or symptoms are cleared, it is recommended that you return every two to three months for periodic treatments and/or homeopathic remedies, much the same way as you keep your automobile in tune. Also, ongoing treatments with herbs and remedies will keep your body functioning smoothly and in balance.

It is important for you to feel safe, so feel free to ask as many questions as you need. There are many different approaches to holistic medicine and each doctor may practice differently based on his or her training, experience, personality, or philosophy. No procedure, herb, or remedy should be used if you do not feel comfortable with it, so be sure to speak up. If you have a preference as to which approach you prefer, your doctor would want to know it.

An effective alliance between doctor and patient is one in which both parties agree to make decisions jointly and share the responsibility for both the process and the outcome.

—Richard Moskowitz, M.D.

I consider healing much too limited a concept; it implies that someone is sick. I prefer to see disease as a dream trying to come to consciousness.

— Stephan Bodian
Yoga Journal
April 1990

Health Journal

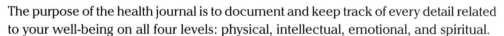

I suggest to all my patients that they begin to keep a journal as soon as possible. On the next page, you will find listings of suggested categories and headings that my patients have found useful. If you use a looseleaf binder and assign a full page to each category, you will be able to keep track of your progress over an extended period of time. As you fill a given page, you can simply add another one. Be sure to label each page with the appropriate headings.

The purpose of the health journal is to document and keep track of every detail related to your well-being on all four levels: physical, intellectual, emotional, and spiritual.

Start today to begin your record-keeping. List any visits to health care practitioners (medical doctors, chiropractors, acupuncturists, physical therapists, psychologists, dentists, nutritionists, as well as any spiritual practices you may be doing or want to be doing in the future). Be sure to obtain copies of blood tests and keep track of any herbs, homeopathic remedies, or dietary supplements you take.

In addition, you may wish to keep a dietary record, record your dreams, or keep poetry or artwork, comics from the newspaper or insights you may have that reflect feelings or insights about your health.

Feel free to add pages or new sections as appropriate to your individual outlook and approach to health. I suggest that you keep them in a three-ring binder so that you can add pages whenever you want. You may also wish to purchase dividers so that you can make each section easier to access. The following sections and headings are a starting place. Feel free to create others, according to what is useful to you at a given time.

Remember the old Chinese saying: "There is opportunity in the midst of crisis."

Your disease or health problem may be just the *opportunity* you have been waiting for—

- ✦ To begin a new personal growth program
- ✦ To start a new positive outlook on life
- ✦ To commence a good exercise program
- ✦ To undertake a new, healthier eating program

Take this opportunity as an opportunity to grow—to move beyond self-limitation.

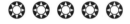

The greatest limitations you will ever face will be those you put on yourself. Only you can stifle your potential.

—*Dennis Waitley*
Being the Best

25

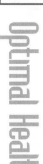

Optimal Health

Herbs and Nutritional Supplements

Always record the symptoms that go with each herb or supplement so that you can go back later and learn why a particular herb or supplement was taken and which worked.

Date   **Symptoms**   **Herb or Supplement Taken**

Homeopathic Remedies

Date   **Symptoms**   **Homeopathic Remedy**

X-Rays

Date   **Place/Doctor**   **Part of Body**   **Results**

Tests

Record all laboratory tests including blood, urinalysis, and hair analysis; always obtain a duplicate for your personal files.

Date   **Place/Doctor**   **Type of Test**   **Results**

Minor or Major Illnesses

Minor illness includes headaches, flu, colds, sprained ankles, yeast or urinary infections, etc. and major illness includes hospitalizations, surgeries, cysts, fibroids, tumors, etc.

Date   **Illness or Problem**   **Solution or Remedy**

You may wish to be exceptionally creative and expect miracles. Additional sections may include:

- ❀ Exercise goals
- ❀ Emotional goals
- ❀ Spiritual goals
- ❀ Record of meditation practice
- ❀ Record of daily or weekly exercises
- ❀ Artwork, visual imagery
- ❀ Dreams
- ❀ Poetry or personal journal writings
- ❀ Insights
- ❀ Fears related to becoming healthy and strong

Phone Calls & Confidentiality

During your ongoing treatment, if you have a question that cannot wait until your next office visit, you should feel free to call your doctor. When in doubt about taking any remedy, it is always better to call than to wait. He/she should usually be able to return your call the same day if it is a day they are working. Otherwise, they should return your call on their next working day.

If the call is an emergency, be sure to tell the office staff so they can immediately notify me to return your call.

Of course, everything you share with your doctor during the process of your treatment is completely confidential.

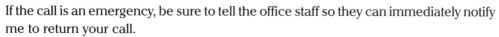

HEALING AND FRUSTRATION

Do you find yourself coasting along fine, feeling great, and all of a sudden you come down with what seems like a bizarre set of symptoms you have never had?

You come to the doctor and expect an instant cure... of course! We live in a culture that expects everything to occur instantaneously, but in most cases it can take time to experience true healing. With time you may become frustrated. Does this scenario sound familiar? Do you get frustrated waiting to get well? Do you want your symptoms to immediately disappear? Do you find your inner voice saying to your symptoms: "Get out of my way. You're interfering with my life!"?

Please try to remember that if you have a simple problem it will be healed quickly, but if you have a complex problem, it may take some time to get rid of it. Symptoms are only the tip of the iceberg. If you want a "quick" solution, go to an allopathic doctor and have your problem cut off or drugged!

If you want *healing*, you need to remember the amount of ice under the iceberg. Your symptoms are only the tip of the iceberg! True and long-lasting healing will take the time it takes to melt down this massive growth under the surface. Your body didn't manufacture symptoms overnight, even if that's how it appears to you, and it might take some time to detoxify and bring you back into balance.

The body naturally tends towards balance. With a little push by the correct herb, acupuncture treatment or homeopathic remedy, your body will come back into balance itself. But patience may be necessary. If you stick it out, later on you will be rewarded with the best health of anyone you know. Let them eat their Hershey bars and drink their Starbucks... you'll have your health!

How to Report Your Symptoms

Think of how often you look out a screened window without ever seeing the screen. This is analogous to habitually ignoring all the physical symptoms you may feel but have learned to ignore. When visiting your acupuncturist or homeopath, it's very important to focus on all the little pieces of "dirt" on the screen and to share as much of this information as possible.

History

❈ Describe the beginning of your troubles. To the best of your knowledge, state how they began, any previous treatments, and the results of these treatments. Be sure to indicate any changes in the symptoms over the years, months, or recent weeks or days.

❈ Be sure to mention all your previous illnesses and problems, including childhood illnesses, even if they seem unconnected to your current problem.

❈ Describe any major emotional or physical trauma, shock, or injury in your life, and what treatments you received.

Mental Function

❈ Report on any abnormal memory problems, recent problems in your overall mental functioning, or changes in your intellectual capability.

Emotions

❈ Mention any odd feelings, conditions, likes, and dislikes that you think set you apart from the norm. Such things as desires, fears, timidity, anxiety, stress, lack of interest, persistent thoughts, discouragement, irritability, being overly critical, confusion, aversion to particular people or work, changeable moods, or dullness of mind are all important.

❈ Describe your state of mind relative to your current problem.

❈ Describe your basic personality and whether it has recently changed much; if so, explain why and how. Are you quiet or talkative? Do you prefer to be alone or with others?

❈ What is your relationship history?

❈ Have there been any major emotional shocks or disappointments?

Appetite

❈ If health wasn't an issue, what foods would your "inner child" crave or dislike?

❈ Do you have much thirst, and what temperature do you prefer food and drink?

❈ Do you now, or have you ever had, have any emotional issues with food—are you overweight, anorexic, bulimic, etc.?

Primary Problems

❈ Clearly state your primary problems so that the doctor knows exactly what you want to be treated for, and in what order of importance.

❈ Are your symptoms always present or how long do they persist? Do they come and go, or alternate with any other symptoms? For instance, do you get headaches only on Sunday, or experience pain only after sex?

Pain

❈ Where do you experience pain?

❈ Is it constant, changing, or alternating with other symptoms?

❈ What things make it better or worse: being inside or outdoors, covered or uncovered, cold or hot packs, walking or exercising, sitting or standing?

❈ What side of the body do your pains occur on, or do they travel back and forth from side to side? Do they start at a certain time of day or after having eaten a particular food or drink?

❈ Exactly what does it feel like? What is the sensation—cutting, burning, stabbing, stitching, aching, dull, sharp, nerve-like, moving around, shooting, drawing?

❈ Describe all sensations, however slight or peculiar, in terms of "It feels *as if . . .*"

Modalities

❈ Begin to pay attention to and be able to report on the time of day, seasons of the year, and the day of the week that your symptoms occur, as well as their intensity.

❈ Do sleep, exercise, baths, showers, eating, or thinking about the problem change its intensity or duration? What exactly makes it worse or better?

❈ How does different weather affect you—dry, cold, heat, storms, thunder, frost, cloudiness, high or low altitudes, or before a storm? Does the full or new moon affect you one way or another?

Skin

❈ Regarding all skin, scalp, or nail troubles, tell the exact location, color, whether it is dry or moist, thick or thin, scaly, pimply, with or without blisters or liquid, warts or growths, and precise appearance and feeling.

❈ Does your skin itch and, if so, when? Does anything make it better or worse, such as the heat of your bed or a hot shower?

Discharges

❈ Describe any discharges—where they are, when they occur, and what they look like. Color and texture are important to note. Do the discharges burn or is the skin around them raw?

Urine

❀ Do you have any pain before, during, or after urination?

❀ Do you urinate frequently? Is your urine colored or odorous?

Bowels

❀ Describe your bowel movements and whether you have any pain, blood, diarrhea, or constipation.

❀ Do you have frequent urging with no stool? Is the stool flat, skinny, large, dry?

Gynecology

❀ How many days occur between your periods? Do you experience pain before, during, or after the period? Do you have heavy or light bleeding? If you experience pain, what does it feel like and where does it occur (thighs, stomach, back, sides)? What relieves or aggravates the pain?

❀ Have you a history of infertility or miscarriage?

❀ How is your sexual desire? High, medium, low?

❀ Any herpes, vaginal warts, HPV, cysts, or tumors?

Men's Issues

❀ How is your sexual drive and "performance?" Any prostate problems, erection or ejaculation problems, or pains?

❀ Any pubic warts, HPV, or herpes?

Sleep

❀ Do you have any problems with your sleep?

❀ Do you have any repeated dreams?

It is the most peculiar and apparently insignificant symptom that is often the one to lead the doctor to the correct diagnosis and remedy. If in doubt, it is better to mention something than to ignore it.

> *People come to the consulting room and lay out a collision of values with great embarrassment and agony. They want resolution but would have something even greater if they could ask for the consciousness to bear the paradox.*
>
> —*Robert Johnson, Ph.D.*

SYMPTOMS: GOOD OR BAD?

Headaches, allergies, TMJ, fatigue, low sex drive, cramps??? Most of us think of our symptoms as problems that we need to get rid of. Understandably, our symptoms make us very uncomfortable, so it's a natural response to want to change and get rid of them. But if you don't mind suspending this way of thinking for just the time it takes to read this article, I can show you another very helpful way to view your symptoms that, if given a chance, will lead you to a higher state of health than you imagined possible.

What would you do when a circuit breaker in your home gets "tripped"? Would you ask your electrician to eliminate the circuit breaker? Remember that the circuit breaker was specifically designed into the electrical system as a way of keeping the circuits from burning out. The circuit breaker was put in your home by its "grand designer" or architect; they are purposely built as the weakest link in the electrical circuit. You need them as a warning that there is something wrong somewhere else in the circuitry.

On the other hand, the circuit breaker doesn't tell you what the problem is. It only tells you what portion of the home the problem is in. Similarly with your symptoms—they do not tell you what is wrong; they only tell you which system in the body has the problem. You must take all the clues and trace the problem back to the source. The homeopath and acupuncturist use your symptoms to trace your problem back to *its* source, as well.

By then treating the energy imbalance and eliminating the source of the problem, the body's circuits will cease to "blow" and your symptoms will decrease or disappear altogether. Just as in your home, every time you overload *your* circuits, a circuit breaker will "blow" again and you will see your symptoms reappear. And this is when you need to see your acupuncturist or homeopath again.

Your symptoms are your gifts from the "grand designer"; they are your "blessings." Honor them. Deal with them with integrity. Respect them and pay attention to their message. Don't cover them up or cut them out. The body was put together with the perfect wisdom of the universe. We are a part of nature and we can function to perfection when we give ourselves the chance and permission to do so.

If you're not now functioning to perfection, it's not the fault of the designer, nor is it the fault of the symptoms (or circuit breakers), nor is it your fault. But you do have the opportunity to take the responsibility to respect, honor, listen to and deal with your symptoms as signals, as signs and as gifts.

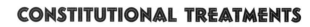

CONSTITUTIONAL TREATMENTS

Patients often ask me what I mean when I say I am treating them "constitutionally," or that I am giving them a "constitutional" homeopathic remedy or acupuncture treatment. Simply defined, a constitutional treatment considers the sum total of your life and has the potential to cause changes in the following areas:

- ❀ Genetic inheritance—what you were born with on a cellular level
- ❀ Mental processes— your intellect, your thinking potential and processes
- ❀ Emotions and how you handle emotional stress and conflict
- ❀ Spiritual attitudes and your ability to assimilate new behaviors and attitudes
- ❀ Physical problems, including your personal and family history
- ❀ Lifestyle and diet, including sleeping and waking patterns, food cravings, and addictions
- ❀ Body type, appearance, weight, immunity, overall health and vitality (i.e., basic energetic appearance and body type)

Constitutional treatment works on all of the above. Different treatments and homeopathic remedies act on different levels at different times during your treatment. Some treatments and remedies focus more on the spiritual or emotional; others work on the physical or your lifestyle. After being treated for a longer period of time, it is possible to affect your genetic inheritance level—to have an impact on what genetic predisposition you may pass on to your offspring.

The Role of Blood Tests in Oriental Medical Diagnosis

Often a patient comes to me for treatment and is shocked to find that I hesitate to treat them without first examining a recent and complete blood test. A common complaint is that they came to me as a homeopath and doctor of Oriental medicine precisely because they distrust or dislike Western medicine and testing.

It is difficult for me to effectively treat the majority of my new patients without first seeing a complete blood panel. The reason for this is simple. If I were living in China a thousand years ago and the only tools I had to diagnose my patients with were the traditional tongue, abdominal, and pulse diagnoses, I would probably be an expert with those methods alone. But why deny many of the benefits of Western medicine and the wonderful diagnostic techniques available? Expertise in Western diagnostic and traditional Oriental diagnostic techniques is my goal. Also, as a primary care health provider licensed by the states of California and Oregon, I am also legally responsible to "flag" any serious or life-threatening disease processes.

Often when I request a blood test from a patient, I am told they recently had one and their doctor said everything was "just fine." When I interpret a blood test, I do so according to traditional Western medical parameters, but I also interpret the results in terms of what they tell me about the individual's *chi*, yin, yang, and various other diagnostic criteria used in Oriental medicine. Blood tests interpreted according to Oriental medical principles can be incredibly interesting, far beyond the normal parameters defined by Western medicine.

Often the results of a blood test will point me to a particular homeopathic remedy, specific herbal regimen, or acupuncture treatment. I often also discover imbalances in a patient's metabolism or endocrine system that may have been overlooked using the normal Western interpretation.

Let's work together to create a truly holistic and complementary form of medicine, the best of the Orient and the West. Let's utilize as many tools and treatments as are appropriate and available, and develop a *synthesis* of East and West.

THE HEALING "AGGRAVATION"

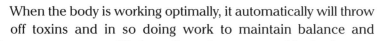

When the body is working optimally, it automatically will throw off toxins and in so doing work to maintain balance and equilibrium. But when you are blocked or get sick, it stops performing this function as well.

When you receive any type of natural treatment or do a fast, the body goes into a kind of "panic" mode to locate and release the stored toxins and blockages. The treatment forces or catalyzes the body to re-check its "circuitry." (For those who are into computers, it is similar to a spell-checker in a word processor, or a utility program that checks an entire computer hard disk, and when it finds a problem, it corrects it automatically.)

Similarly, when the body finds a problem it immediately works to eliminate it; this is what symptoms are. But if you have suppressed your symptoms inadvertently over the years, then when you take a homeopathic remedy or receive a strong acupuncture treatment or begin to fast, your body will throw off more than your fair share of symptoms. While it's doing so, you are apt to feel a lot worse for a time, but then you will feel better and BE better, too!

SELF-EMPOWERMENT:
THE OPPOSITE OF CODEPENDENCE

Taking care of your health may not be your primary mission in life, but my ultimate goal is to support, teach, and encourage you to do just that. In fact, my goal is to eventually put myself and other doctors out of business! I know that I am the happiest and most satisfied when I take care of myself, so I would like to teach you to do it, too.

I encourage you to reach out and give your health practitioner a call when you're unsure of how to treat yourself. He/she should want to develop an interdependent relationship with you. The difference between an interdependent relationship and a codependent relationship is self-empowerment. The relationship I am encouraging is based on self-empowerment.

The components of a self-empowering relationship with your doctor should include the following:

❀ Mirroring—allowing your doctor to become a mirror of your ills so that you can more objectively "see" what is really going on.

❀ Learning the language of holistic medicine so that you can effectively communicate with your doctor and accomplish your own research.

❀ Becoming familiar with your constitution and its unique strengths and weaknesses. This will require an initial complete diagnosis and examination using either Oriental medical diagnosis or "miasmic" homeopathy. When you are familiar with your constitutional type, you can determine your exact nutritional needs and assume an active role in obtaining "tune-up" treatments.

❀ Asking for help and clarification when needed.

In summary, self-empowerment is a simple process of taking charge of your health. My goal is to help you do this.

A great deal of healing occurs as soon as you take control of your own disease and wellness process. It is through this philosophy and conviction that I educate each patient that a visit to the doctor is not meant to "get rid" of a particular illness. It is to work together as a healing team to create personal balance.

Balance rather than cure is the rule in holistic health. Process rather than product is the way in which we achieve balance.

Curing disease is an illusion. There will always be a new set of symptoms to replace the ones you remove. If you are brought into balance, true health and equilibrium will be maintained despite environmental stress and pollution.

It is not the end product of wellness we are striving for; rather, it is becoming involved in the *process* of wellness that creates balance and health.

The process of achieving wellness can at times feel confusing, frustrating, and difficult. It does get easier, and with practice it can be a lot of fun to team up with your doctor.

> *Everything is connected to everything else. This is the one statement that embodies the spirit of holism more than any other. The statement itself connects with many other important concepts: all is one; I am connected to you; America is connected to China; things that are connected can be put into balance.*
>
> —*Peter Albright, M.D.*

SPEAK UP! EMPOWER YOURSELF!!!

Your medical practitioner is the first person you should see to discuss any fears or worries you may have about any of your medical problems. If necessary, he or she can then help to direct you to an appropriate specialist. When talking to your practitioner, here are a few guidelines to follow:

1. Write down your questions ahead of time. The doctor's consultation room is not the place to try to recall every concern you've had since your last visit. Keep a health journal and label one section for questions. Bring your questions, pen and paper to each visit.

2. Always have a pen and paper with you when you call your doctor. Don't expect the doctor to wait while you run and get them. Also have your homeopathic remedies, herbs and questions by the phone when you call; keep them with you so when the doctor returns your call, you don't keep him or her waiting. Write all instructions down while on the phone so you don't have to call back. Be succinct. A busy doctor is usually calling back many patients and he/she needs you to be businesslike and to the point.

3. Be as specific as possible with your questions. You'll learn more by asking, "Can I eat apricots?" or "What can I eat instead of sugar to satisfy the cravings?" than by asking, "What should I eat?"

4. Listen carefully and take notes. If the doctor uses a word you don't understand, ask him or her to spell it out and to clarify its meaning.

5. Understand your treatment. Try to memorize the names of the homeopathics and herbs you are taking so that you can become a more informed and empowered participant in your own health care and healing process.

6. Know which symptoms constitute an emergency or at least merit a call or office visit. Study and read as much as possible about your condition and the type of treatment you are receiving.

7. Ask for recommendations of books, magazine articles or pamphlets to read. This book will help answer many of your questions and is a great place to begin your studies. The reference section at the back of the book lists additional resources you can read next.

IS THE CAUSE OF MY PROBLEM PSYCHOLOGICAL OR PHYSICAL?

This is a question I'm constantly asked, and the answer isn't ever very simple. As you can see from the graph below, some people's problems are considered more emotional and some more physical. Two different people can have the same health issue and the cause for one may be emotional and for another physical.

Each of us is born constitutionally unique. Depending on the genetic imbalances, our childhood, lifestyle, diet and ability to cope with and manage stress, we will generate different diseases. Whether the cause of these disease processes is emotional or physical will vary from individual to individual.

Every disease process is caused by components that are both emotional and physical. There is no disease which is exclusively caused by emotional or exclusively by physical causes. Here are a couple of examples:

Fay, a 27-year-old woman, comes to my office to be treated for severe eczema of the hands. In taking Fay's history, I discover she was bulimic throughout high school and college. The bulimia began just after she was sexually violated by a second cousin.

Question: Is the eczema caused more by emotional causes or is it physically induced? She has no history of eczema in her family. In this case, the eczema is due primarily to malnutrition, and from the body not being able to absorb and assimilate the proper nutrients to build healthy skin.

The breakdown of her digestive system began with the eating disorder, but the eating disorder began as a direct result of the emotional trauma from the sexual abuse from age 8 to 12. So, in this case, the majority of the eczema problem is emotionally-based, a result of the trauma experienced in childhood. But the treatment will be aimed primarily at strengthening the digestive system, since this is now the most immediate cause.

Fay has already spent many years in therapy working out her emotional issues, so for her the emotional element is no longer the cause. We could say that for Fay, her problem is about 85% physical and 15% emotional at this point.

Another example: Rodney, a 32-year-old man, comes in for treatment of severe psoriasis. Its cause is primarily genetic. His father also has it and they both began to get psoriasis at around age eight. So we could say that Rodney's psoriasis is strictly physically-based. But if we probe further, we see from his family history, that his father, as well as Rodney, is severely emotionally suppressed.

Rodney began experimenting with recreational drugs while he was in college, and he had a "nervous breakdown." This resulted in him coming back and living with his parents, and at this point he got involved in a strict religious order. The religious order helped him put his life back together, but he never then worked on resolving the existential issues that were "waking up" in him in college and on drugs.

Rodney is a very anxious and nervous young man, always in a hurry to get in and out of the office quickly—very impatient, lacking in self-introspection, and heavily relying on the religious order for answers to life.

We would say that in Rodney's case, his skin disease is caused about 50% emotionally and 50% physically. It is not uncommon for a patient to assume that the cause of a disease is genetic, as in this case, because his father has the same disease when actually there are also strong emotional components. Rodney not only inherited his father's psoriasis, but also his father's emotional "model" for coping with his feelings. As such, he has never explored his "inner dimensions," and this has subsequently become a component in his psoriasis.

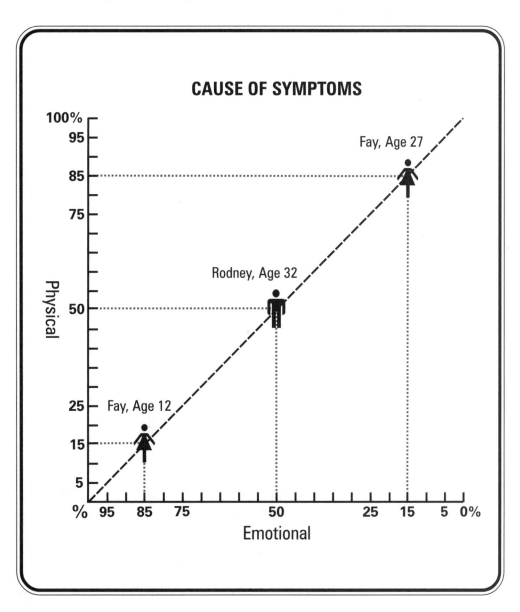

CAUSE OF SYMPTOMS

ARE YOU READY FOR OPTIMAL HEALTH?
IT CAN BE YOURS!

I'm very excited to share with you what I think is the type of news we all hope and wait for. Over the past 24 months, I've been witnessing some miraculous results in my practice with many of my patients, family members, friends and associates. No, this isn't another network marketing product. I invite you to please read on ...

What I've discovered is a great combination of treatments which, when followed conscientiously for over a period of at least one year, produces astounding and even miraculous results in health, vitality, feelings of well-being, emotional stability and centeredness. Of course, results will vary tremendously, depending on your level of health when starting the program, your current lifestyle and genetic background.

So if you're serious about wanting to achieve Optimal Health, please give the following program a serious look. You really owe this to yourself. If you're able to invest just one year of your life in working on your diet, monitoring your blood chemistry, and staying on a homeopathic remedy, I can almost guarantee that you will look back and say to yourself at the end of the year: "I really can't believe how much better I feel," and friends will say, "I can't believe how much younger you look."

Enough said. Here's the program we use and exactly what it would require from you:

1. Constitutional Homeopathy. See the section beginning on page 104 for a definition of Classical Homeopathy. In terms of time, this involves office visits every four to six weeks over a period of one year. At each visit, we evaluate what has taken place in your life since your last visit, both physically and emotionally. For this to be effective, you must be open and interested in doing two things: (a) keeping track of changes in your physical symptoms and (b) sharing with the doctor the emotional and lifestyle changes that have taken place since your last visit.

2. The Health Equations Program (HEP). This is the most comprehensive, cutting-edge blood analysis program I have ever seen! Up until I discovered the HEP in 1997, I'd been evaluating blood based on Chinese and Western medicine only. The HEP has the additional ability of assessing the functional capacity of the body to utilize the various minerals and electrolytes in the bloodstream. Your blood is like soil. If the soil is full of all the right nutrients in the proper proportions, the tree (your body) will grow strong. The purpose of the HEP is to adjust your blood chemistry to have all the right nutrients in the proper amounts and proportions. Once your "soil" is strong and balanced, your health will improve and you will look and feel younger.

3. The Body Type Diet Plan. This first involves filling out a three-page questionnaire to determine your Body Type (see page 142). We then combine this information with your blood type and your Five Element

Body Type Analysis from Chinese Medicine. Some people may have additional needs, such as Food Allergy testing. In some cases, we also have to consider other specific health needs, such as cholesterol problems, high blood pressure, PMS, chronic fatigue syndrome, colitis, candida, diabetes, hypoglycemia, compulsive over- or under-eating, or vegetarian dietary requirements. We integrate all these special health needs into an individualized dietary program. This program is a process of our working together to modify your existing diet until we find, together, exactly what works best for your metabolic type, your personal lifestyle, and *you*.

Your entire commitment to this program requires one monthly office visit for a period of 12 months. If you should need acupuncture, however, this will usually require more frequent visits. Additional tests may also sometimes be needed and may include: Adrenal Function, Allergy Tests, Bone Density, Hormone Levels, Heavy Metal detection through Hair Analysis, Urine Tests to detect Oxidative Stress, Liver and Kidney Functioning, or the Stool Purge Test to rule out Candida and parasites.

Get started now! Optimal Health and Optimal Energy are your birthright!!!

Remember the Patient

Somewhere lost in the complexities of chartomegaly, information glut, electronic medical records and medical legal hysteria, is a patient who simply wants your attention. Sit close. Listen intently. Practice tenderness. Give a hug. Pray with him. Cry with her. And never underestimate the unsurpassed, God-ordained, therapeutic power of empathy.

—Author Unknown

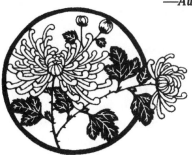

It is a true blessing as a health practitioner when you get a patient who is an advocate for his own health because you can learn so much from these individuals.

—Anonymous

De-fin-i-tions
(to be definite; to know; understanding)

Classical Homeopathy: The most effective, deepest acting treatment; uses minuscule amounts of plant, animal or mineral substances to stimulate the body to heal itself; the prescription is based on a complete evaluation of all physical, emotional, intellectual and spiritual patterns in an individual. In Classical Homeopathy, we use the emotional symptoms to point us in the direction of where to treat the imbalance in the body. Symptoms become metaphors or symbols for where imbalances are, either emotionally or spiritually. For example, asthma might be used as an indication of some long-standing unresolved grief or loss; urinary tract infections, a symbol of suppressed anger or resentment; low back pain could be a sign of fear or feelings of being overwhelmed, etc.

Your physical symptoms will all eventually be cured using Classical Homeopathy, but as a part of the process, you will also feel much better and happier emotionally. This type of treatment will take from six months to two or more years. Training to become a Classical Homeopath takes many years of study and is highly specialized. Most good Classical Homeopaths study for at least five years before getting good results. Few homeopaths have the patience to dedicate their lives to this type of intensive in-depth study and discipline.

Constitutional Homeopathy: Similar to Classical Homeopathy, but in some homeopathic circles, this term is used to describe a method where only one single remedy is used throughout one's lifetime. In reality, each person has many constitutional layers and requires many remedies in their life. Constitutional Homeopaths use only one dose of one remedy. In reality, as we evolve, we often need to move from one remedy to the next, (even though in some cases, we may need to stay on only one remedy for a number of years,) and may need to take the remedy daily.

Acute Homeopathy: In acute homeopathic prescribing, we don't place an emphasis on the emotional factors involved in disease. Rather, we directly treat and place our emphasis on removing the physical symptoms as quickly as possible. We do, however, look at the causal factor, which in many cases *does* include an emotional component. For instance, did the cold or flu begin from the emotional stress of a broken relationship, when out in a cold rain or wind, or was the cause from lack of sleep and reduced resistance to infection? Is the constipation caused from a difficulty in letting go, a craving for meat, or from not drinking enough water? Acute homeopathy will treat every physical symptom known to man, treat it quite effectively, and in most cases very quickly. But it won't be a long-term cure, as in Classical Homeopathy.

Oriental Medicine: This encompasses many disciplines and treatment types, including acupressure massage, acupuncture, Chinese nutritional medicine, Chinese manipulation (similar to chiropractic) and Chinese herbal medicine. There are many different ways to practice Oriental medicine, including Five Element Theory, Yin/Yang

Theory, acute prescribing and Korean constitutional prescribing. I use TCM, or Traditional Chinese Medicine most, and place an emphasis on the pulse and tongue diagnostic methods. I do not believe in the use of highly technical computer analysis, but use the more traditional techniques of facial observation and Five Element analysis which have been effectively used for thousands of years to diagnose and treat illness.

Chinese Herbal Medicine: This method of herbal medicine is based on the diagnostic methods described in the paragraph above on Oriental medicine. In this case, however, we use herbs, in addition to or instead of acupuncture, to create the most dramatic and quick curative action that is possible. Chinese herbology usually utilizes formulas containing many different herbs rather than just the individual herbs used in the Western approach. This method is very effective in treating chronic illness and preventing future illness from occurring. There are wonderful Chinese herbal formulas for almost every type of illness, ranging from high blood pressure, menopausal symptoms, high cholesterol, migraine headaches, PMS, ADD, insomnia, colitis, allergies and many other illnesses that plague modern society and which have no known cure in Western medicine.

Western Herbal Medicine: This approach to herbal medicine uses herbs primarily found on the North American and European continents. This method generally uses single herbs in order to achieve very specific results. There are wonderful single herbs such as Vitex, Dong Quai, Echinacea, Astragalus, Goldenseal, White Willow Bark, Milk Thistle and others, which can be used to build immunity, balance hormones and eliminate many types of pain.

Five Element Acupuncture: This method of diagnosis and treatment utilizes the Five Elements of Earth, Fire, Water, Metal and Wood. The Five Elements are a metaphor for the five primary organ functions in the body: spleen/stomach, heart/small intestine, kidney/bladder, lung/large intestine, and gall bladder/liver. Each organ and grouping of organs has an emotional component as well. Utilizing this type of understanding, we can treat constitutionally as well as symptomatically.

Acute Acupuncture: This method utilizes specific acupuncture formulas that are designed to treat the acute problems you want to treat. This is the type of acupuncture that most medical doctors study, since it only requires a few weekends of study. It requires many years of concentrated study to practice the deeper-acting Five Element and Constitutional forms of acupuncture.

Constitutional Acupuncture: This method utilizes the tongue and pulse diagnoses to assess and then design a treatment plan to treat from a deeper, more holistic framework than the Acute Acupuncture approach. Many very serious and even life-threatening health problems can be totally cured using this method.

Biochemical Nutritional Analysis: This method of analysis utilizes the Health Equations Program to assess the functional status of your electrolytes and minerals. We start from a Chem Panel and CBC and then do a comprehensive analysis utilizing the basic data from your blood tests.

Optimal Health

Body-Type Nutritional Analysis: There are many types of Body-Type Analysis. Just a few of the possibilities are Yin/Yang and Five Element Analysis, Endocrine Organ Analysis and Metabolic Typing, among others.

Five Element Nutritional Analysis: This is based on the Five Element Analysis discussed above.

Yin/Yang Nutritional Analysis: This is based on assessing your balance of yin and yang and working with the diet to change the imbalance in yin and yang. If your yin and yang are in proper balance, it's very hard for you to become ill. Balanced yin and yang is the foundation and cornerstone of balance and Optimal Health.

Vitamin/Mineral Supplementation: In our culture, most people need vitamin and mineral Supplementation because very few of us eat properly. In addition, most of us operate on such a high level of stress that we need more of certain vitamins and minerals than in times past. The soil our food is grown on is also almost totally depleted of organic minerals and because of this we need to supplement our diets. Even most organic food is not as complete as in times past.

The fact that we are totally unable to imagine a form of existence without space and time by no means proves that such an existence is itself impossible.

—Carl Jung

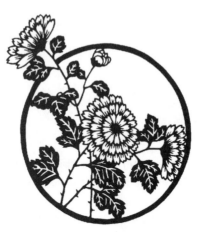

Six of the nations' leading medical schools received awards of $10,000 to teach students how to incorporate spirituality into clinical care. Polls conducted by USA Today and Time Magazine indicate that more than 70 percent of patients believe spirituality, faith and prayer helps in recovery from illness and that physicians should address spiritual issues as part of their care and should pray with patients if they request it.

BRAIN, MIND, AND CONSCIOUSNESS: A HOLISTIC MEDICAL MODEL

In discussing the brain, mind, and consciousness, it's crucial to first define what is meant. Spiritual, emotional, and intellectual aspects are all to be considered. One way to approach the discussion, from a medical point of view, is to examine what are "problems of consciousness" within the context of a "naturopathic" or holistic medical model. We will discuss this from a spiritual, emotional, and intellectual point of view.

A spiritual problem can be defined as an inability to "connect" to oneself, to other people, and in a larger sense to the universe as a whole. If one is open and flowing on a spiritual level, he or she should be able to channel and focus energy freely and at will.

An aspect to be included in this definition is the ability to effectively connect to and relate on each chakra level at will. The concept of chakras will be discussed below within the context of how acupuncture treatment is used to expand consciousness.

Another "problem in consciousness" involves emotional blockage. This can manifest as compulsive behavior, obsessive thought, phobia, obsession, excessive fear, being stuck in grief or anger, or perhaps being shut down emotionally without the ability to respond in a healthy way to other people and their expressions of feelings or love.

Intellectual blockage involves unclear thinking, foggy thought processes, forgetfulness (forgetting words, events, or people's names), or not being able to clearly focus on, plan ahead, and follow through with a task in front of you.

All these "problems in consciousness" can be effectively influenced using a holistic or naturopathic approach to health. This can include manipulation of the body's naturally occurring neurotransmitters/endorphins, Classical homeopathic medicine, traditional Chinese medicine and acupuncture, herbal medicine, diet therapy, and amino acid supplementation.

Endorphins and Their Effect on Mood and Behavior

Holistic health care can affect consciousness and the mind by manipulating the body's naturally-occurring endorphins. Endorphins are the body's own naturally-occurring opiates. They relieve pain, provide a feeling of serenity, and relax you when you're uptight. It's possible for the body to naturally release endorphins in times of stress or when exercising. That is why it feels so good to do aerobic exercise.

When endorphins are released into the body, we become relaxed and feel at ease. Falling in love is also said to release endorphins; thus we see people craving the excitement and endorphin release that is experienced in a new relationship. Certainly that feeling of "natural high" during the initial stage of a love affair feels wonderful. But, because the positive addictive aspect of endorphins manifests itself in falling in love, many people in our culture now go from relationship to relationship to score that natural high—which results in a negative addiction.

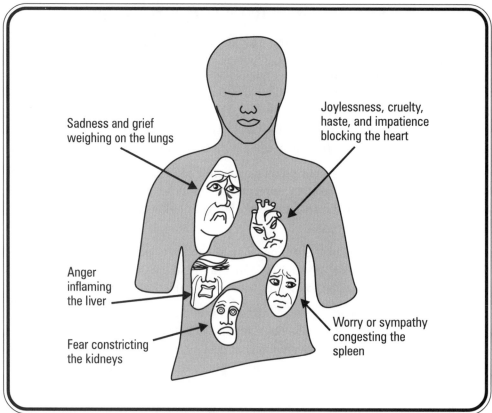

Sadness and grief weighing on the lungs

Joylessness, cruelty, haste, and impatience blocking the heart

Anger inflaming the liver

Fear constricting the kidneys

Worry or sympathy congesting the spleen

A similar destructive addiction includes smoking. Nicotine performs a role similar to endorphins in the body; thus, smoking causes a relaxation response like endorphins. The big problem starts when a person stops smoking. Endorphin production stopped when the person started smoking because, chemically speaking, nicotine effectively replaced the endorphins. The lack of endorphins creates intense craving in the patient.

Acupuncture, Chinese herbs, and amino acid supplements can be used to reestablish the flow of natural endorphins in the body (and overcome nicotine addiction and most other forms of drug addiction). Specific types of supplements and herbs can also used be to treat codependents, adult children of alcoholics, and compulsive overeaters.

One doesn't need to be addicted to substances to receive endorphin-stimulating benefits of acupuncture. There are specific acupuncture points known to release endorphins. Those who have received acupuncture for pain control already know of these effects.

The Homeopathic Approach to Altered States of Consciousness

Let's look at homeopathic medicine and how it helps create an altered state of brain, mind, and consciousness.

Homeopathic medicine began in Germany about 200 years ago. It uses minute amounts of plant, mineral, or animal substances to balance energy fields and boost immunity. Homeopathy can be used to help cure almost any problem on a physical level, but what you may not know is that it's also extremely effective in changing energy on spiritual and emotional levels.

As an example, let's look at a patient of mine, a man in his twenties who can't seem to move his life forward. He is in perfect physical health, but on an emotional level he can't decide whether to continue in his mundane, boring job as a box boy or go back to school to earn a degree in architecture—thus fulfilling his dream of working in an artistic and creative profession.

After weeks of talking with this young man, I discover that there is an emotional impasse due to a long-time wound imparted by the parents when the man was very young. The man is given an appropriate homeopathic remedy *(Nat. mur)*. Over the next few months his life begins to move forward. He enrolls in classes at a local junior college and gains a new sense of confidence in himself.

In another case, a woman in her thirties has experienced years of inexplicable compulsive anxiety and fear in crowds. Her fears are paralyzing just before her menstrual period. In this case, a homeopathic remedy called *Sepia* gave this woman a newfound sense of calmness and serenity. For the first time in years, she did not experience fear and anxiety before her period.

Many homeopathic "cures" are not this simple. Some require a number of different homeopathic remedies over a period of months, depending on how deep the physical, emotional, intellectual, and/or spiritual blocks are.

Homeopathic remedies can also be used to treat symptoms including insomnia, jet lag, or performance anxiety. In treating minor problems such as these, it is often possible to treat yourself. You may want to purchase a couple of homeopathic reference books and begin to experiment. However, if you have more complex symptoms, you will want to rely on the expertise of a trained homeopath.

Bach Flower remedies work just like homeopathic remedies and create holistic balance. The difference is that Bach remedies are prescribed solely based on emotional and psychological symptoms, whereas homeopathic remedies also take into consideration physical symptoms.

Bach Flowers are actually a subgroup of homeopathic remedies and the two are not usually used together; there are times when one or the other is most appropriate. Gem Elixir remedies and Flower Essences are similar to Bach Flower remedies. All have a valid and important place in the healing equation.

Traditional Chinese Medicine and Consciousness

Homeopathic medicine and traditional Chinese medicine have a lot in common—they treat the whole person. This type of holistic approach always acknowledges emotions, intellect, and physical complaints.

Within traditional Chinese medicine there are a number of healing models and systems. Each one arrives at a diagnosis and treatment program in its own way. The paradigm in traditional Chinese medicine that most completely deals with the mind, emotions, spirit, and consciousness is called the Five Elements. It is somewhat similar to astrological analysis.

According to the Five Elements paradigm, we each contain within ourselves parts of each element—Fire, Earth, Metal, Water, and Wood. If one or more of these are too strong (dominant) or weak (diminished), it opens us up to develop illness and disease.

Each element has an array of correspondences that helps your doctor determine where the dominance or weakness is centered. For instance, the Wood element corresponds to the emotions of anger, resentment, or "stuck" emotional energy; its corresponding spiritual quality is a desire or will to live. Symptoms that can arise due to an imbalance of the Wood element include feelings of panic, desperation, lack of control, or feelings of emotional or spiritual vulnerability or weakness.

Other correspondences for the Wood element include the color green, the sense organ of the eye, the body tissue of muscle, ligament, and tendon, and the associated organs of the liver and gall bladder.

A skilled doctor can determine which of the Five Elements is out of balance by making a thorough diagnosis. This is determined by talking with the patient in much the same way a counselor or best friend talks with someone. As much personal information as a person is willing to share will become material for the diagnosis.

In addition, the doctor may use Oriental face, eye, tongue, and pulse diagnoses and abdominal palpation to determine a patient's specific "holding pattern." Treatment uses acupuncture and/or herbal medicine. Each treatment is targeted to specific blockages along the affected acupuncture meridians. As energy begins to flow more smoothly along the meridians, the treatment will be altered to reflect the new symptom picture.

Another distinct way Oriental medicine can be used is to diagnose a person as either predominantly yin or yang. People who are predominantly yin in nature tend to be more right brain (quiet, artistic, feeling, lower in energy, and emotionally receptive). Yang individuals tend to be more left brain (outgoing, intellectual, active, high energy, aggressive).

Although these are broad generalizations, the diagnostic procedure makes it possible to clearly distinguish between these two basic constitutional types. Depending on which type you are, there are distinct acupuncture points, treatments, and Chinese herbs that are used to balance yin with yang. According to theory, when yin and yang are in balance there is perfect health on all levels.

The chakras or energy centers make up a conceptual and energetic system in the body which is said to control much of our physical and emotional energy. There are seven primary chakras and many lesser ones. These energy centers correspond to acupuncture points. Depending on which energy centers are weak, acupuncture can be used to stimulate and balance the overall system. According to this system of medicine, when the seven chakras are in balance optimal health will follow.

Using Amino Acids to Affect Consciousness

The use of specific amino acids, the "building blocks" in your body, is becoming very popular. Seventy-five percent of the human body is comprised of proteins. Amino acids are the building blocks of all proteins.

Amino acids must be supplied fresh daily. They cannot be stored in the body. Of the 22 amino acids, 9 are called *essential* because they must be supplied through a daily intake of food and supplements.

Perhaps the most significant recent event involving amino acids was when tryptophan was taken off the market. Now it's apparent that the tryptophan was not at fault. A poison contaminated a particular batch of Japanese tryptophan during the manufacturing process.

Another amino acid, L-tyrosine, plays an important role in brain functions. L-tyrosine is a nonessential amino acid found in food and in supplement form. Recent biochemical research indicates that in some cases, low moods may be associated with a brain deficiency of L-tyrosine. L-tyrosine creates norepinephrine, which has been identified as the human body's natural mood enhancer.

Other amino acids have also been identified with specific effects on both emotional and physical problems. For instance, DL-phenylalanine can be used to control pain and combat eating disorders.

A combination of DL-phenylalanine, L-glutamine, and L-tyrosine can be used to reduce stress, treat alcoholism, and treat addictions to sugar, crack cocaine, nicotine, caffeine, and prescription drugs. In addition, some researchers suggest that adult children of alcoholics and codependents have an innate deficiency of these amino acids.

Herbal Medicine and Consciousness

People have been using herbs for thousands of years. Over the last ten years, the consumption of herbs for a variety of problems has increased in popularity. There are many herbs that affect the brain and act on our energy levels and mental abilities.

Though the amino acid tryptophan has been taken off the market, there are many other herbal formulas that treat insomnia, depression, and nervousness.

The following herbs effectively take the edge off depression, lack of concentration, or low energy: Ginseng, Licorice, Ginger, Gotu Kola, and Damiana. Often herbs are combined into formulas for maximum effectiveness. Formulas in the form of teas or capsules can be obtained over the counter at most health food stores.

Herbs to "take the edge off," to act as "downers," and to help people unwind include the following: Skullcap, Valerian Root, Passion Flower, and hops. Skullcap is a good herb for nervous fear or irritability. Muscle twitching or nervous weakness following illness may also be an indication for this herb.

Valerian Root has been used for 500 years to promote sleep without the aftereffects commonly produced by narcotics. It has a quieting and soothing effect. Passion Flower has been used since the early 1800s as a sedative and is especially good for restlessness and insomnia.

Hops are generally associated with ale and beer and are a prime ingredient in those drinks. The oil extracted from hops has been used to induce sleep and combat restlessness or overactive mental processes.

Food and Its Effect on Mind and Mood

Most people are unaware of how the body, mind, and thought processes are controlled by the foods they eat. Eating certain foods has been shown to significantly alter thought patterns. The chemicals, sugars, additives, and amino acid composition of food can drastically influence thinking processes and emotional moods.

Common food allergies will often cause foggy and unclear thinking. Everyone has particular foods they're sensitive to, but the primary foods that affect a large number of people are citrus fruits, refined sugar, caffeine, dairy products, beef, wheat, rye, oats, chocolate, and eggs.

Many people are chemically sensitive and experience foggy thinking or low energy after ingesting such things as MSG, residual pesticides on fruits and vegetables, and preservatives or colorings in processed foods.

It has also been shown that eating protein stimulates thinking processes, while eating carbohydrates releases serotonin, an amino acid precursor that is a relaxant and soporific.* High protein foods include fish, beans, chicken, and beef; carbohydrates include grains, starchy vegetables, and pastas.

Of course, sugar and caffeine affect energy and thought with an immediate rush of energy. Then they cause an even longer period of depression and low energy that leads to an even greater need for more stimulant. Nicotine has a similar stimulating effect, which is followed by an even longer period of "down time."

Conclusion

There are many types of natural approaches to holistic health. People can play a large role in improving their physical, emotional, and spiritual harmony by using some of the techniques and tools discussed here.

Remember that you are in control and can alter your thought processes, consciousness, and energies. Awareness of the tools discussed in this article is a good first step. Now it's up to you!

You Decide

Educating yourself, knowing which modalities you want and are most interested in, defining your treatment goals, and knowing what you are willing to do to get there,

---

*Soporific—a substance which induces sleep

are **all** invaluable components of becoming healthier and **overcoming the obstacles** to losing weight, exercising, eating right and joining in partnership with your health care team. You decide which treatment options are right for you.

Find out what a person fears most and that is where he will develop next.
—*C.G. Jung*

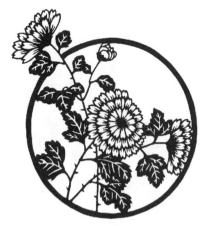

…the sacred is immanent—it's present right here and now, in nature and in ourselves. And by "sacred" what I mean is not a great something that you bow down to, but what determines your values, what you would take a stand for. And when you locate that principle in the world, rather than beyond it, you also see that everything has its own inherent value.
—*Starhawk*

ORIENTAL MEDICINE

Yin and Yang

Chi, or life force energy, is divided into *yin* and *yang*. The concept of yin and yang is a way of looking at life. The two are flip sides of the same coin, two halves of the whole. In Eastern cultures, seeing the yin and yang in everything is a state of mind, but in the West we are more used to seeing everything as black or white, good or bad, male or female.

Creating a balance between yin and yang is the Asian ideal of health. When either is out of balance, whether as abundance or deficiency, disease occurs. Part of the basis for traditional acupuncture theory and practice is distinguishing between the yin and yang components of a person's constitution and illness.

In nature, the summer and spring seasons are yang and winter and autumn are yin. The opening of a flower is yang, and the winter hibernation of a bear is yin. On an emotional level, too much aggressive energy or anger can create an imbalance of yang and too much passive energy or depression, apathy, or sadness can create a predominance of yin.

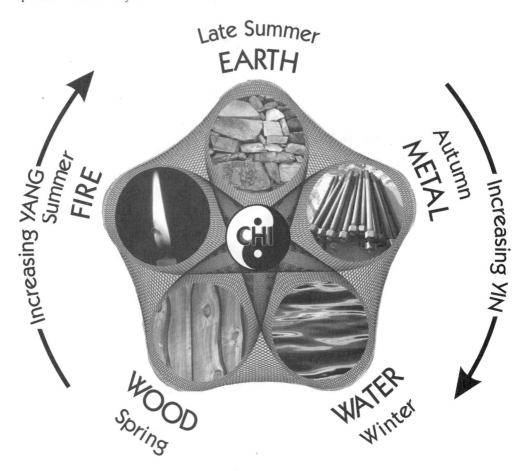

YIN   YANG

RIGHT BRAIN	LEFT BRAIN
Controls left body	Controls right body
Subdominant	Dominant
Inner focus	Outer focus
Images	Linear
Dreams	Thought
Instinctive	Rational
Unconscous	Conscious
Synthesis	Analysis
Cycle	Sequence
Association	Logic
Music	Speech

Yin embodies such qualities as cold, dark, reflective, intuitive, right-brained, artistic, contractile, receptive, and "data input." Yang has the opposite and complementary qualities of hot, light, active, left-brained, logical, expansive, and "data output."

Tarzan is yang and Jane is yin. A macho football player is yang and a quiet, reserved artist or intellectual is yin.

In terms of medical problems, overly yin people might have anemia, hypoglycemia, dizziness, confusion, diarrhea, low blood pressure, or pain that is relieved by pressure and heat. Yang people are more likely to get constipation, vascular headache, restlessness, Type A behavior, high blood pressure, be easily excited or "wired," and have pain that is relieved by ice and made worse by pressure or massage.

Being overweight is most often an excessive yin problem; being anorexic or thin is excessive yang or an extreme lack of yin. Yin is considered feminine and yang masculine, but we each have both the feminine and masculine energy within us, just as modern medicine has shown that men naturally have a small amount of female hormones and women naturally have a small amount of male hormones.

Within the general framework of yin and yang, it is possible to determine whether a person's constitution or illness is predominantly yin or yang and to treat the person accordingly. For instance, if a football player comes to an acupuncturist complaining of headaches and constipation, eats a lot of red meat and salty foods, and discovers he has hypertension, he would be treated by choosing acupuncture points to reduce yang and stimulate yin. In addition, more passive or yin activities such as meditation may be suggested to balance the overly active yang component in his life.

By contrast, if a pale, anemic-looking computer programmer came to the same acupuncturist complaining of low energy, hypoglycemia, and dizziness, and upon further examination he was found to have an excessive yin and deficient yang condition, specific yang acupuncture points and dietary and lifestyle recommendations could be used to boost his yang.

In theory at least, whenever our outgoing, male, yang energies or our inward, receptive, female, yin energies become blocked, we may begin to experience ill health. In the real world, the yin-yang diagnosis and treatment is more difficult than this, because everybody has components of both yin and yang. It is only with much study and experience that an acupuncturist can determine which treatment will best correct the particular imbalance in each person.

Using modern psychological theory to explain yin and yang, we find that an introverted person is considered to be more yin and an extroverted person is more yang. Yin people tend to be more quiet, introspective, meditative, and self-absorbed. Yang people tend to be more outgoing, active, assertive, and concerned with worldly events.

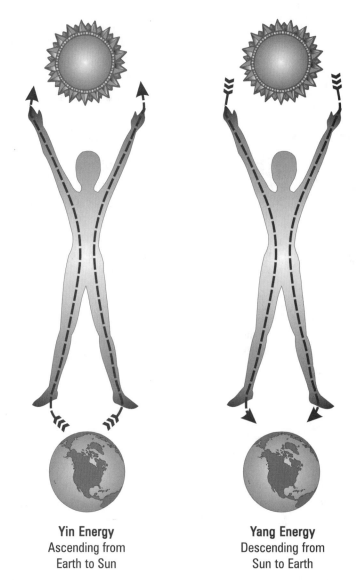

Yin Energy
Ascending from
Earth to Sun

Yang Energy
Descending from
Sun to Earth

In Western medicine, the parasympathetic nervous system is considered yin; the sympathetic nervous system (the fight-or-flight response) is yang. One is passive or relaxed, and one is active. In terms of metaphysics and the theory of *chakras* or body energy centers, yang people tend to be more grounded and centered, fixated in their lower chakras, while yin people tend to be more aware of (or "stuck" in) their upper chakras. In terms of astrology, yin people are more Air and Water, and yang people are more Earth and Fire.

Often yin is thought of as dark and negative, and yang is thought of as light and positive. Since yin is also feminine and yang is masculine, many people think of the feminine element as a negative, but this is a misinterpretation. We each have feminine and masculine energy within us in varying amounts. The ideal is for each of us to nurture and explore the feminine (yin) and the masculine (yang) within.

Carl Jung talked about the need for men to explore and accept their anima/yin portion and for women to explore and accept their animus/yang side. He proposed that if you do not develop a sensitivity to the opposites within yourself, they will grow to be very powerful and begin to unconsciously control your behavior. Jung called the less-dominant side the "shadow" side. By accepting the shadow within each of us, actions and inner feelings can be more fully integrated.

In terms of a global viewpoint, our country and the rest of the Western world are traditionally yang, while China and the Eastern part of the world are yin. This changes as communication and integration between the two viewpoints ensues.

Looking at the yin-yang sign, we can see that there is yin within the yang and yang within the yin. Yin and yang cannot exist without each other. There is no value judgment with regard to either yin or yang. They are interdependent, symbiotic, and both oppose and reflect each other.

To create a better balance of yin and yang in your life, there are some techniques you can use. One very common acupuncture treatment called the *Four Gates* balances the yin and yang energies and is safely used on almost everyone. This treatment consists of four acupuncture points: two on the hands at *Hoku*, and two on the feet called *Tai Chong*. In terms of Western medical theory, this treatment has been shown to be very effective in balancing the sympathetic and parasympathetic nervous systems.

Diet is perhaps the easiest way to alter your yin-yang balance. If you are too yin, eat more yang foods, and vice versa. You can also pick the appropriate exercise to complement your imbalance. If you are very yin by nature, try more yang or active forms of exercise such as swimming, jogging, bicycling, etc. If you are too yang by nature, include exercise which calms you down and stretches your muscles. Try tai chi chuan, aikido, walking, meditation, or listening to classical music.

You can use acupressure and herbs to help create an inner balance. Visual imagery is also an excellent way to create balance. There are many books available that will teach you how to accept within yourself those attributes which are suppressed or unexpressed.

Within our global community, we have already made great strides in drawing a balance between yin and yang by increasing contact and encouraging communication and economic interdependence between our eastern neighbors. The more communication and contact, the more we will be able to internalize differences in others as unexplored parts of our own selves. This is true on the global and personal levels.

A nonjudgmental attitude, an acceptance of differences and opposites, and an attempt at understanding and integration promote balance and health. Yin-yang theory is a holistic way to look at life. Once it is mastered, it can provide you with many insights about yourself and your environment.

Yin and Yang Checklist

This checklist is not meant to be definitive or diagnostic, but it will give you a rough idea as to whether you tend to be more yin or yang.

Do not assume that you definitely fall into these categories simply because you check a lot of the items in that category. If you go through these lists carefully and place a mark next to each characteristic you have or which you feel identifies you, it will enable you to have a richer understanding of the complexity of this type of medical diagnosis. You may also have a lot of fun trying to see which category sounds most like you! Place a check next to each characteristic you identify with.

Yang Checklist

Yang Physical:

❏ Constipation
❏ Heavy menstrual flow
❏ Urination is dark
❏ Craving for salt
❏ Restless
❏ Face is red or flushed
❏ Craving for red meat
❏ Hyperactive
❏ Stomach ulcers
❏ Burning feet
❏ Hotter than others
❏ Never cold
❏ Rapid pulse
❏ Warm body
❏ Prefer contact sports

❏ Menstrual cycle less than 28 days
❏ Clotted menstrual flow
❏ Thirsty and drink a lot of fluid
❏ Prefer cold drinks instead of hot
❏ Pains are violent and stabbing
❏ Sweat a lot when exercising
❏ High blood pressure
❏ History of gall bladder or liver problems
❏ Hyperacidity of stomach
❏ Sleep with little covers
❏ Grind teeth
❏ Like winter the best
❏ Fever for no apparent reason
❏ Get a headache in the sun

Yang Emotional:

❏ Talkative
❏ Rage at others
❏ An idea person
❏ Extrovert
❏ Bully
❏ Pushy
❏ Manipulative
❏ Nervous
❏ Very assertive
❏ Witty
❏ Difficulty meditating
❏ Left-brained person

❏ Anger easily and express it
❏ Gregarious and outgoing
❏ A natural salesperson
❏ Like math and science
❏ Lead other naturally
❏ Hard to accept criticism
❏ Cry very easily
❏ Do not hold in feelings
❏ Like more active sports; has needed endurance
❏ At a party, go up to others and talk
❏ Difficulty taking directions, letting go of control
❏ In nature, like to keep moving, not meditating

Yin Checklist

Yin Physical

- ❐ Diarrhea
- ❐ Light menstrual flow
- ❐ Lack of thirst
- ❐ History of anemia
- ❐ Like the hot sun
- ❐ Crave sugar
- ❐ Crave fruit
- ❐ Hard to get started
- ❐ Fatigue
- ❐ Adrenal weakness
- ❐ Hands and feet cold
- ❐ Left-handed
- ❐ Sleep curled up
- ❐ Weak hearing
- ❐ Low blood pressure
- ❐ Chronic indigestion
- ❐ Weak muscles
- ❐ Dizziness
- ❐ Pale face

- ❐ Menstrual cycle more than 28 days long
- ❐ Urination clear and very frequent
- ❐ Like hot drinks
- ❐ Pains are dull and aching
- ❐ Like summer the best
- ❐ Headaches in the morning
- ❐ Hypoglycemia
- ❐ Like to be alone and quiet a lot
- ❐ In nature, like to sit and be contemplative
- ❐ Night sweats
- ❐ Right-brained person
- ❐ Sleep with lots of blankets
- ❐ Always colder than others
- ❐ Slow pulse naturally without a lot of exercise
- ❐ Lack of appetite
- ❐ Loose stools or diarrhea often
- ❐ Ringing in the ears
- ❐ Premature ejaculation in men
- ❐ Decreased sex drive or disinterest in sex

Yin Emotional

- ❐ Quiet
- ❐ Receptive
- ❐ Very organized
- ❐ Passive
- ❐ Withdrawn
- ❐ Psychic
- ❐ Worrier
- ❐ Tightness
- ❐ Fatigue
- ❐ Hard to assert self
- ❐ Introvert
- ❐ Inner focus

- ❐ Difficulty generating ideas
- ❐ Artistic
- ❐ Difficulty following through with ideas
- ❐ Hard to get started
- ❐ Low spirits, depressed easily
- ❐ Intuitive
- ❐ Emotions often get stuck, rerun over and over
- ❐ Constriction
- ❐ Angers easily, but does not show it
- ❐ Like solitude
- ❐ Like relaxing, new age music
- ❐ At party, walk to corner to observe others

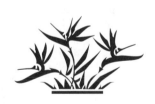

THE FIVE ELEMENTS

In this section I will explain how every common physical or emotional problem you could have can relate in some way to one of the five "elements" of Oriental medicine. These are Fire, Metal, Earth, Water, and Wood. They are poetic or metaphorical ways of looking at our health—or physical and emotional body and mind.

Study of the Five Element theory in Oriental medicine yields many insights into our body/mind imbalances and the source of many of our problems. Because so much of the theory is metaphorical, it leaves a lot to be desired in terms of scientific explanation. However, it has survived thousands of years and is still widely practiced in China, Japan, most of the Eastern, and some of the Western world, so there must be something to it.

Five Element theory is a very exciting way to view the body and mind, and allows you to delve deeply into spiritual blocks as well as the physiological pathologies behind a given problem.

All five of the elements are within us to some degree, so you will likely experience characteristics of all of the groups at one time or another.

If you experience four or more of the characteristics of a particular element much of the time, you may be predisposed to be that "type" of person. Most likely we inherit this typology from our parents, but there is much you can do to treat and control predisposition.

The Five Element system can also be a model for understanding health and treating disease. Once you have identified which element(s) address your particular set of problems at a particular time, you can treat yourself effectively.

Treatments call for specific herbs and acupuncture or acupressure points to unblock and move the flow of energy through the particular affected organ and meridian. With appropriate treatment, you can counter a genetic predisposition or heal disease. For children, treatment can ensure a much healthier, happier, and more balanced childhood.

These are but brief summaries of each element:

Fire

The Fire Element relates to the small intestine and the heart. Common problems relating to this element include insomnia, unsettled sleep, waking too early, palpitations in the chest, sweating for no reason, anxiousness or discomfort in one's environment, being "spaced out," lack of emotional groundedness, forgetfulness, impatience, emotional distance from others, heart problems, or any assimilation problems having to do with the duodenum. Often the Fire Element person will move very quickly and have a round face, broad cheeks, horizontal facial lines, and a high and cracking voice.

Metal

The Metal Element relates to the lungs and large intestine. Common problems may include shortness of breath, asthma, chronic bronchitis, frequent colds, dry coughs, hoarseness, or a dry nose or throat. Dry skin can also be a Metal problem. Psychologically, a person with Metal problems suffers from accumulated grief, hurt, sadness, weariness, and the need to replenish after the strain of losing something. When recovering from a loss of any kind, the lungs or Metal Element may be affected. This can include holding on, or the inability to let go manifested as emotional or physical constipation.

Earth

The Earth Element relates to the stomach, pancreas, and spleen. Common problems include abdominal distention, bloating, chronic weak digestion, loose stools, diarrhea, nausea, or lack of appetite. Other problems can include a "wasting away" of the muscles, inability to gain weight, chronic tiredness, fatigue, or weakness. On a psychological level, one may feel unable to get involved with oneself or others, unable to undertake projects, or be especially pessimistic or lacking perseverance. Other qualities include being overly self-aware, unable to make moves because of the risks, obsessiveness, indecision, pessimism, and an inability to nurture oneself and others. The Earth type of person may have thick thighs, a square face, yellowish complexion, heavy body movements, and a thick, tall back. They may also crave sweets.

Water

The Water type of person may have problems related to their kidneys or bladder, such as chronic urinary infections. Other problems may include sexual problems such as premature ejaculation, low sexual energy, pain during intercourse, uterine bleeding, or prostate problems. Other Water Element problems include low back pain, sore legs, knee pain, or dryness of the eyes, skin, hair, eyes, or mouth. This person may be agitated or nervously uneasy, unable to sit still with no inner calm, fearful, have a lack of faith or willpower, searching but never arriving, uneasy, emotionally tired, lazy, and lacking assertiveness. They may stammer and have a shriveled or dry appearance and be thirsty all the time.

Wood

The Wood Element person will have problems with the liver and gall bladder and may suffer from headaches, dizziness, and fatigue, and stiffness in particular joints, tendons, or all over. Chronic Fatigue Syndrome usually involves the Wood Element. This person may feel very fatigued even after a nap or a good night's sleep. A woman with Wood problems may get PMS; a man may have testicular pain. Other problems include gas, distention, difficulty in digesting fats, or bloating. There may be a certain emotional edginess, moodiness, agitation, resentment, feelings of separation from the environment, negativity, or anger. The body of a Wood person may be somewhat angular, rigid, uneasy or especially taut.

The Five Elements in Traditional Chinese Medicine

EARTH
LATE SUMMER
MOIS-TURE
YELLOW
SYM-PATHY
STOMACH
TASTE
SING
SPLEEN
MOUTH
7 am-11 am
SWEET
CENTER

FIRE
SUMMER
HEAT
RED
JOY SORROW
SMALL INTESTINE
SPEECH
THREE HEATER
HEART CIRCULATION SEX
TONGUE
LAUGH
11 am-3pm 7-11 pm
BITTER
SOUTH

METAL
AUTUMN
DRY-NESS
WHITE
WORRY GRIEF
LARGE INTESTINE
SMELL
CRY
LUNGS
NOSE
3 am-7 pm
PUNGENT
WEST

WOOD
SPRING
WIND
GREEN
ANGER
LIVER
SIGHT
SHOUT
GALL BLADDER
EYES
11 pm-3 am
SOUR
EAST

WATER
WINTER
COLD
BLUE BLACK
FEAR
KIDNEYS
HEAR-ING
GROAN
BLADDER
EARS
3 pm-7 pm
SALTY
NORTH

ELEMENT
SEASON
CLIMATE
COLOR
EMOTION
YIN ORGAN
SENSE
SOUND
YANG ORGAN
SENSE ORGAN
TIME
TASTE
DIRECTION

Key to the Diagram Above

FIVE ELEMENT SELF-EVALUATION

This checklist is just a sample of Five Element criteria used in diagnosis. You can use it by simply checking off those categories that pertain to you and then adding up the results. The results will be a superficial yet somewhat reliable calculation and diagnosis. Complete diagnosis requires careful observation by a trained Doctor of Oriental Medicine, tongue and pulse diagnosis, and a complete family and personal health history.

FIRE ELEMENT

Overall: Anxiety, mood swings, burnout, heartbeat irregularities, insomnia, difficulty connecting to people, excessive or inappropriate laughter, predisposition to heart problems, difficulty in assimilating and digesting food, rumbling in the stomach

- ❏ emotionally a very warm person
- ❏ emotionally very protected
- ❏ difficulty getting close to people
- ❏ always laughing or giggling
- ❏ heartburn
- ❏ flatulence a few hours after eating
- ❏ dislike or love for heat of summer
- ❏ stuttering
- ❏ perspiration: too much or not at all
- ❏ like or dislike for the color red
- ❏ red car
- ❏ wear red clothing a lot
- ❏ emotional problems
- ❏ dreams of fire, laughing, or blazing flames
- ❏ red complexion
- ❏ hot flashes
- ❏ poor circulation
- ❏ cold more often than others
- ❏ high blood pressure
    Total Fire _____

WATER ELEMENT

Overall: Emotionally isolated, depression, fear, despair, pessimism, grouchiness, apathy, low sex drive, prostate problems, kidney or bladder infections, yeast or urinary infections, low back pain, arthritis, hearing problems, fatigue, low energy from 3 to 5 P.M.

- ☐ tired 3–5 P.M.
- ☐ hypoglycemia
- ☐ crave salt
- ☐ crave a "meat and potatoes with gravy" diet
- ☐ like or dislike for the color dark blue or black
- ☐ have a black car
- ☐ wear predominantly black clothes
- ☐ urinary tract infections
- ☐ little sex drive
- ☐ premature ejaculation
- ☐ prostate inflammation
- ☐ prostate cancer
- ☐ dark circles under the eyes
- ☐ poor hearing
- ☐ dizziness
- ☐ afternoon headaches
- ☐ low energy in general
- ☐ need to snack frequently
- ☐ fear is a primary emotion or motivating factor in life
- ☐ fear change
- ☐ fear sexual contact
- ☐ fear the dark
- ☐ claustrophobia
- ☐ weak or painful knees
- ☐ losing hair
- ☐ dislike for cold or rainy weather
- ☐ vaginal discharge
- ☐ vaginal pain
- ☐ painful sexual intercourse
- ☐ menstrual difficulty
- ☐ poor will power and follow through
- ☐ difficulty sticking to your diet
- ☐ dream of drowning people, plunging into water, or of boats

    Total Water _____

METAL ELEMENT

Overall: Stiffness, fragile, prone to over-rigidity or passivity, prolonged grief or sadness, chest tightness, asthma, chronic bronchitis, breathing difficulties, frequent colds or flu, chronic skin problems such as psoriasis or eczema

- ❏ pale face
- ❏ white skin
- ❏ white automobile
- ❏ wear white clothing a lot
- ❏ look good in white
- ❏ allergies
- ❏ lots of colds and flu
- ❏ hay fever
- ❏ constipation or diarrhea a lot
- ❏ must use laxatives
- ❏ chronic bronchitis
- ❏ asthma
- ❏ skin rash
- ❏ eczema
- ❏ psoriasis
- ❏ dry skin
- ❏ often very sad
- ❏ constantly dwelling on the loss of a loved one
- ❏ cry at the drop of a hat
- ❏ never cry
- ❏ difficult to feel any emotions
- ❏ grieving over a recent sad event
- ❏ like hot and spicy foods
- ❏ like or dislike the color white
- ❏ worry a lot
- ❏ shortness of breath
- ❏ emphysema
- ❏ smoker, or got a lot of passive smoke growing up
- ❏ sigh a lot
- ❏ acne
- ❏ boils
- ❏ post nasal drip
- ❏ dream of white objects, cruel killing, crying, flying in the air
- Total Metal _____

WOOD ELEMENT

Overall: High blood pressure, cramps, muscle spasms, tension in neck and shoulders, impulsive or volatile behavior, headaches, nerve pains, sciatica, allergies, acne, hay fever, feels worse during Santa Ana winds, gets a lot of energy late at night

- ❏ dislike of the wind, especially Santa Ana winds
- ❏ airborne allergies or hayfever
- ❏ anger easily, often resentful
- ❏ fly off the handle
- ❏ like or dislike for the color green
- ❏ like fatty or fried foods
- ❏ crave cheese
- ❏ flatulence/burping
- ❏ heartburn
- ❏ poor eyesight or wear glasses
- ❏ like or dislike for sour foods (vinegar, pickles, sauerkraut)
- ❏ voice is of a shouting nature
- ❏ family history of liver or gall bladder problems
- ❏ acne
- ❏ alcoholic mother or father
- ❏ drink too much alcohol yourself
- ❏ menstrual cramps
- ❏ premenstrual symptoms
- ❏ insomnia, can't get to sleep, or hyper between 11 P.M. and 1 A.M.
- ❏ an "idea" person
- ❏ start projects easily, but trouble following through
- ❏ arthritis or joint pain
- ❏ pain in the right shoulder blade
- ❏ pain in the right shoulder
- ❏ pain in the right eye or left eye radiating from the back of the head
- ❏ nightmares of being trapped
- ❏ feelings of being smothered
- ❏ overly organized
- ❏ difficulty planning
- ❏ difficulty making decisions
- ❏ muscle spasms
- ❏ epilepsy or convulsions
- ❏ Multiple Sclerosis
- ❏ cystic breasts
- ❏ warts/moles/freckles

(continued)

- ❐ cysts/fibroids
- ❐ family history of cancer
- ❐ dream of mountain forests or trees
  Total Wood _____

EARTH ELEMENT

Overall: Over or underweight, dry skin, water retention, chronic fatigue, flatulence, bloating, feeling overwhelmed, compulsive or obsessive, worried a lot, menstrual problems, craves sweets

- ❐ feel connectedness with the earth
- ❐ very grounded
- ❐ stubborn
- ❐ overweight
- ❐ underweight
- ❐ anorexic
- ❐ bulimic
- ❐ homesick or difficulty leaving home
- ❐ constantly think about the past
- ❐ obsessive/compulsive
- ❐ feel alone a lot
- ❐ feel a sense of disconnection from life in general
- ❐ like or dislike the color yellow
- ❐ yellowish complexion
- ❐ stomach pains
- ❐ ulcers
- ❐ stomach gas right after eating
- ❐ constant stomach troubles
- ❐ hypoglycemia
- ❐ fatigue after eating
- ❐ diabetic
- ❐ inability to receive sympathy
- ❐ monotone voice
- ❐ singing voice
- ❐ likes to sing a lot
- ❐ belching after eating
- ❐ dislike for dampness
- ❐ arthritis which is worse in damp weather
- ❐ dream of lack of food or drink, singing, or building buildings
- ❐ crave sweets or dislike for sweets
  Total Earth _____

THE FIVE TYPES OF PEOPLE

According to Oriental medical theory there are basically five types of people. Because we inherit these "types" from our parents, there is not a whole lot you can do to avoid them. But there is a lot you can do to treat and change them. The five types and their keynote symptoms are the following (Note that if you experience four or more attributes of any type, you may have this particular weakness.):

1. **Earth Type:** overweight or underweight, dry skin, water retention, chronic fatigue, flatulence, bloating, feeling overwhelmed, compulsive or obsessive, worried a lot, menstrual problems, crave sweets.

2. **Water Type:** feel emotionally isolated, depression, fear, despair, pessimism, grouchiness, apathy, low sex drive, prostate problems, kidney or bladder infections, yeast or urinary infections, low back pain, arthritis, hearing problems, fatigue, low energy from 3–5 P.M.

3. **Wood Type:** high blood pressure, cramps, muscle spasms, tension in neck and shoulders, impulsive or volatile behavior, headaches, nerve pains, sciatica, allergies, acne, hay fever, feels worse during Santa Ana winds, gets a lot of energy late at night.

4. **Fire Type:** anxiety, mood swings, burnout, heartbeat irregularities, insomnia, difficulty connecting to people, excessive or inappropriate laughter, predisposition to heart problems, difficulty in assimilating and digesting food, rumbling in the stomach.

5. **Metal Type:** stiffness, fragile, prone to over-rigidity or passivity, prolonged grief or sadness, chest tightness, asthma, chronic bronchitis, breathing difficulties, frequent colds or flu, chronic skin problems such as psoriasis or eczema.

The treatment for each type is to use acupuncture points and traditional Oriental herbal formulas to treat the weak meridian(s). With appropriate treatment, you can counter your genetic predisposition to getting the same problems your parents or grandparents have had. For children, treatment can assure a much healthier and happy childhood.

Children usually respond best to homeopathic and herbal treatment, since most kids don't like the idea of needles. For adults who don't like needles, homeopathic and herbal treatment is also extremely effective in changing the genetic predisposition to ill health.

THE CHINESE FIVE ELEMENTS AND NUTRITION

There are many different types of diets available today. Some promise to help you lose weight, others say they'll help you to score with the women by helping to "pump you up." Many of us are choosing diets based on our politics or ethics, such as John Robbins' recommendation, and still others are choosing diets for optimal energy, such as Barry Sears' Zone diet.

So what I'm about to propose may seem weird to you, but according to the Chinese philosophy of the Five Elements, your diet should not be selected based on your goals, nor on some recent fad, but should be based on the best diet for your particular constitution.

The Chinese Law of Five Elements is based on ancient concepts that were first observed in nature. These natural laws evolved over hundreds, if not thousands, of years and eventually led not only to the medical system which includes acupuncture and herbs, but also a complete theory of nutrition and diet.

According to Chinese theory, if you eat according to your constitution, you will more easily be able to *stabilize* your weight, optimize your energy, have better brain power and also be in closer synch and integrity with nature.

So how do you determine your constitution? The five elements are Fire, Metal, Earth, Water, and Wood. They are poetic or metaphorical ways of looking at our health and our physical and emotional health. Each of us has pieces of each of each of the five elements within ourselves. Your underlying constitution and which foods will work best to optimize your health can be determined from a careful analysis of the elements. Read each paragraph and see the checklist to see which element seems most like you!

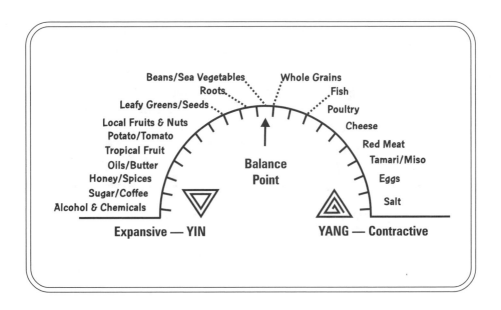

THE FIVE FLAVORS

According to Chinese medicine there are five flavors, which correlate with each of the five elements. Some people love sweets, others love sour foods and many of us love sweets. Depending on which foods you love the most, we can diagnose which of your meridians and organs are weak and strong.

Sour corresponds to the Wood element (liver, eyes, and gall bladder) and includes foods such as sweet tarts, lemons, pickles, vinegar, and sauerkraut.

Bitter corresponds to the Fire element (heart and small intestine) and includes foods such as greens, cranberries, coffee, unsweetened chocolate.

Sweet corresponds to the Earth (stomach and spleen) element and includes sugar, pastries, candies, and fruit.

Spicy corresponds to the Metal element (lungs, skin, and large intestine) and includes curries, cayenne pepper, pungent sauces, ginger.

Salty corresponds to the Water element (kidneys, bladder) and includes pretzels, chips, seaweed.

To maintain your health you must eat foods corresponding to all five food groups. This will keep all the organs and meridians in your body in balance. A little of each food group will tonify and feed the element it is associated with. On the other hand, if you eat too much of any one group you will begin to weaken the element it is associated with.

Sometimes if you note a change in your preference for foods from one of the groups, it can be an "early warning" signal of changes on a deeper level in your body. If you suddenly crave sweets, it's an indication of your spleen becoming weakened. On the other hand, if you always crave sweets, this is an indication of a deeper weakness in the spleen that has been with you for a longer time.

If you have a weakness in a particular meridian and organ, sometimes the treatment will be to eat a little more of the flavor that relates to that particular organ and sometimes the treatment will be to abstain from the flavor corresponding to that organ. Acupuncture and herbal medicine are also used to treat the imbalance reflected by the food craving.

If people pay attention to the five flavors and blend them well, chi and blood will circulate freely and breath and bones will be filled with the essence of life.

—*Nei Jing*

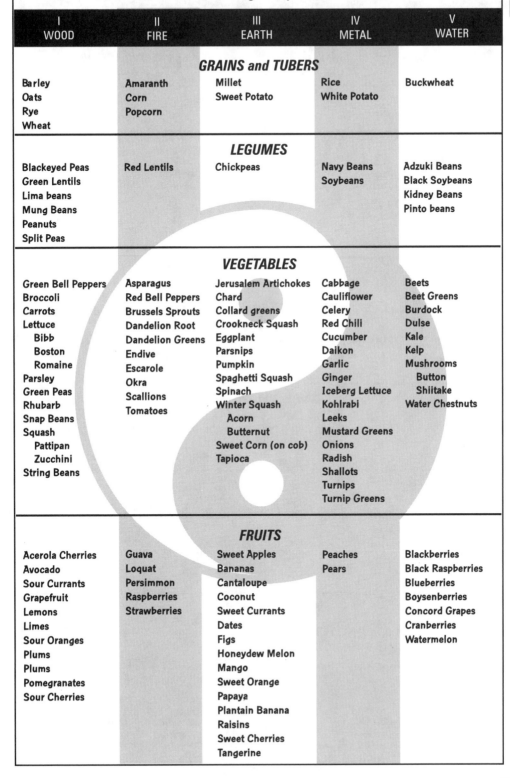

FIVE ELEMENT FOOD CHART
Use this chart to strengthen your weak element!

I WOOD	II FIRE	III EARTH	IV METAL	V WATER

GRAINS and TUBERS

I WOOD	II FIRE	III EARTH	IV METAL	V WATER
Barley	Amaranth	Millet	Rice	Buckwheat
Oats	Corn	Sweet Potato	White Potato	
Rye	Popcorn			
Wheat				

LEGUMES

I WOOD	II FIRE	III EARTH	IV METAL	V WATER
Blackeyed Peas	Red Lentils	Chickpeas	Navy Beans	Adzuki Beans
Green Lentils			Soybeans	Black Soybeans
Lima beans				Kidney Beans
Mung Beans				Pinto beans
Peanuts				
Split Peas				

VEGETABLES

I WOOD	II FIRE	III EARTH	IV METAL	V WATER
Green Bell Peppers	Asparagus	Jerusalem Artichokes	Cabbage	Beets
Broccoli	Red Bell Peppers	Chard	Cauliflower	Beet Greens
Carrots	Brussels Sprouts	Collard greens	Celery	Burdock
Lettuce	Dandelion Root	Crookneck Squash	Red Chili	Dulse
Bibb	Dandelion Greens	Eggplant	Cucumber	Kale
Boston	Endive	Parsnips	Daikon	Kelp
Romaine	Escarole	Pumpkin	Garlic	Mushrooms
Parsley	Okra	Spaghetti Squash	Ginger	Button
Green Peas	Scallions	Spinach	Iceberg Lettuce	Shiitake
Rhubarb	Tomatoes	Winter Squash	Kohlrabi	Water Chestnuts
Snap Beans		Acorn	Leeks	
Squash		Butternut	Mustard Greens	
Pattipan		Sweet Corn (on cob)	Onions	
Zucchini		Tapioca	Radish	
String Beans			Shallots	
			Turnips	
			Turnip Greens	

FRUITS

I WOOD	II FIRE	III EARTH	IV METAL	V WATER
Acerola Cherries	Guava	Sweet Apples	Peaches	Blackberries
Avocado	Loquat	Bananas	Pears	Black Raspberries
Sour Currants	Persimmon	Cantaloupe		Blueberries
Grapefruit	Raspberries	Coconut		Boysenberries
Lemons	Strawberries	Sweet Currants		Concord Grapes
Limes		Dates		Cranberries
Sour Oranges		Figs		Watermelon
Plums		Honeydew Melon		
Plums		Mango		
Pomegranates		Sweet Orange		
Sour Cherries		Papaya		
		Plantain Banana		
		Raisins		
		Sweet Cherries		
		Tangerine		

Oriental Medicine

FIVE ELEMENT FOOD CHART—SUPPLEMENTARY FOODS

I WOOD	II FIRE	III EARTH	IV METAL	V WATER
SPROUTS				
Barley Alfalfa Mung	Corn Sunflower	Millet	Celery Radish Rice	Buckwheat
SEEDS				
	Sesame	Caraway Pumpkin		Chia Black Sesame
HERBS				
Alfalfa Root	Hops	Anise Licorice Shepherd's Purse	Basil Bay Leaf Cardamom Cayenne Cinnamon Clove Coriander Dill Fennel Horseradish Nutmeg Black Pepper Thyme	
NUTS				
Brazil Cashew Lychee	Pistachio	Almond Filbert Pine Macadamia	Walnut	Chestnut
DAIRY PRODUCTS				
Butter Cream Mayonnaise Sour Cream Sour Yogurt		Cottage Cheese Ice Cream Fresh Milk Sweet Yogurt	Cheese Egg Whites	Egg Yolks
SEAFOOD				
Fresh Water Clam Trout	Shrimp	Anchovy Eel Salmon Sturgeon Swordfish Tuna	Cod Flounder Haddock Halibut Herring Perch Scrod	Abalone Bluefish Catfish Clams Oysters Crab Lobster Sardine
MEAT & POULTRY				
Beef Liver Chicken Chicken Liver Lamb Liver	Lamb	Rabbit	Beef Turkey	Pork Duck
MISCELLANEOUS				
Nut Butter Vegetable Oils Olives Vinegar Wheat Bran Nutritional Yeast	Beer Coffee Chocolate Catsup Liquor Tobacco	Honey Barley Malt Maple Syrup Relish Rice Syrup Sugar	Mint Mochi Peppermint Spirulina Tempeh Tofu	Decaffeinated Coffee Gomasio Miso Salt Tamari Bancha tea

PULSE DIAGNOSIS

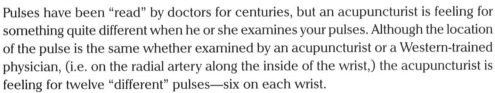

What are you doing when you "take my pulses"?

Pulses have been "read" by doctors for centuries, but an acupuncturist is feeling for something quite different when he or she examines your pulses. Although the location of the pulse is the same whether examined by an acupuncturist or a Western-trained physician, (i.e. on the radial artery along the inside of the wrist,) the acupuncturist is feeling for twelve "different" pulses—six on each wrist.

Each of the twelve acupuncture meridians has a particular "spot" or "position" on the wrist, and each can be diagnosed separately. The object is for all twelve pulses (and meridians) to be in perfect balance, but this is never the case; there is always some work to be done on balancing the meridians.

The pulses are also used to determine the relative yin and yang in the body/mind/spirit. When your yin and yang are in perfect balance, then you will be in perfect health. But everyone has some relative deficiency in either yin or yang. An excess of nervous energy or hyperactivity is usually due to a yin deficiency; fatigue is usually due to a relative deficiency of yang.

The pulses will help the acupuncturist to confirm the symptoms you have discussed with him or her as well as give more information that you might not be aware of. For instance, if you have mentioned symptoms of weak Kidney energy such as poor memory, fatigue, thinning hair, frequent urination and low sexual drive, then your doctor will check the Kidney pulses to determine if they are a bit weak.

If you have difficulty with digestion, menstrual problems, PMS, anemia, headaches, or spend a lot of time thinking and ruminating, or have "teeth marks" on the edges of your tongue, the doctor will want to check your Spleen pulse for weakness.

Reading the pulse is only one part of traditional Chinese diagnosis, along with tongue diagnosis, color and facial diagnosis, listening to the voice, and observing the posture and body type. Most contemporary Doctors of Oriental Medicine will also perform blood tests, X-rays, hair analysis and other tests as necessary.

Within the field of Oriental medicine, there are many different techniques for examining the pulses. Some doctors check the pulses with the patient lying down, others with the patient sitting up. Some will examine both wrists at the same time and others will check each wrist separately. As with all medical practices, this will differ based on the doctor's training and philosophy.

Sometimes the pulse can stay the same for several treatments and at other times the pulse will be different each time you come for treatment. Some doctors will only check your pulse at the first visit and others will use it more often to check the progress of treatment. Some doctors will not examine the pulses if they have not had specialty training in this diagnostic technique.

Ask your doctor which diagnostic techniques he or she relies on in their treatment. If he or she is focusing more on homeopathic medicine they may rely mostly on your behavior and on subjective symptoms as described by you in your own words.

No single diagnostic technique is better or more accurate than any other. You must find a doctor whom you can trust and remain with him or her long enough to see long-term results, usually for at least six months and often for up to a year or more.

COMMON QUESTIONS ABOUT TONGUE DIAGNOSIS

Why are you looking at my tongue?

The tongue shows the condition of the organs in your body. By looking at your tongue, I can determine the health of your liver, lungs, kidneys, heart, stomach, spleen, gall bladder, and intestines. In addition, the tongue tells whether you are in balance in terms of yin and yang, hot and cold, and damp and dry.

What exactly are you looking at?

I am looking at the shape, color, and coating, and whether the tongue has any cracks, bumps, dips, or other irregularities.

Does it matter that I brush my tongue?

Yes, most definitely! Please do not brush your tongue the day you come for treatment, as this will affect the diagnosis. Be sure to tell me if you *do* brush your tongue. Brushing will affect the true color and coating, and may change other aspects as well.

Does it matter if I eat just before you look at my tongue?

Not really—as long as what you eat does not substantially discolor the tongue. Foods that discolor the tongue include coffee, candies, and tea. Remember that if you are receiving acupuncture treatments, it is better to not eat for about an hour before and half an hour after your treatments.

I feel embarrassed because my tongue is "ugly."

You have nothing to be ashamed of. I am not comparing your tongue to anyone else's. In fact, everyone has a unique-looking tongue. There is no such thing as a "perfect" tongue. Everyone's tongue reflects the imbalances going on in their particular organs.

What do the different colors mean?

A pale tongue indicates a deficiency, which can be a deficiency of yang energy or of blood circulation, or it can indicate anemia.

A bright red tongue indicates an excess condition, whether too much yang or heat in the body, or not enough yin or nutritive energy in the body.

Depending on other parts of the tongue, the deficiency or excess can be pinpointed to specific organs in your body. For example, a bright red tip indicates internal heat, heart problems, or emotional disturbances. A red tongue with a purple center indicates heat in the stomach. A reddish-purple tongue may indicate heat or liver yin deficiency. A blue tongue indicates internal cold. A blue tongue in a pregnant woman may indicate the danger of miscarriage. A scarlet red tongue may indicate a lung yin deficiency or heart yin deficiency.

What do the cracks on the tongue indicate?

Depending on the area on the tongue, the direction of the cracks and their depth, the color of the tongue, and the type of tongue coating, the cracks can mean a lot of different things. Interpreting cracks can be fairly complex and takes years of study and practice.

For instance, a deep crack running from the center to the tip means you may have some disturbance in the heart or *shen*, which we interpret as emotional stress. If the tongue color is a light pink, this crack may not indicate a disease process at all. If the tongue color is red with a redder tip, the crack may indicate "heart fire" with deep emotional problems. If the tongue color is red with no coating at all, the crack may indicate a yin deficiency of the kidneys leading to heat in the heart.

Little cracks just behind the tip of the tongue may indicate lung diseases such as childhood pneumonia, tuberculosis, or long-standing lung yin weakness.

A crack running along the center and dividing the tongue in half means you have what is called "stomach heat," or a deficiency of stomach yin. This could be experienced as an insatiable appetite, poor assimilation of food, or a lack of yin, depending on other factors.

Little cracks on the sides indicate heat in the liver, or a deficiency of spleen yin, and a lack of yin and fluid assimilation in the body. Irregular small cracks may indicate a general deficiency of stomach yin and body fluids, depending on the area they occur in and the color of the tongue.

What does the tongue coating show?

The main thing the coating shows is the condition of digestion. A "normal" tongue, if there is such an animal, should have a thin, slightly white, moist coating. A thick white coating indicates poor digestion or the beginning of a cold or flu.

A thick yellowish coating indicates more severe indigestion, constipation, or a fever or heat somewhere in your body. Depending on the area of the tongue that has the yellow coating, we can determine which organ systems are overheated or congested.

A thick yellow coating on the rear of the tongue, for example, can indicate either constipation or congestion in the urogenital system. This could be either prostate problems in a man or uterine fibroids, ovarian cysts, vaginitis, or a urinary infection in a woman.

How many different shapes are there?

There are two primary shapes and a lot of variations on them. If the tongue is flabby and big, and shows teeth marks, it indicates too much dampness in your body or not enough "fire" or yang.

Depending on which parts of the tongue are swollen or enlarged, we can tell which organs in your body have imbalances and need to be treated. For example, if the sides are swollen it indicates a liver or spleen problem.

A thin tongue may look pointed and dry; this generally indicates a depletion of yin, blood, and fluids in the body. If the tongue is elongated or thin with a central crack, and swollen on both sides of the central crack, it may indicate a heart problem.

If the tongue goes to one side when it is extended, it may mean there is "internal liver wind." If the tongue doesn't stop moving when extended it may mean there is heart fire and a deficiency of spleen yin. Tooth marks on the sides usually have something to do with a spleen deficiency.

How accurate is tongue diagnosis?

It is extremely accurate. The tongue changes according to your inner health over months of treatment. You can expect the tongue to change very slowly as your health improves and you experience more balance, vitality, and optimal health.

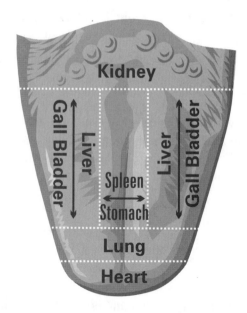

Therapy, any type of therapy, is the space created by and for healing, existing somewhere between resistance (i.e. the stuck place in the patient) and the helping (i.e. the therapist). Often the resistance is created in the interaction and is not clearly a result of the patient's resistance. Both the archetypes of resistance and helping simultaneously exist in the patient and the doctor. The doctor's job is to catalyze and nurture the healing/ helping response in the patient.

—Dr. Randy Martin

THE ROLE OF STOOL TESTS IN ORIENTAL MEDICAL DIAGNOSIS

Stool tests are an invaluable addition to the diagnosis and treatment of most health problems. The stool test can point out many problems that are hard to diagnose with any other means. Included in this list are parasites, various types of yeast (including *Candida albicans*), leaky gut syndrome, disbiosis,* lack of favorable bacteria, etc.

According to the theory of Chinese medicine, the gut, or stomach, must be in good shape in order for our health to be strong. The stool analysis is an inexpensive way to determine the overall health of the entire digestive tract.

But remember—there are different types of stool analysis, and the only one that will give you accurate data is the stool purge, which uses a laxative before the stool sample is taken. The regular sample taken in the doctor's office is not sufficient to detect the parasites and other harmful organisms.

Another important point to remember is that there has been a lot of talk recently about parasites and the harm they can cause in your body. This is the exact reason it's so important to have a stool test done. But on the other hand, everyone has some small parasites and yeasts in their body most of the time. The main thing is to strengthen the digestive tract. The stool sample is one of the many tools we can utilize to do this. But your digestive tract is never going to be totally free from harmful bacteria, yeasts and parasites.

HOW MUCH SHOULD A DOCTOR OF ORIENTAL MEDICINE REVEAL TO THEIR CLIENT?

Using pulse and tongue diagnosis, a Doctor of Oriental Medicine can often tell a lot about the state of health of his patient. But how much of this is it ethical to tell the patient? Most people come for treatment to alleviate an acute pain or for some other acute problem. All too often, they don't really care too much about their long-term health.

There are many tools a Doctor of Oriental Medicine has at hand, but most of these tools are much more effectively used for prevention than for the treatment of acute problems. When diagnosed properly, Oriental/Chinese medicine can increase one's health dramatically. But a patient doesn't always want to hear the real truth of what the doctor may have to say. Some of the unpleasant findings I have to commonly confront my clients with are the following:

❋ When tongue color is extremely purple, there is a severe liver condition. If untreated, this will lead to gall bladder disease, PMS, anxiety, severe depression, etc.

---

*Disbiosis—a disfunction of the digestive tract, which leads to symptoms such as candida overgrowth, belching, bloating, flatulence, burning, fatigue and other digestive problems.

❋ A deep crack in the tongue, in the center section, indicates long-standing stomach and digestive problems; if untreated, this will lead to stomach ulcers, colitis or irritable bowel syndrome. It also points to a patient who has had years of very poor eating habits and food choices.

❋ Severe indentations on the tongue with lots of white coating: a patient comes in with endometriosis or cysts and wants them removed using acupuncture. But the overall condition of the body is so weak and "damp," as indicated by the tongue, that I know it'll take at least a year or more to create a positive change.

❋ There is a deep crack in the tongue, going all the way to the tip, and the tongue is dry with many small cracks. This can indicate what we call in Oriental medicine a "shen" disturbance. In Western terms, it can indicate a long-standing emotional problem. If a patient is coming to my office for treatment of psoriasis or sciatica, they probably don't want to be told they might have an emotional problem that in some way has created the skin disorder.

❋ Blood test results often show such things as a low protein count, anemia, high liver enzymes, low calcium, low sodium or high cholesterol. Patients have often been told by their medical doctor that their blood test results are all normal, but through more precise interpretation using Oriental medical theory as applied to blood tests, I can often see problems before they develop. Protein malnutrition is one of the more common problems, and many patients are not open to hearing this diagnosis, nor open to changing their diet to effect a change.

❋ Some people can handle more information than others and some people are more open to change than others. A good example of this is someone whose pulses, according to Oriental pulse diagnosis, show that they have what is called a "low or weak blood" problem, even though the complaint they come in for is low back pain. They may only want treatment for the low back pain, even though the "low blood" condition, if left untreated, will cause problems later on.

❋ Some patients may be open to looking at some of their eating habits or emotional patterns and others may not. As a Doctor of Oriental Medicine, it can be very tricky to decide how much to share with a patient about some of these patterns and problems, when they are only coming to the doctor for the treatment of their immediate pain.

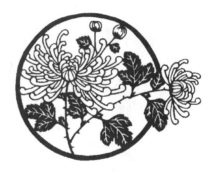

ACUPUNCTURE

Introduction

Acupuncture is about 3,000 years old and is used to treat everything from pregnancy and childbirth to head colds, headaches, arthritis, back pain, facial wrinkles, cysts, fibroids, PMS, and colitis. It is based on removing energy blocks in the body which keep people from functioning optimally. These energy blocks are removed by stimulating *energy meridians* or paths in the body with very tiny, surgically sterile, stainless steel needles or filaments.

There are a variety of theories why acupuncture works. Recent research points to its effect on brain chemistry and how it affects the body's immune system and hormone levels. Other research indicates that acupuncture increases endorphins. Certain acupuncture points can increase sex drive, combat infertility, increase digestive enzymes, decrease inflammation or fever, boost immunity, improve memory, or aid in the reproduction of red or white blood cells. Acupuncture balances yin with yang energies, thereby creating balance and increased energy. It can also reduce stress, overcome addictions, clear up skin problems, and eliminate most types of pain. I'll elaborate on all of these concepts more fully later in this chapter.

Is Acupuncture for You? The Most Common Questions Asked by the New Patient

What is the origin of acupuncture?

Thousands of years ago in China, it was noted that soldiers wounded by arrows in battle sometimes recovered from illnesses which had afflicted them for many years. Eventually doctors began to correlate certain points with certain effects.

The earliest writing on acupuncture appeared about 2,000 years ago in the *Nei Ching (The Yellow Emperor's Classic of Internal Medicine)*. This book contains writings on acupuncture, diet, spinal manipulation, massage, hydrotherapy, herbalism, sun and air therapy, and exercise.

Traditional Chinese medicine quickly spread to the rest of Asia. In the 1600s, it spread to Europe after a Frenchman published the first book on acupuncture ever written in the Western world.

Former President Nixon's visit to China heightened public awareness of the effectiveness and acceptability of acupuncture as an alternative medical treatment in the U.S.

How is an acupuncturist licensed?

Each state has its own licensing procedure. In California, the first licensing exam was in 1978. The title L.Ac. (Licensed Acupuncturist) is awarded by the California Board of Medical Quality Assurance when an individual has from three to four years of education and training, and passes a rigorous written and oral exam given by the state board.

How does acupuncture work?

Research demonstrates that acupuncture produces definite physiological reactions in the body such as changes in heart rate, blood pressure, intestinal activity, and blood chemistry. How these effects occur still remains unclear; research is currently being conducted throughout the world.

The ancient Chinese believed that *chi*, a basic life force or energy, is present in all living things. All cultures have a name for this energy. The Hindus calls it *prana*; a Western doctor named Wilhelm Reich called it *orgone energy*; some metaphysicians call it the "vital force" or "life force." *Chi* ("chee," as it is pronounced in Chinese) or *ki* ("kee" in Japanese), is the energy that vibrates all around us. Without chi, all life would cease to exist.

Chi is divided into *yin chi* and *yang chi*. Yin and yang chi are further divided into chi that circulates along specific invisible energy pathways in the body, called *meridians*. We have good health when our yin and yang chi are flowing smoothly throughout the meridian system, like a river flowing downstream. We succumb to disease when our chi becomes blocked, or when there is too much or too little chi flowing through any individual meridian.

The existence of meridians can now be verified with specific devices that scientists and some acupuncturists now use to measure areas of lower electrical skin resistance. These instruments, called *electro-acupuncture devices,* are used by some acupuncturists to diagnose and treat the meridians that are out of balance.

When the flow of chi is interrupted or blocked, there is a disruption in an individual's health that results in pain or disease. By stimulating the appropriate acupuncture points along these meridians, the blocked energy is released and health restored. The science of acupuncture is to locate these blockages and use needles to stimulate and restore the normal flow of energy through the meridians.

The Chinese do not differentiate between mental, physical, or spiritual chi. When a blockage occurs, it is likely to cause an obstruction on any or all of these levels

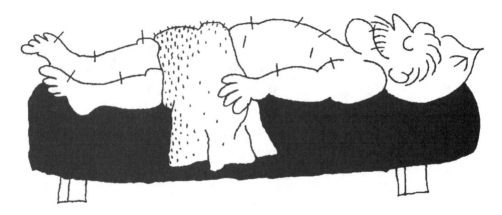

simultaneously, or it may fluctuate between levels. Depending on the predominant level where the blockage occurs, the acupuncturist will be able to determine the most effective type of treatment.

A more Western theory states that acupuncture works to reduce or eliminate pain by releasing endorphins, the body's naturally occurring sedatives. Experiments proved that people with a high threshold for pain also have a higher concentration of endorphins flowing through their body.

Another theory states that acupuncture creates a new or distracting sensation which allows the brain to forget the old sensations.

What are meridians and acupuncture points?

There are 12 primary acupuncture meridians and another 8 "extra" meridians. There are a total of approximately 360 primary acupuncture points and another 400 supplementary points.

The acupuncture meridian is an invisible channel of energy which transmits electrical current from one acupuncture point to another. Experiments show that the body cells located along the meridians have up to ten times more sodium and potassium compared to cells lying outside the meridians. This makes the meridians excellent conductors of electrical current.

Individual acupuncture points act as miniature receptor sites, attracting or repelling electrical current. The insertion of needles into these points has the net effect of "telegraphing" bioelectrical energy to certain areas within the body along the meridians.

How do you find the acupuncture points?

Points are like doorways. They are specific areas on the body where we can gain access to the chi and affect its movement. The exact placement of the points varies slightly from person to person. Usually there is a small depression or dip in the skin at a point. Part of an acupuncturist's training is to learn to precisely locate these points.

How do you know they really exist?

There are machines, ranging from inexpensive to thousands of dollars each, that actually measure the points and show precisely where they are on the body.

What is an acupuncture examination like?

A typical initial examination will take about an hour. Most of the exam is spent talking to the prospective patient about all aspects of his life, including emotions, thoughts, fears, apprehensions, hopes, etc. A complete history is taken, including childhood illness, family background, and emotional history.

An acupuncturist may also carefully examine the face and body, features, nails, skin temperature, and skin color. The physical exam may include blood pressure readings, traditional tongue diagnosis, pulse diagnosis, and abdominal palpation. Each acupuncturist works differently and finds different information valuable for a diagnosis.

Oriental Medicine

I often use Western diagnostic techniques such as blood tests, urinalysis, stool tests, or hair analysis.

Some acupuncturists use an electronic device or computer to diagnose your meridian imbalances. I believe in the more traditional approach and find the electronic equipment to be unnecessary—an impediment to obtaining a deeper connection with, and understanding of, my patients.

How many different types of acupuncture are there?

There are at least six types of acupuncture treatments:

1. *Stop smoking/addiction control/stress relief.* This type of treatment releases endorphins. Many people under a lot of stress find this type of treatment very relaxing. In itself it can be addictive, but it is a positive addiction. This treatment also promotes a good night's sleep.

2. *Pain control.* This type of treatment controls pain with the release of endorphins. It is very effective in tennis elbow, sciatica, carpal tunnel syndrome, neck and shoulder pain, back pain, athletic injuries, arthritic pain, slipped disc, and tendonitis.

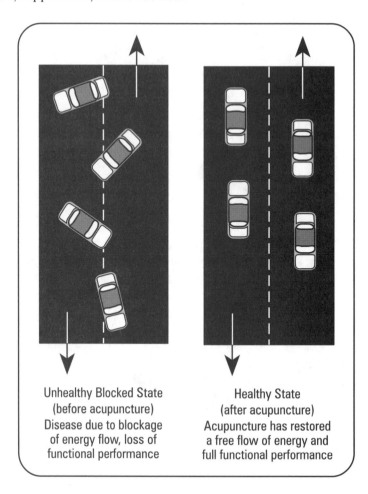

Unhealthy Blocked State
(before acupuncture)
Disease due to blockage
of energy flow, loss of
functional performance

Healthy State
(after acupuncture)
Acupuncture has restored
a free flow of energy and
full functional performance

3. *Acute problems.* This treatment is for a specific problem of short duration such as PMS, migraine headache, bronchial asthma, allergies, stomach ulcers, sour stomach, constipation, diarrhea, head cold, flu, or ovarian cysts. If the problem is more long-standing, then it is considered systemic treatment.

4. *Systemic treatment.* This is for chronic or long-term problems. It is effective when treating the same types of problems as those in Number 3, but the treatment methods penetrate deeper into the body and have a greater effect. This treatment takes a longer time because it focuses on particular systems in the body which have been out of balance for a long period of time. The focus is on treating whatever body system is out of balance, such as the urogenital system, the cardiovascular system, or the gastrointestinal system.

5. *Electro-acupuncture.* As I stated above, this is not a type of acupuncture I am attracted to personally. It uses very sophisticated electronic equipment to diagnose blocked meridians. Some acupuncturists treat patients with electronic as well as other methods. I have known many people to receive tremendous benefits from this type of treatment.

6. *Constitutional treatment.* This is my personal favorite to receive and to give. If acupuncture had an ultimate way of being performed, this would be it! The Worsley School of Acupuncture and those trained in the Worsley Method perform only this type of acupuncture. They claim that all other forms are superfluous and inferior. This type of treatment is based on a complete history of the patient, along with body type, diet analysis, emotional issues, family history, lifestyle issues, pulses and tongue diagnosis, skin temperature and coloration. It is the most complete form of diagnosis and treatment. This type of treatment does not address any particular or acute problem directly; rather, it treats the whole person, and in doing so the acute or chronic problems eventually heal. The primary purpose of constitutional acupuncture is to promote your long term optimal health.

There are no negative effects from acupuncture.

What part do the emotions play in diagnosing and treating my problem?

It depends. In some cases, the emotional component may play a major role; in others, a relatively minor one. The emotions are only one aspect of health and must be integrated into a diagnosis which also uses the tongue, pulse, and complete history of physical symptoms.

How do I know which type of acupuncture I need?

If you are patient, the best type of treatment is constitutional. However, in many cases you may want to begin with acute treatments—especially if you are in a lot of pain or discomfort. After your initial problem is under control, you can begin constitutional treatment. It is best to discuss your treatment needs with your doctor and to decide together on the best type of treatment for you.

Traditionally, Oriental physicians in China and Japan used diet, exercise, and lifestyle changes to heal their patients before the use of herbs or acupuncture. Acupuncture was the final resort and only used if herbs, diet, and counseling techniques failed to effect a cure. But here in America, where the quick fix to healing is what most people understand and expect, acupuncture usually starts with the initial treatment.

How many treatments will it take?

Constitutional treatment takes longer, and the treatments are spread out over a longer period. One treatment each month is the average. After you are in balance, it is recommended you have one treatment four times a year—at each change of season. For acute problems and for addiction withdrawal, it is common to be treated two or three times a week for an average of four to five weeks, and then undergo another evaluation.

What is a typical acupuncture treatment like?

An acupuncture treatment usually consists of the insertion of stainless steel needles through the skin at specific acupuncture points. Eighty percent of the points are located around the wrists and ankles, arms, and legs. Other points located on the ear, stomach, face, back, neck, or shoulders may be employed, depending on the type of problem being treated.

The acupuncture needles are extremely thin, and the patient feels only the slightest sensation on insertion. When the needle reaches the acupuncture point under the skin, a characteristic sensation of heaviness, tingling, numbness, or dull aching may be felt. Most often there is very little or no sensation at all.

After insertion, the needles may be carefully turned to provide extra stimulation. The needles are usually left in place for approximately 10 to 40 minutes, after which time they are gently and easily removed, usually without any sensation at all.

In constitutional acupuncture, only two needles might be used. Other types of treatment may use 10, 20, or 30 needles in a single treatment. Of course, all needles are completely sterile, used once, and then discarded.

Most patients report feeling slightly light-headed or even euphoric after a treatment, and many describe a pleasant sensation of relaxation or general well-being which usually lasts for 24 hours or more.

How do I know if acupuncture will cure my particular problem?

It is important to know that acupuncture treats the patient as a whole, not just the individual parts of his body. Mind and body are considered interconnected and inseparable. Accordingly, the patient should not be surprised if s/he feels healthier overall from the treatment.

Every person is unique and will respond to treatment in a unique way. It is impossible to predict how quickly the treatment will work on your particular problem. Although two people may have the exact same problem, the cause of that problem may be entirely different. It is essential that you have patience.

What about the use of herbs and homeopathic remedies during my treatment?

In general, most acupuncture treatments will include the use of herbs and/or homeopathic remedies to help tone and balance the body's energy. Herbs and homeopathic remedies will continue to provide you with care between your acupuncture treatments. If you are given a constitutional homeopathic remedy, it is important that your acupuncturist be alerted, as some types of remedies can be antidoted by acupuncture treatment.

Rules to Follow When Receiving Acupuncture Treatments

The most important thing to remember during treatment is to relax. Concentrate on your breathing if you like—and relax. This will help the body perform its own healing process more efficiently. Balance is the result of a free mind and flowing energy.

Many people are a bit nervous about the possible discomfort associated with acupuncture treatment. There is no reason to be concerned about this, as pain is rarely ever experienced. There are two sensations you will experience during acupuncture—the needle penetrating the skin experienced. There are two sensations you will experience during acupuncture—the needle penetrating the skin (which doesn't hurt; it may feel like a slight pinch or prick, or you may not feel it at all), and what the Chinese call *ta chi* or "getting the chi." This refers to the needle contacting the meridian and moving the chi within the meridian. It may feel like a numbness, tingling, throb, or electrical sensation.

You can best participate in the treatment by being vocal. When you experience the *ta chi,* let your acupuncturist know. Some specific rules for acupuncture treatments are:

✧   Refrain from eating 1 hour before or after treatment.

✧   Take a short or long walk or a nap after the treatment. It is best not to go back into a stressful situation immediately.

✧   Do not shower, bathe, or swim for 2 hours after the treatment.

✧   Do not be surprised if you feel a little "funny" during or after your treatment. Different emotions or sensations may unexpectedly surface. Some people experience profound relaxation, sadness, anger, or euphoria after a treatment. Some people don't experience anything in particular.

✧   Some people have immediate relief from their symptoms after the treatment and others may take up to a week to feel the effects. Each person's body is different and responds in its own way.

✧ Be sure to report new symptoms or changes in symptoms to your doctor on your next visit. Keep a health journal and bring it with you so you don't forget to share everything you experience.

✧ Get well … think positive … and relax. You deserve it!

The three figures that follow show some of the most commonly used acupuncture points and their indications. In actuality, each individual acupuncture point can be used for many different problems. Some points might be used to treat as many as one hundred different problems.

When points are combined with other points, their purposes may also change significantly, so that the entire treatment "formula" is what really counts in most treatments, rather than each particular point being used. This synergistic effect of the points is part of what makes the practice of acupuncture so complex and also so difficult to explain to the newcomer. After you have received a number of treatments, you will probably begin to see the patterns of points being used to treat you.

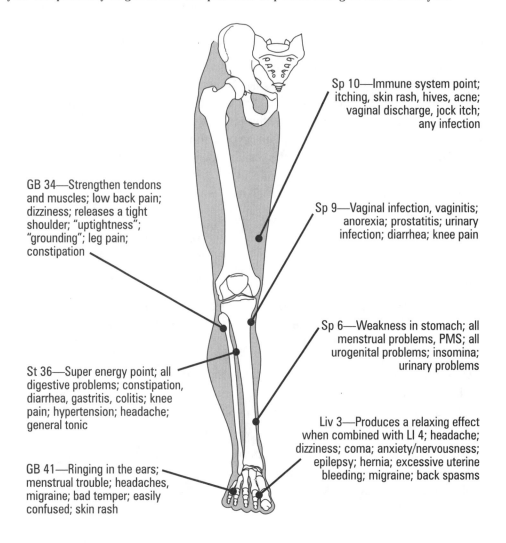

Sp 10—Immune system point; itching, skin rash, hives, acne; vaginal discharge, jock itch; any infection

GB 34—Strengthen tendons and muscles; low back pain; dizziness; releases a tight shoulder; "uptightness"; "grounding"; leg pain; constipation

Sp 9—Vaginal infection, vaginitis; anorexia; prostatitis; urinary infection; diarrhea; knee pain

Sp 6—Weakness in stomach; all menstrual problems, PMS; all urogenital problems; insomina; urinary problems

St 36—Super energy point; all digestive problems; constipation, diarrhea, gastritis, colitis; knee pain; hypertension; headache; general tonic

Liv 3—Produces a relaxing effect when combined with LI 4; headache; dizziness; coma; anxiety/nervousness; epilepsy; hernia; excessive uterine bleeding; migraine; back spasms

GB 41—Ringing in the ears; menstrual trouble; headaches, migraine; bad temper; easily confused; skin rash

Most Commonly Used Acupuncture Points

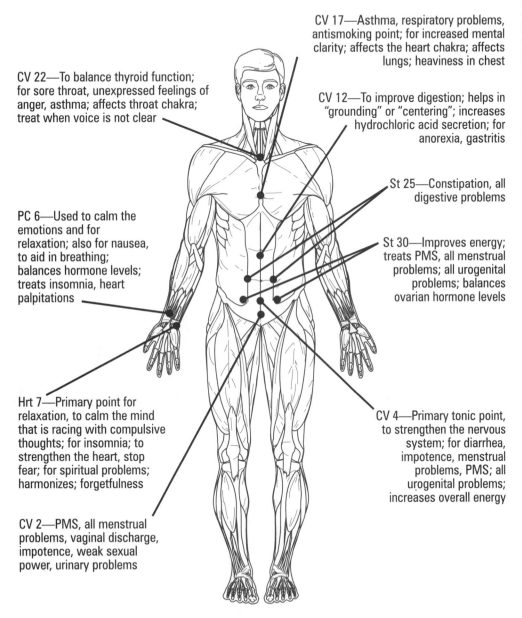

CV 17—Asthma, respiratory problems, antismoking point; for increased mental clarity; affects the heart chakra; affects lungs; heaviness in chest

CV 22—To balance thyroid function; for sore throat, unexpressed feelings of anger, asthma; affects throat chakra; treat when voice is not clear

CV 12—To improve digestion; helps in "grounding" or "centering"; increases hydrochloric acid secretion; for anorexia, gastritis

St 25—Constipation, all digestive problems

PC 6—Used to calm the emotions and for relaxation; also for nausea, to aid in breathing; balances hormone levels; treats insomnia, heart palpitations

St 30—Improves energy; treats PMS, all menstrual problems; all urogenital problems; balances ovarian hormone levels

Hrt 7—Primary point for relaxation, to calm the mind that is racing with compulsive thoughts; for insomnia; to strengthen the heart, stop fear; for spiritual problems; harmonizes; forgetfulness

CV 4—Primary tonic point, to strengthen the nervous system; for diarrhea, impotence, menstrual problems, PMS; all urogenital problems; increases overall energy

CV 2—PMS, all menstrual problems, vaginal discharge, impotence, weak sexual power, urinary problems

Most Commonly Used Acupuncture Points

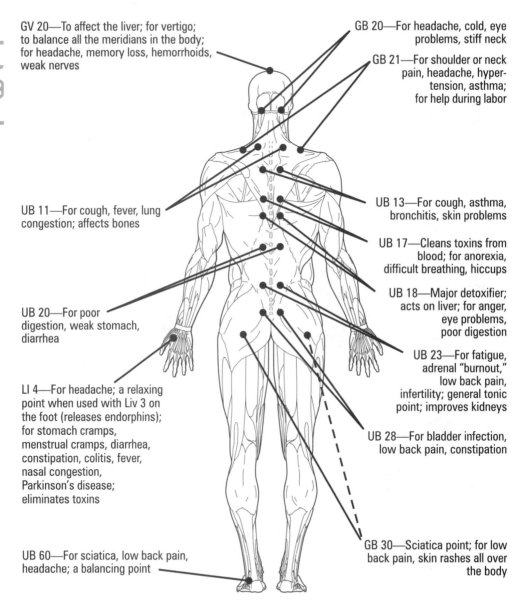

GV 20—To affect the liver; for vertigo; to balance all the meridians in the body; for headache, memory loss, hemorrhoids, weak nerves

GB 20—For headache, cold, eye problems, stiff neck

GB 21—For shoulder or neck pain, headache, hyper-tension, asthma; for help during labor

UB 11—For cough, fever, lung congestion; affects bones

UB 13—For cough, asthma, bronchitis, skin problems

UB 17—Cleans toxins from blood; for anorexia, difficult breathing, hiccups

UB 18—Major detoxifier; acts on liver; for anger, eye problems, poor digestion

UB 20—For poor digestion, weak stomach, diarrhea

UB 23—For fatigue, adrenal "burnout," low back pain, infertility; general tonic point; improves kidneys

LI 4—For headache; a relaxing point when used with Liv 3 on the foot (releases endorphins); for stomach cramps, menstrual cramps, diarrhea, constipation, colitis, fever, nasal congestion, Parkinson's disease; eliminates toxins

UB 28—For bladder infection, low back pain, constipation

GB 30—Sciatica point; for low back pain, skin rashes all over the body

UB 60—For sciatica, low back pain, headache; a balancing point

Oriental Medicine

The choice of which points to use is based on the school of thought that the acupuncturist has been trained to use. Some acupuncturists, like myself, are eclectic and have studied many different systems. I tend to pick and choose between acupuncture systems, depending on the particular problem of the individual patient. There are, at a minimum, about six to ten currently popular acupuncture systems being taught to American acupuncturists.

Note that the indications listed for each point on these figures do not directly apply if your acupuncturist is performing Five Element (or Worsely) acupuncture. Five Element acupuncture utilizes a somewhat different explanation for what each point does.

WHY ACUPUNCTURE DOESN'T ALWAYS WORK

There are a number of reasons why the application of acupuncture doesn't always work. Here are just a few of the possible reasons:

1. Misdiagnosis: Usually, diagnosis is done from the point of view of Oriental medicine, and this can be a fairly complex process, taking time for the practitioner to perform. It may involve reading the pulse and/or tongue diagnosis and if the diagnosis is wrong, the treatment can go awry.

2. Another type of misdiagnosis is when the patient enters into acupuncture treatment with an incorrect Western diagnosis. Here's an example: A patient comes for acupuncture treatment for what she is told are ovarian cysts, but it turns out she is actually suffering from endometriosis or P.I.D. (pelvic inflammatory disease.) This misdiagnosis will complicate and possibly lengthen the acupuncture program. Expected results will not occur, and the patient will have to be sent back to their medical doctor for a new diagnosis.

3. Sometimes if a patient is on prescription medications, it is hard to get an accurate reading on the pulse and tongue diagnosis. We never have a patient stop their prescription medications, but the medications may sometimes complicate the acupuncture treatment to some extent. This is an unfortunate circumstance that cannot be changed, since we rarely will advise the patient to discontinue his Western medications in favor of acupuncture. The two modalities are complementary and can be used together very successfully

4. Another example is when a patient is taking a lot of pain relievers, antihistamines or is on a daily regimen of antidepressants. Again, this makes the Oriental diagnosis more difficult because the medications can distort the diagnostic picture somewhat.

5. Lack of adequate treatment: Often a person has come to expect, through Western medicine, instant results. With Oriental medicine, including acupuncture and herbs, it can take a longer period of time to get results,

since the treatments are much more subtle than what the person may have come to expect with Western medicine. Some people stop treatment before giving acupuncture an adequate opportunity to work.

6. Frequency of treatments are inadequate: For acute, severe pain, it's necessary to have acupuncture twice weekly. In fact, if we lived in China, one would receive treatments daily, or even twice daily when in severe pain. If a person chooses to have treatments only monthly, for example, and they have acute pain, it makes it much harder for the acupuncture to work.

7. Nutritional imbalance: I have seen many people with chronic neck, shoulder, back or leg pain who do not respond to acupuncture until adding the missing nutritional supplements to the diet. The most common nutrients missing in people's diets are usually sodium, potassium, silica, calcium and magnesium. These nutritional needs can be easily determined by blood testing and/or hair analysis.

8. Clients do not properly follow recommendations: Often I'll prescribe Chinese herbs to complement the acupuncture treatment. If the patient doesn't take them, it lessens the effectiveness of the acupuncture treatments.

9. Unrealistic Expectations: Some people have had problems or pains for months or even years, and expect the problems or pains to be resolved very quickly, as if one were taking a prescription drug, but acupuncture can take longer. Also, the effects of acupuncture can be more subtle than most of us are used to.

The important thing to remember is that there are many different acupuncture techniques. Please don't give up. If one technique doesn't work, ask you doctor to try another technique, or to try another type of treatment altogether, such as Chinese herbs, homeopathy or nutritional supplements. If a doctor cures 95% of his patients, it would be unfair to him or his future patients to discontinue his practice because of the 5% who do not respond. One would hope that there is some other method or practitioner who is better suited for this client.

I have never liked needles. In fact, I was always so afraid of needles I considered myself a needle-phobic. But after my first acupuncture treatment I realized it was just a breeze. It was just the thought of needles that bothered me, but they were so small I never felt anything!
—D.R. Financial Analyst

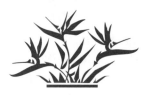

GROWTH

As one of my patients was getting up from the acupuncture table the other day, we began chatting about our personal growth. She said, "You know, if we're not growing, we're dying."

I've always had a problem with the idea of growth for growth's sake. "If something's not broke, why fix it?" I'd often say to myself. But I see now how true my patient's simple, profound statement really was. There's got to be constant expansion and growth in at least some aspect of our lives, or stagnation occurs. And stagnation is the first step in the process of disease and eventual premature death.

I know this to be a fact when I see so many patients with a "Stagnant Liver Chi" or "Blocked Heart Chi" who have chosen to ignore the condition and watch it turn into more serious diseases like cancer, heart attacks, depression, panic attacks, deteriorating eye sight, spinal problems, etc.

To prevent this type of deterioration in your health, you must focus beforehand on your expansion and growth. Here I'm talking about both external and internal health and growth. The two cannot be separated. One person may be working to expand their meditation time while another may be working to expand their exercise program to tone themselves. Another person may be taking a night class in calligraphy or ballroom dance. One might be starting a program of walking twenty minutes twice per day, reading a book on spiritual growth before bed, or learning to pray before a meal or on waking in the morning. Others may realize their marriage is stagnating and encourage their partner to enter couples therapy or to take a couples massage class together.

Each of us needs to decide for our own self what area of our life is stagnant and stuck and then develop a plan to expand beyond our "comfort zone" in this area. Our lives are too valuable and too sacred to waste in a stagnant pool of fear. No one can do this important work for us. No psychic or psychologist or best friend has the answers for us. We each must decide where we need to place our focus and our intensified energy to break out of our personal place of stagnation.

Let us each commit to making that extra special effort to not let ourselves die. Let us each commit to reaching out, to moving through, to stretching beyond our comfort zone in at least one area of our life at all times. Death doesn't become us. Together, let us reach for the stars, with the faith that this is not only exactly what we need to do and are meant to do, but also with the faith that we are being called upon to move forward as an example and inspiration to our fellows.

USING ACUPUNCTURE TO HELP STOP SMOKING

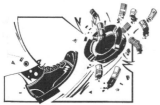

Do you smoke?

Do you want to quit?

If your answer to both of these questions is an emphatic YES, then read on.

How will acupuncture help me quit?

If you've ever tried to quit smoking on your own, you know how difficult it can be. Your body is chemically and physically addicted to nicotine. Acupuncture can help you overcome this addiction. It does this by increasing the level of *endorphins* in the body.

Endorphins are themselves addictive, but in a positive way. That is why joggers and people who aerobicize regularly are so enthusiastic—because their bodies release endorphins as they exercise.

What do endorphins do?

Endorphins kill pain and give you the feeling of a "natural high." They also reduce body tension, eradicate anxiety, and can induce a state of euphoria. To put it in simple terms, when produced in sufficient quantities, these morphine-like substances make you feel good.

The body stops producing endorphins under certain circumstances—such as when the endorphins are replaced by an addictive substance that competes with them. Nicotine is one such substance.

How does nicotine replace endorphins?

Within your body, endorphins and nicotine occupy the same spot at the end of a nerve cell. When this specific location is occupied by an endorphin, you feel relaxed. When you smoke, nicotine "wins out" over the endorphins and takes their place at the end of the nerve cell. The result? Rather than being relaxed, your nerves are more excitable; you may feel nervous, tense, stressed, and irritable.

In long-term smokers, nicotine takes the place of endorphins, because the body actually becomes lazy and "forgets" how to produce them.

Why do I crave cigarettes?

When you stop smoking, you cut off your supply of nicotine and your body is unable to manufacture endorphins so your nervous system becomes very anxious and overly excited. Your body then begins to crave a supply of either nicotine or endorphins to calm it down.

Since your production of endorphins has stopped and nicotine is easier and quicker to obtain, there is a big risk that you may simply resort to smoking because nicotine is the most readily available way to end the craving and relax your body. Unfortunately, you may never stop smoking long enough to allow your body the chance to begin producing endorphins again.

What does acupuncture do?

Acupuncture replaces the need for nicotine by stimulating your body to produce endorphins. Nicotine turns off your body's production of endorphins. Acupuncture turns your body's production of endorphins back on, even if you have been smoking for 20 years or more.

How many treatments will it take?

In general, it takes at least six acupuncture treatments to reactivate the natural production of endorphins in your body. Because each person is physiologically different, some people may need a few additional follow-up treatments.

Participating in a regular aerobic exercise program will make it easier to stop smoking by increasing the release of endorphins. You will also be given specific herbs, homeopathic remedies, and nutritional supplements to help curb your cravings, more quickly detox your lungs and liver, and boost the power in your adrenal glands.

How long will this work?

Once you have stopped smoking, your body and mind both need a chance to adjust to the new behavior. If you are like many people, you may have a tendency to try a cigarette now and then just for the fun of it. A problem will occur, however, if you are under stress and simultaneously start smoking. When you are under stress, your body stops the production of endorphins. If you smoke under stress, your body will become lazy and stop producing endorphins again. You risk becoming dependent on nicotine.

You must make a commitment to yourself. If you are under stress and tempted to start smoking again, come in for a couple of tune-up acupuncture treatments. These will enable you to balance your body and reactivate the release of an adequate supply of endorphins. (A good diet and adequate exercise are also musts during times of stress.) This is true whether you have been off cigarettes for two months or two years.

Is acupuncture for you?

The way out of nicotine addiction is easy for some and difficult for others. Acupuncture treatment offers substantial help if you already have the determination to quit and you don't want to suffer through it on your own.

If you have decided you are going to quit, you can get support for your decision through the same acupuncture treatments, herbs, homeopathic remedies, and nutritional supplements that have proven effective for so many of my friends and patients.

Personal testimonies

"Acupuncture is the only way to quit smoking. It was so easy! I felt absolutely no withdrawal symptoms and felt fantastic!"   —H.B., *Airline Attendant, Actress*

"Without your acupuncture treatments, I doubt we would have ever stopped smoking. We had a two packs a day habit for over nine years. After your treatment, we walked away from smoking and (seven years later) have never inhaled again."

—S.S., *Attorney*; M.S., *Therapist*

Oriental Medicine

STUCK

by Dr. Randy W. Martin

When you are stuck
    it's because you are hung up on content instead of process.
You have lost contact with life force.

When you are hurting
You are too *into the form* instead of the essence.

When you are in your symptoms and believing they and you are the same,
When you feel you *are* your symptoms,
You are in constriction.

All this discomfort,
All this dis-ease,
    comes from cutting off—
Putting down the *self*
    the deeper sense of what is and what we are.

Denial of the self
    of the interconnectedness of all
Denial and Denial and more Denial
    ...it's very deep

For instance
you hear something
you feel something
uncomfortable
And constrict as a result—
    ouch ! ! !

The meridians block,
Causing a dam across the stream of life (across the shoulder, or in the stomach, or colon, or in the throat, or wherever it is that your chi tends to block)

Perhaps it is your Liver chi that blocks at point Liver 3, the "Great Thoroughfare"
Or your heart (spirit-Shen) chi blocks at Heart 7, called "Spirit Gate"
Or perhaps your Yin gets constricted and blocks at Conception Vessel 4, which is the Dan Tien and also called "Hinge at the Source"
Or your Yang chi blocks at Governing Vessel 1, "Lasting Strength."

You go in for an acupuncture treatment
and a few acu-needles inserted in a few strategic spots unblocks the chi
and you're
    ...suddenly unstuck !

THE SECRET OF ACUPRESSURE MASSAGE

Acupressure* uses the gentle pressure of your hands and fingers to stimulate specific acu-points (the same points that are used in acupuncture) on the body. The secret to acupressure massage—and what is usually not taught in classes—is that the best acupressure is done "from the inside out." By this I mean that you must *feel* what you are *touching*.

No teacher can make you "good" at acupressure. A teacher can teach you the location of the points and how to use the points for various problems, but it is up to you to learn to feel the chi and to feel the energy coming from your hands and from the body of the person you are working on.

Try to be sensitive to whether they want and need a heavier or softer touch, and longer or shorter stimulation of points. These are all things you will discover for yourself as you begin to work on yourself and others.

There is no right or wrong way to give a massage. Find what suits you and work on exploring your own techniques.

---

*Acupressure—a type of Oriental medical treatment involving the use of finger pressure; uses the same points as acupuncture

Acupuncture and Cancer
Acupuncture was effective for nausea caused by cancer chemotherapy drugs, surgical anesthesia and pregnancy, and for pain resulting from surgery, according to a panel convened by the National Institutes for Health.

Acupuncture and Osteoarthritis
In another study, acupuncture was shown to be very effective for treating osteoarthritis of the knee. In all 57 patients with osteoarthritis, acupuncture was shown to significantly reduce pain and improve physical function when received twice weekly for 8 weeks.

Acupuncture and ADHD
According to pediatrician and child psychiatrist Neil Sonenklar, MD of the Virginia Treatment Center in Richmond, Virginia, acupuncture proved effective in a double blind study for three out of seven youngsters with ADHD. Both behavior and concentration improved when needleless acupuncture in the ear was used. He said more research was needed but in the meantime acupuncture might be a useful adjunct to the standard medical procedures.

Generally, each of the points can be massaged or "held" from 5 seconds to 10 minutes, depending on the strength of the person doing the massage and the chi of the person receiving the massage. To stimulate more, massage for longer periods; to stimulate less, massage for less time. The shorter the time, the less intense will be the treatment. If you or the person you are working on is weak or in a weakened state, then do each point for a shorter period of time. If you or the person you are working on has a strong constitution, then massage the points for longer periods of time.

There is one exception to this rule: If the person you are working on has a strong constitution or if the particular problem the person has is particularly stubborn (for instance, a severe muscle spasm), then working longer on this person will sedate, or disperse, the "stuck" chi.

For your technique, you can use either your thumb, fingers, elbow, or anything else you want. The object is to give maximum stimulation, with minimum stress and tension on your body. You want to learn to give many massages and save your energy and chi, and also not to weaken your own muscles giving the massage. Generally, you want to rub in a circular motion with a gentle pressure or with a vibrating feeling, or you can "hold" a point by making contact with the point and intuitively feeling what is going on beneath your fingertip. Always do the massage on both sides of the body evenly, unless one particular area needs extra work. If you work harder on one particular area, it's always a good idea to go and work a bit on the opposite side in the same area.

It's a good idea to balance the treatment by treating points at a distance from the area you are working on while remaining on the same meridian. For example, if you are working on gall bladder points on the neck and shoulders, then end the massage by doing a few gall bladder points on the legs or feet.

If you do the 20 points outlined below on a daily basis, or even twice weekly on yourself, you will quickly begin to feel the effects of a more relaxed body, be able to cope with stress more easily, and feel more balanced. After a week or so of practice, you should be able to perform the whole 20-point regimen in about 5 to 10 minutes. If you want to take 30 minutes, you will feel even stronger effects.

If you perform the neck release and the 20 points on another person, they will have deep and lasting effects that you both will be able to see. Massage generally works better if someone else is doing it on you. But if this is impossible, do not hesitate to do it on yourself.

Go ahead and experiment. And good luck—you can expect to have a lot of fun with the massage points. In fact, you will probably begin to experience the release of endorphins, which are our bodies' own naturally-occurring opiates.

The only possible side effects of the massage are that you may feel sore if you have pressed too hard, or you might experience diarrhea or other cleansing reactions if you have a lot of stored toxins. If you have any previous health conditions, you should always consult with your health practitioner before doing the massage.

Also, if you are receiving constitutional acupuncture or homeopathic treatments, you should first check to ensure that the acupressure will not negate any of the treatment you are already receiving.

The Neck and Shoulder Release

This exercise is easy to perform on anyone. Most of the acupuncture meridians go through this area of the body, so under stress the body forms major energy blockages here.

Refer to the diagram below. Here's how to do it:

The receiver sits in a chair or lies on a massage table or bed. The receiver needs to guide the giver to the most sensitive spots as the massage is performed.

The giver begins by applying pressure to the first points on the diagram (point A), left hand on left side and right hand on right side. Pressure should be varied depending on what the receiver prefers. Each point can be held from 1 second to 5 minutes, depending on how deep you want to go.

The giver and receiver should both breathe deeply throughout the entire process.

If the receiver feels dizzy, stop the massage immediately.

Proceed to the second point (point B). Try to find the tight spots and spend more time on these. Let your fingers and the receiver's feedback be your guide as to the amount of pressure to apply.

And so on, from points A through F on the diagram.

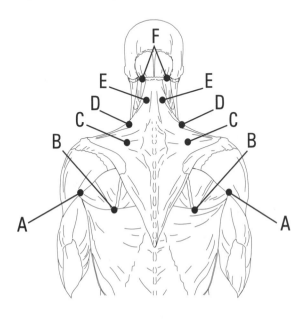

The Twenty Most Common Acupressure Points

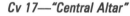

Oriental Medicine

Cv 17—"Central Altar"

One inch up from the bony end of the sternum, this point relieves tension and the feeling of heaviness in the chest; it frees breathing and opens the heart chakra, influences the spirit and calms the emotions. Useful for stage fright. Use Cv 17 with P6.

Cv 12—"Center Reunion"

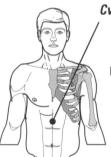

Promotes digestion and relieves stomach congestion. Cv 12 is halfway between the navel and the bony end of the sternum, directly over the stomach. Massage gently—do not press deeply. On inhale, press gently; on exhale, press harder. Good after overeating.

LI 4—"Hoku" or "The Great Eliminator"

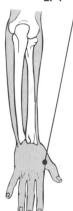

Hoku is the most famous and commonly used point. It promotes regular elimination and prevents tension buildup in the shoulders, neck, and face. Like aspirin, it is good against headaches, toothaches, sore throat, constipation, colds, and fever. Hoku helps to build general body strength. **Note:** Press across toward the other side, not down. Hoku should **NOT** be used on pregnant women.

Lv 3—"Happy Calm"

Strengthens the liver, clears the head and thinking, and mellows the spirits of the quick-tempered. Good for lowering blood pressure and to relieve a fever. Also useful for establishing equilibrium after a plane, car, or boat trip. With LI 4, it is said to retune the body clock and harmonize the descending and ascending energies. Helpful in treating jet lag or a general feeling of imbalance. Further, these points help prevent or relieve some types of headaches.

Cv 4—"Hinge at the Source"

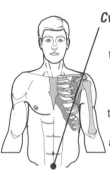

Located three fingers below the navel, Cv 4 is the center of the body's energy. This point builds strength, replenishes the body's energy, and clears the mind. Because it increases circulation in the lower abdomen and pelvis, this point is traditionally closely related to sexual functioning. The "hara" is located internally to this point.

UB 62—"Spirit of the Pulse"

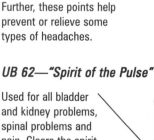
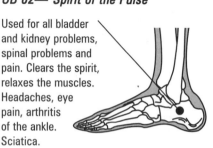

Used for all bladder and kidney problems, spinal problems and pain. Clears the spirit, relaxes the muscles. Headaches, eye pain, arthritis of the ankle. Sciatica.

The Twenty Most Common Acupressure Points

K 16—"Vitals Associated Point"

Strengthens kidney function and imparts renewed strength to the body. K 16 helps regulate water balance in the body; it influences the condition of reproductive organs, improves bladder and large intestine function, and boosts the function of the digestive tract. Point is located half an inch from the navel.

Gb 20—"Wind Pond"

Clears thinking and relieves feelings of frustration and stress. Traditionally used for all head, eye, ear, nose, and mouth conditions.

Gv 20—"Hundred Meetings"

A tonic for the whole body, Gv 20 is said to be a very spiritual point through which we can receive vibrations from the Infinite. It affects and balances the hypothalamus, is good for headaches, and influences brain concentration, "spacing out," and hemorrhoids. Tibetan monks meditate on this point opening up.

K 1—"Courage" or "Gushing Spring"

An excellent first aid point for unconsciousness, this point stimulates and builds adrenal reserves and balances the appetite. By strengthening courage and willpower, K 1 helps to overcome fear. Located just beyond the ball of the foot, K 1 also energizes the entire body, builds sexual endurance, and increases resistance to disease.

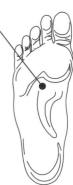

B 67—"Reaching Yin"

This tonic point strongly influences the reproductive organs in men and women. It helps prevent prostate problems and difficult or premature menopause. B 67 strengthens the bladder, regulates blood circulation, builds good quality blood, and keeps the head light and clear. Press straight into the bone.

SP 4—"Grandfather-Grandson"

This is the body's "generation gap" point. It adjusts the flow of energy to fill deficiencies and eliminate gaps in body function, especially between top and bottom. Good for digestion and excellent for circulation, including cold feet. Especially good for women.

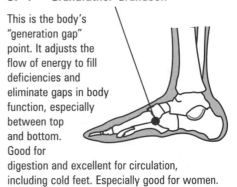

The Twenty Most Common Acupressure Points

Oriental Medicine

S 36—"Foot Three Miles"

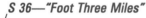

The most popular point in the Orient for longevity, this point is a special strengthening point that is used for general lack of energy, to promote digestion, improve muscle tone, and to promote long and healthy life. It is often used by athletes. Go across the muscle 8 or 9 times to stimulate this point.

Lu 1—"Middle Mansion"

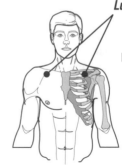

This point releases vast amounts of energy into the body. It is an area of emotional holding—when its tension is released, the feeling is of a great burden having been thrown off. Cheers the spirit and prevents depression and melancholy. Brings a sense of freedom.

L 9—"Absorption of the Spirit of Good" (inside wrist)

Adjusts blood, energy, and prevents depression. Opens lungs, strengthens respiration, and all lung-associated functions. Traditionally used for insomnia. Strengthens the pulse and makes it smooth.

Lv 14—"Gate of Hope"

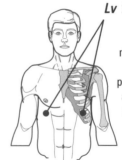

Influences the diaphragm muscle, which must be in good shape for full respiration. This point aids digestion. It is said to add robustness to living and to relieve snoring and hiccoughs.

UB 23—"Ambitious Room"

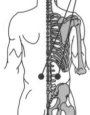

Strengthens lower abdomen, renal, and bladder function. Relaxes lower back tension; helps prevent sciatica, lumbago, and genital problems. Strengthens testes and uterus.

K 6—"Joyful Step"

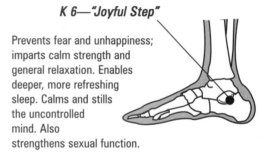

Prevents fear and unhappiness; imparts calm strength and general relaxation. Enables deeper, more refreshing sleep. Calms and stills the uncontrolled mind. Also strengthens sexual function.

The Twenty Most Common Acupressure Points

Tw 5—"Outer Gate" (Outside)

P 6—"Inner Gate" (Inside)

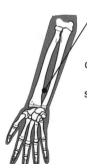

Traditionally used to release the arm, elbow, shoulders, and neck; also relieves pain in these regions. Used for cold, flu, headache, fear, or extreme flight. Used in conjunction with P 6.

Historically reputed to improve circulation, reduce nausea, brighten the spirit of the heart, promote easy and sound sleep, and reduce pain anywhere in the body. Good for stage fright or for nervousness.

THE CHINESE SYNDROMES

In Chinese medicine, syndromes are the diagnostic categories and definitions given to disease states; this is somewhat similar to a diagnosis in Western medicine. They are based on the grouping of various symptoms. If you have a particular grouping of symptoms, along with specific food cravings, a particular pulse and tongue picture, then you may fall into a particular syndrome.

Rarely are these syndromes absolute. Most people fall into more than one syndrome and most people do not "fit into" a syndrome completely. You need not have all the symptoms and findings in the syndrome classification for it to apply to you. This is because of the complexity of the human mind/body organism. But the syndromes are still very useful in diagnosing and treating disease.

Remember that in Chinese medicine, we are always treating the whole person and not the name of a particular disease or syndrome. So the following syndromes are discussed for the sake of convenience only. This is only a small sampling of the syndromes. These are the most common ones, but there are many more than these and there are also quite a few subcategories and combinations of the syndromes that are too complex to go into here.

Kidney Yin Deficiency: The Kidneys are the source, or "seat," of chi (life energy). The Yin is the feminine, introverted, nurturing aspect of the chi. We have both Yin and Yang Chi in the Kidneys.

Kidney Yin Deficiency will manifest as low back pain, knee pain, teeth problems, and dryness of skin, hair, eyes and mouth. There may be excessive thirst, stammering, excessive heat, dark complexion, thick eyebrows, ringing in the ears, vision problems, hair loss, hyperthyroidism, hypertension, urinary problems, premature ejaculation or pain during intercourse.

Emotionally there may be agitation, nervousness, insomnia, excessive fear, lack of faith and direction, inability to stick to a plan and difficulty in "turning it over" to a higher authority.

The pulse picture may be thin, deep and rapid and the tongue may be red, small, dry or excessively cracked.

Kidney Yang Deficiency: This type may have weak adrenal glands, asthma, chronic fatigue syndrome, low sexual desire, shortness of breath, sore back and weak knees, frequent urination, edema, a dislike for cold weather, congestion anywhere in the body, infertility, confusion, indecisiveness, paralysis emotionally or physically, laziness, hopelessness or lacking in motivation.

The pulse picture may be deep, weak, thin, and slow and the tongue may be "large" or "flabby" and unusually moist.

Stagnant Liver Chi: This one of the most common presentations in Western culture and may show up in combination with any number of other syndromes. The reason is poor diet composed of refined foods and sweets along with too much stress. Because the Liver is in charge of the free flow of chi and energy in the body, any blockage may be due to Stagnant Liver Chi.

Some of the most common symptoms are PMS, headaches, migraines, sour taste in the mouth, diabetes, hypoglycemia, poor eyesight, frequently pulled tendons, muscles or sprained ankles, dizziness, chronic fatigue, stiff neck and sore upper back or difficulty getting pregnant.

Almost any and all menstrual irregularities and problems may be due to this syndrome, including painful menses, breast distention, depression and chocolate cravings. Digestive symptoms may include gas, distention, pain, diarrhea or constipation.

Emotional characteristics may include agitation, insomnia, anxiety, anorexia, phobias, aggressiveness or an inability to assert oneself in a healthful way, anger, haughtiness or excessive sexual desire.

The pulse may be wiry and excessive in the liver and gall bladder positions, and the tongue will show abnormalities on the sides with a purple color throughout.

Spleen Damp Cold: The spleen performs the function of astringent to the dampness in the body and has a lot to do with immunity, digestion and the menstrual cycle. Wherever there is excessive dampness or phlegm, the spleen is involved, whether it's in the vagina, prostate, sinus, lungs or stomach. If it's a damp cold condition the phlegm will be clear or white and if its a damp heat condition the discharges will be darkened yellow or brown.

Typical symptoms of Damp Cold Affecting the Spleen may be bloating, gas, distention, fatigue, obsessive compulsive disease or excessive thinking, difficulty in competing with others, excessive sputum, obesity or anorexia, coughing, nasal discharges, mucus in the stool, headaches, numbness, tumors, cysts, excessive worry, excessive empathy or poor emotional boundaries, emotional confusion with a lack of centeredness or heart palpitations.

Chronic weak digestion will be common with loss of appetite or an excessive craving for sweets, cold or frozen foods.

The tongue may be flabby and thickly coated white with teeth marks on the sides. The pulse will be tight, slippery and excessive in the spleen position.

Damp Heat: Specific signs might include excessive urination and thirst, prostatitis, burning urination, vaginitis, yeast infection, diarrhea, headaches, red eyes, itching and skin rashes, cysts, tumors and fibroids, swelling, foul odor, too frequent seminal emissions, discharges, conjunctivitis, ear infections and sore or strep throat.

Emotional characteristics may include a combination of Liver and Spleen problems such as volatility, arrogance, anger, agitation and a lack of grace and peacefulness or centeredness.

The tongue may be red and "flabby." The pulse may be floating an fast and excessive in either the spleen or liver positions.

(**Damp Heat in the Lower Burner** refers to symptoms of damp heat which manifest anywhere below the umbilicus. There are three "burners" in the body. The upper burner is anything above and including the chest area; the middle burner is the center, or digestive area, including the stomach, spleen, liver and gall bladder; and the lower burner includes the reproductive organs, small and large intestines.)

Congealed or Stagnant Blood: Stabbing pain or gastric ulcer are two common symptoms, as are lumps, tumors and palpable masses; or heavy, clotted menses with irregular cycles or lack of menses. On an emotional level there may be suspicion, frustration, anger, resentment, depression, egotism and a poor connection with oneself or ones surroundings.

The tongue may show red or purple dots and have a dark purplish color with a yellow coating. The pulse may be tight, weak and wiry.

Wind-Cold: Primary symptoms of Wind-Cold may be those typical to the initial stages of the cold or flu; another manifestation may be skin eruptions and rashes or a wide variety of musculoskeletal problems. Symptoms may include chills, low-grade fever, stuffy nose, headaches, stiff neck and shoulders, sore throat, bronchitis, mumps, strep throat, hives, measles, boils and other acute skin problems, even including poison oak. Wind-Cold syndromes exist on the superficial level of the meridians. If the disease process forces its way to a deeper level, it is no longer defined as Wind-Cold. This usually occurs if a cure is not achieved within the first forty-eight hours of the disease process.

Lung Heat: This syndrome is usually seen as a deficiency in Lung Yin. The onset is most commonly seen in chronic smokers, but it can also be present during a severe cold, flu or respiratory illness. Typical symptoms are smoker's cough, dry throat, nose and skin, hacking coughs, hoarseness, tickling cough and difficulty breathing.

On an emotional level, some of the common pictures may be the desire to withdraw, lack of hope, grief or silent prolonged grief, sadness or an inability to cry.

The tongue will be very dry and cracked and the pulse will be fast and weak in the lung position.

Disturbed Shen: In Chinese medicine, Disturbed Shen is the term given to many different emotional problems. According to Chinese medicine, the Heart is said to rule the emotions, so Disturbed Shen applies to Heart problems. Common symptoms may include hypertension, palpitations, insomnia, anxiety, obsessive compulsive problems, phobias, worry, scattered thinking, excessive sweating, difficulty forming lasting relationships, many upsets in relationships, forgetfulness or difficulty concentrating. More in the extreme, this syndrome may manifest as bipolar disorder or borderline personality.

The tongue will usually have a bright pink tip and the pulse may be fast.

Deficient Blood: In Chinese medicine, Blood is a metaphor for the "Yin" of the Yin. It has much more meaning than what we in the West think of as blood. A Deficient Blood pattern may include symptoms of dizziness, thin body, spots in the visual field, poor vision, lots of wrinkles, dry hair, skin, low back pain, poor appetite, habitual miscarriage, difficulty conceiving or difficulty recovering from a pregnancy.

Chronic fatigue is usually associated with Deficient Blood as is anemia, insomnia, palpitations and cracked fingernails. Psychologically, one may feel brittle, awkward, hesitant or shy. The tongue may be pale and the pulse picture will be deficient, small and thin, lacking in overall strength.

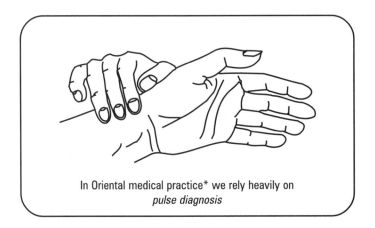

In Oriental medical practice* we rely heavily on
pulse diagnosis

* Chinese medicine vs. Oriental medicine—Chinese medicine refers to a system of medicine discovered and evolved in China; Oriental medicine includes the Chinese system, in addition to Japanese and Korean methods.

HOMEOPATHY

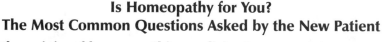

Is Homeopathy for You?
The Most Common Questions Asked by the New Patient

What is the origin of homeopathic medicine?

Homeopathy is a therapeutic system of medicine developed by Dr. Samuel Hahnemann, M.D. almost two hundred years ago in Germany. Homeopathic medicine was still very popular and taught in medical schools in the United States until the late 1930s, when growth of the drug industry replaced it (at least temporarily). Homeopathic medicine has remained popular however, and is still widely practiced today in Mexico, England, France, Germany, and India. It has remained dormant in the United States and has just recently begun to experience a tremendous resurgence in popularity.

How does homeopathy work?

Homeopathy works by stimulating the body's own defense mechanisms, much the same as an allergy shot, flu or polio vaccination. In a healthy person, the body successfully fights disease on its own. For example, when attacked by germs, the body produces its own antibodies to kill the germs. Our body can also raise its temperature and send special blood cells to stop infection. It may cause vomiting and diarrhea to get rid of poisons in our stomach and intestines.

Because of the stressful lifestyles most people live today, and because of the less than perfect diets we eat, it is common for our defense mechanisms to break down and to stop working effectively. When we get a cold, flu, or any other infection, it is because our body could no longer successfully fight off the disease on its own.

Homeopathy is based on the principle of "similia similibus curentur" or "like is cured by like." This means that a substance that causes a disease in healthy people can actually cure the same kind of disease in a sick person. This is because the sick person is very sensitive to such a substance and just a little bit of it can stimulate his or her defense mechanism to make a greater effort to promote a cure.

What are homeopathic remedies?

Any substance occurring in the universe might be used as the source of a homeopathic remedy. Most of the common remedies are made from the naturally occurring substances of vegetable, animal or mineral sources. These substances are then broken down into minute molecular quantities and mixed in either a lactose, sucrose or alcohol base.

The way in which homeopathy differs from other types of medicine, and also the reason it is so controversial, is because of the amount of the original substance used to make the remedy. The homeopathic pharmacy employs only the smallest amounts of the substance. The amount of the original substance may not even equal one molecule by the time the process is completed.

The Three Types of Homeopathic Remedies: Animal, Plant, and Mineral

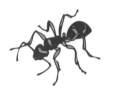

Animal: The Ant
(*Formica Ruta*)

Plant: Parsley
(*Petroselinium*)

Mineral: Silica
(*Silicia*)

When you purchase a homeopathic remedy it is identified by a name and a number. The number is followed by an "X" or a "C." The 1X potency contains $1/10^{th}$ part of the original substance. The 3X potency contains $1/1000^{th}$ part of the original substance, the 6X potency, $1/1,000,000^{th}$ part of the original substance, and so on. You can see that very little of the original substance is left in the final homeopathic remedy.

If the remedy you purchase has a number followed by a "C," it means that the remedy is being diluted by a hundred times instead of ten times, at each step of the process. For example, a 1C potency contains $1/100^{th}$ part of the original substance, and so on.

The homeopathic higher potencies, such as the 200th, 1M, 10M, 50M, contain the most minute amounts of the basic substance. The less of the original substance, the "higher" the potency and the "stronger" is the remedy.

How do we know homeopathic remedies really work?

To determine the usefulness of a remedy, it is administered in repeated doses to healthy people and its effects are scientifically noted in detail. Eventually, after having "proved" its effects on healthy people, a complete list of the symptoms thus produced by the remedy are written down for comparison with the symptoms of a sick person.

The remedy symptoms produced in healthy people which most closely resemble the symptoms of the sick person is called the "similimum" (or most similar). This similimum is then administered to the sick person to catalyze their own defense mechanism to fighting off the particular symptoms and disease.

A homeopathic doctor does not cure a disease. The correctly chosen homeopathic remedy stimulates the individual's body to cure itself.

How is a homeopathic remedy selected?

The homeopathic remedy is selected on the basis of the patient's subjective symptoms, with some symptoms receiving greater weight than others. For example, mental or physical symptoms which refer to the patient AS A WHOLE are considered more important than symptoms which apply to a LIMITED part of the person. EMOTIONAL symptoms are of more importance and given more weight in long term treatment than are PHYSICAL symptoms. But in short term treatment of more acute problems, physical symptoms are weighted more heavily than emotional symptoms.

Each person has an extremely complex, sensitive and intricate set of personal "Bio-detectors." For this reason, the most valuable information in homeopathy comes from the patient him/herself, in his or her own words.

If a person feels pain, it is important to know exactly what type of pain sensation they are experiencing: tearing, burning, sharp, cutting, sore, bruised, etc. Also, it is extremely helpful to know the "modalities." For example, is it better or worse by moving the affected part, by walking into a room or into open air, by standing, sitting, or lying down? Is it altered by eating or drinking, by speaking to others, by coughing or by any other action? What time of day or night does it usually occur, and what other peculiar characteristics are associated with it?

The foregoing questions are only an example of the types of information that is helpful in homeopathic prescribing. The dependence of homeopathy on the patient's subjective symptoms is not a limitation but a recognition of the extreme sensitivity of each individual and their own perceptions of their disease process.

Many medically trained homeopaths also use blood tests and other Western diagnostics techniques in determining the correct remedy. My training in Oriental medicine allows me to incorporate traditional Chinese medical techniques in diagnosis into my choice of the correct homeopathic remedy.

Are there ever any homeopathic side effects?

Since the remedies are administered in very small quantities, usually there are no side effects. The effect is only to strengthen the body's own healing mechanism.

But occasionally the body will produce a "healing reaction" or what homeopathic medicine calls an "aggravation." Since homeopathy heals from the inside out, it can release stored toxins to the surface of the body. The skin or areas of mucus membranes are usually the primary areas to receive healing aggravations.

A healing aggravation is the body's own defensive mechanism trying so hard to rid the body of disease symptoms that it kind of goes into "overdrive" temporarily. The aggravation is always short-lived.

One can never exactly tell what reaction will occur after the correctly indicated remedy is found — it depends largely on the vitality of the individual in question. But the homeopathic patient must be willing to persevere and have patience in the short term, in order to experience a more optimal state of health in the long term.

True prophylaxis [prevention] does not exist in the form of a pill. The only true form of prophylaxis is health, in the broadest sense, of the patient. Health can be defined as the dynamic balance of vital force in and between mind, body, and spirit.
—Stephen Silver "Homeopathy in the Treatment of AIDS and HIV Related Illness"
Journal of the Society of Homeopaths, No. 51

ARE YOU READY FOR CLASSICAL HOMEOPATHY?

What is homeopathy?

Homeopathy uses very small doses of either plant, animal or mineral substances to stimulate the body and emotions to heal. Homeopathy is not to be confused with the use of acupuncture, nutrition or herbs. Homeopathy is about 200 years old and originated in Germany. Homeopathy is very scientific in nature and was very popular all over the world until the early 1900s when drugs became popular.

What is Classical Homeopathy?

Classical Homeopathy is not practiced by very many homeopathic doctors. The training takes many years, and includes formal training as well as many hundreds of hours of study. There are also different types of homeopaths calling themselves "Classical."

Classical Homeopathy focuses on the emotional and spiritual aspects of a person's health and uses only one remedy at any given time. Although the physical problems you may have are very important to evaluate when choosing a homeopathic remedy, the physical symptoms are evaluated and integrated into the person's entire emotional case history.

Choosing a homeopathic remedy following the principles of Classical Homeopathy is sometimes an easy and sometimes an extremely difficult task. It can take only a few minutes in some cases and at other times can take many hours of research. At each appointment, you will want to share the most intimate details of your emotional life, as well as all the physical problems you have been experiencing. Classical Homeopathy is the most effective and long-lasting of any and all healing methods, but it is also the most difficult path for the patient. It may take longer than you expected and you may have to go through several healing aggravations along the way.

The use of herbs or acupuncture may be much faster, but will not be as long-lasting. I may also use herbs or acupuncture as a part of your Classical Homeopathic treatment, but at times it will not be appropriate to combine methods. This will depend on what homeopathic remedy you are taking at any given time.

How does Classical Homeopathy differ from other types of homeopathy?

There are many different ways to use homeopathy. Some doctors use computers to evaluate your condition and then use combination remedies to heal you. This method is much easier to utilize, since all one must do is be trained in using the computer. I am more attracted to Classical Homeopathy because it relies on human interaction and the emotional, spiritual and soul connection between the patient and doctor. It is also the basis upon which homeopathy was discovered and **all** homeopathic literature was created. It is only recently that homeopathy has been somewhat distorted to include other forms, which don't rely on the basic healing principles upon which homeopathy was founded.

Combination homeopathic remedies also do not target the core of your disease process. They are a shotgun approach to homeopathy. Many people experience improvement using this method, but its long-term effectiveness and ability to help promote deeper changes in a person's psyche and spirit is limited.

Another type is acute homeopathy. This uses the remedies to treat problems such as flu, colds, headaches, etc. This form of homeopathy is not bad; it is just very limited in scope. I sometimes use this form of homeopathy with my patients who are not interested in the Classical approach. It will not help to deeply strengthen the immune system over the long-term, nor will it help on an emotional level over the longer term. But it is effective in boosting immunity when we compare it to Western pharmaceuticals, and I would always choose to use acute homeopathy instead of antibiotics, antidepressants or antihistamines.

What will be expected of me if I am treated by Classical Homeopathy?

If you should choose Classical Homeopathic medicine as your modality of choice, you should expect to experience some profound changes in your life, physically, emotionally and perhaps spiritually.

You will also need to follow specific rules, such as abstaining from mint and commercial toothpaste, coffee, decaf, **raw** garlic or **raw** onions.

O.K. Doc, I'm ready. I've decided. Now how do I start?

Find a good homeopath and go for it!

THE HOMEOPATHIC AGGRAVATION: WILL IT GET WORSE BEFORE IT GETS BETTER?

Many of my patients want to know what they can expect when taking a homeopathic remedy. I am always reluctant to answer this question. WHY? Because there is just NO simple answer!!!

In one person a homeopathic remedy may cause no aggravation at all. In fact, in many cases a person's symptoms and problems will just disappear after taking a single dose of a single homeopathic remedy. But in other people, an aggravation may take place, and in some cases it may be quite severe.

The severity of a homeopathic aggravation is usually an indication of the amount of drugs taken in the past to suppress symptoms. The severity may also be a rough indication of the amount of toxicity in your body.

In most cases, if there is a homeopathic aggravation, it will be very minor and only a temporary worsening of the already existing symptoms. But in some cases, an aggravation may cause other problems to appear, usually symptoms that had occurred some time ago in the past of a person's health history.

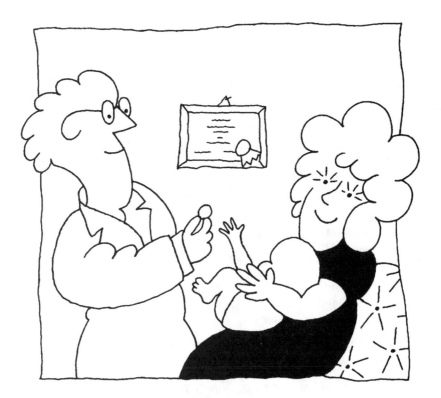

An aggravation is basically the body's attempt to throw off an old state of disease, in order to arrive at a new, healthier state of balance, equilibrium and happiness. For example, let's take the case of someone who has a long history of taking antibiotics for sore throats, flu, strep throat, etc., and who comes for treatment of premenstrual syndrome (PMS). It is a very real possibility that a homeopathic remedy given for the menstrual problem may cause a healing aggravation that resembles a return of the throat problems. This person may think, "Oh, I'm getting the flu again!" but actually it is only a temporary aggravation from the homeopathic remedy.

Another example: A person comes for treatment of recurrent knee pain while jogging. I give her a homeopathic remedy and two days later she gets a severe urinary infection. When she calls me to discuss her pain, it turns out that she has had a long history of urinary problems, all suppressed by antibiotics. I tell her that before her knees will heal, she must live through the short return of what resembles her old urinary infections.

A person who has taken a lot of aspirin for headaches may likewise experience a short return of these headaches while taking homeopathic remedies for an ulcer. A person being treated for eczema or psoriasis may experience the asthma they had as a small child.

Being treated homeopathically takes a great deal of patience. I often tell people they must be somewhat of a masochist to be a good homeopathic patient. Anyone who knows me personally will remember the terrible aggravation I went through in 1991 after taking a dose of Arnica for a sprained back. The Arnica caused my body to send toxins out for about a month which resulted in irritability and huge yellow, pussy facial eruptions.

Homeopathy works. And for the person who is committed to experiencing optimal health, it is well worth suffering through the return of minor symptoms.

It is always impossible to predict whether an aggravation will occur. In many cases it never does, and the healing is painless and fast. If an aggravation does occur while you are taking a homeopathic remedy, immediately stop taking it and call me, or your homeopath. Whenever you are unsure if it is, in fact, an aggravation, it is always better to stop taking it until we have a chance to talk.

If an aggravation occurs and you take drugs to suppress the symptoms (and this includes aspirin), it is not the end of the world. It will, however, take longer to strengthen your system and to cure your problems. Remember that in the long run drugs tend to weaken the body's own immune system and defense mechanism, while in the short run, they are very effective in removing (suppressing and covering up) uncomfortable symptoms.

Homeopathy may or may not be as effective in the short run, but in the long term, it is well worth its weight in gold. So I beg you to have patience. Ill health did not occur overnight. Neither will the cure…

> *For each homeopathic aggravation you go through, you get to live another*
> *ten years.*   *—Vega Resenberg*

CLASSICAL HOMEOPATHY, THE HEALING AGGRAVATION, HERBS AND INTEGRITY

I've had a very active and somewhat difficult winter season. I had to miss work to allow time for a deep-acting homeopathic remedy to work itself through my system. It was a kind of self-imposed sickness that allowed the body-emotions-soul to go to a deeper level in order to clear out old "stuff," to integrate, and to plant new seeds for future growth. The old "stuff" which needs time to "come out" can be in the form of toxins that accumulate in an organ such as the liver, lungs or kidneys, or the "stuff" can be in the form of old "stuck" emotions—anger, grief, sadness, confusion, indecision, etc.

Often we don't have the time, don't know how, or simply don't allow ourselves the luxury of feeling our emotions as they arise in our daily lives. Our emotions become suppressed and lodge deeply in our body tissues. They may take the form of muscle spasms, headaches, indigestion, diarrhea, constipation, menstrual problems, cysts, fibroids, sinus problems, endometriosis, or any number of other physical ailments.

On a deeper level, we may become depressed by not allowing ourselves to feel the full expression of our emotions. What is depression but "de-pressing" or "pressing-down" feelings and holding them back, so they can't surface.

When we take a well-chosen homeopathic remedy, these suppressed emotions and physical "toxins" will resurface, causing the "homeopathic healing aggravation." When this occurs we always immediately stop taking the remedy; but the aggravation may continue for some time.

I chose not to utilize any herbal products or acute homeopathics to help me through my healing aggravation. Although herbal products will boost the immune system and shorten the time of the healing aggravation, they will also sometimes antidote (lessen the effectiveness of) the homeopathic remedy. Without the help of herbs, the homeopathic aggravation will last longer and go deeper. As a result, this winter was a soul-searching time for me.

In our culture when we become ill, we all want a fast solution to the discomfort. We often don't want to feel our bodily discomfort or our emotional discomfort. Television ads and billboards are filled with "solutions" for ridding us of feeling any discomfort at all. But during the homeopathic aggravation, the object is the opposite: "conscious, self-imposed suffering." It's not for everyone.

But now, having come through it and having experienced deeper levels in myself, I feel more authentic and prepared to help guide my patients through some of their deeper levels. True healing is not easy and there is no particular time line for how long it should take, but the rewards are hopefully a deeper sense of well-being, health, and being closer to one's essence or essential self. *That* can be very satisfying!

I am very interested in hearing from other classical homeopaths who "ride the fence" between utilizing herbal or vitamin supplements, chiropractic or acupuncture, and how they have integrated their practice of classical homeopathy into their knowledge and use of these other modalities.

USING HOMEOPATHIC MEDICINE TO TREAT EMOTIONAL IMBALANCES

You may have never considered the use of homeopathic medicine for opening up to and expanding upon your emotional or spiritual awareness. Most people think of joining a church or synagogue, meditating or going to a therapist when it comes to emotions and spirituality.

But homeopathic medicine is an important adjunct to consider when your goal is increased emotional and spiritual growth and self-awareness. In my life, some of the most profound emotional work and spiritual insight has come on the heels of taking the correct homeopathic remedy. One of the first constitutional remedies I took opened me up to meeting a soul mate with whom I spent three important and growthful years of my life. Another well-timed remedy opened me to my feminine side and the ability to cry and express my deep sadness and grief.

The net effect of taking the correct constitutional homeopathic remedy will be to open you to a deeper level of awareness and emotional integration. The remedies will never cause you to experience anything in particular, but if you are ready to evolve in a new direction, they may be the catalyst you need to get you started. In another instance, the correct remedy may help you to deal more effectively with the death of a loved one. In one case this may mean it will enable you to cry, yet in another person who can't stop crying it may help them to feel more centered.

Below, I will discuss just four homeopathic remedies from a psychological perspective. Remember that there are many more remedies to choose from and that this is just a small sample.

Homeopathy

Lachesis: Lachesis is composed of the venom from the bushmaster snake and the dream life of a person who could potentially benefit from taking this particular remedy is sometimes full of snakes. (Another remedy type that may dream of snakes is *Lac can*). Other dream images of the Lachesis type are sexuality, anxiety, business matters, past events, and symbols of the serpent.

The emotional issues occurring within a person who might respond to Lachesis may revolve around repressed or unconscious energy manifesting as a feeling of constriction anywhere in body, but particularly in the throat or stomach areas. Difficulty in swallowing and/or a dislike of jewelry or anything tight around the neck are common characteristics of the Lachesis type.

The Lachesis constitution may have trouble falling asleep because on a conscious level they know they feel worse on waking up. But they also have a subtle fear of going unconscious and of needing to remain in control. They like to talk a lot.

Another typical situation in which Lachesis is prescribed is at the time of menopause. It is a great hot flash remedy. It is also used a lot for PMS and its associated symptoms. The Lachesis personality often can repress their true feelings without being conscious they are doing so. Then they may suddenly lash out at you. It is often a remedy which is useful when treating people who are addicted to drugs or alcohol.

Typical physical and emotional symptoms that respond well to the Lachesis remedy include tumors, cysts, anemia, bitterness, jealousy, suspiciousness or resentment. Most symptoms in the Lachesis type will generally be worse on the right side of the body.

Pulsatilla: This homeopathic remedy is made from the meadow anemone, a plant of the Ranunculus family which grows in the plains and pasturelands of Central and Northern Europe and is commonly known as the "wind flower." The plant is small and delicate, with a flexible stem that bends one way or the other depending on the way the wind is blowing.

The emotional issue most prevalent in the Pulsatilla personality is a feeling of neediness. This person may want a lot of emotional support and attention, may cry easily when given a shoulder to cry on, have a great deal of sadness, a changeable mood or be quite timid. They may easily take on the energy or issues of others around them, not feeling grounded enough to make up their own mind or to take any assertive action themselves.

The Pulsatilla person may have blond hair with blue eyes, a preference for cold or open air, pains that are erratic and changing, swollen glands, flatulence and bloating, cough or other respiratory problems with gastric upset after eating rich foods.

Sepia: This rather unusual remedy is composed of the inky juice of a cuttlefish. The "ink" is excreted to give her enemy a false "smoke cloud" image so that the fish can more easily run and hide when it is in fear. The typical dream images of the person who may respond well to the Sepia remedy include dreams of being chased, threats of physical abuse, confusion or accidents.

A common example of when Sepia is given to a person in actual practice might be with a woman who feels very emotional and insecure before her menstrual period and wants to be left alone to cry. She may feel she is "in an emotional cloud," apart from others, and actually feel a strong dislike for those she ordinarily would love the most. A Sepia man may experience fear of intimacy with constant psychological dodging when a potential intimate partner gets too close.

A Sepia person feels fine as long as they are involved in vigorous physical activity, such as dancing, bicycling or jogging. This is their love. Some common physical problems may include the sense of pain or plug sensation in the throat, stomach or rectum, a craving for acid foods such as pickles or sauerkraut, chronic bladder infections, flatulence with headaches, constipation or many moles and/or warts.

Natrum muriaticum: This homeopathic remedy is made from common table salt and a common symptom of a person needing Nat. mur. is a craving for or intense aversion to salt and fish from the sea. They may also experience an aversion or desire for being at the ocean. They may dream of robbers, being taken prisoner, being thirsty or have a lot of fear in their dreams.

Usually, the Nat. mur. type of person is very sensitive and emotional although them may not show their feelings to others. They usually will not talk about their problems because to do so makes them feel even worse. They are often the "wounded healer" types: nurses, clergypersons, teacher or helpers of one kind or another.

Their emotional and physical problems often date back to a time of intense grief that was repressed and not adequately grieved. Typical physical complaints may include migraine headaches, oily skin with acne, water retention, fatigue, fever blisters or herpes, eczema at the bends of limbs or margin of the scalp, and generally feeling worse around ten in the morning.

According to homeopathic theory, strong emotional reactions or physical symptoms are the body putting up defense mechanisms to shield itself from pain or pathology on some deeper level. So by understanding the "secret code" of the body's symptoms, and interpreting this code into the correct homeopathic remedy, we can prevent illness or imbalance from proceeding to a much deeper level.

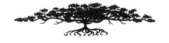

CONSTITUTIONAL TREATMENT

Patients are always asking me what I mean when I say I am treating them constitutionally, or that I am giving them a constitutional homeopathic remedy or acupuncture treatment. A simple definition is that constitutional treatment is the sum total of and has the potential to cause changes in the following areas of your life:

1. Genetic inheritance; what you were born with on a cellular level;

2. Mental process; intellect; your thinking potential and processes;

3. Emotions and how you handle emotional stress, conflict, etc.;

4. Spiritual attitudes and your ability to assimilate new behaviors and attitudes;

5. Physical problems, including your personal and family history;

6. Life style and diet, including sleep/wake patterns, food cravings and addictions;

7. Body type, appearance, weight, immunity, overall health and vitality. Each person's basic energetic appearance and body type is a reflection of his or her inherited constitution.

Constitutional treatment works on all the above levels. Different treatments and homeopathic remedies will act on different levels at different times during your treatment. Some treatments and remedies will focus more on the spiritual or emotional and others on the physical, diet cravings or lifestyle. After being treated for a longer period of time, it is possible to affect your genetic inheritance level as well.

The other day a patient of mine, an attorney, who worked for a large firm, asked what her constitutional homeopathic remedy was for and what she could expect it to cure. I told her it was like bringing an efficiency expert into her law firm to investigate how to help the entire company run more smoothly, more effectively and more efficiently.

Here's the thing: if the Board of Directors for the law firm was aware that there was a problem in a certain department or a problem with some of the clerical staff, the Board could decide simply to fire a few of the problem secretaries. But the better remedy and more effective option over the long run would be to look at the entire structure of the company and to take whatever action would be necessary to improve overall company performance, from the bottom upwards.

This is what a constitutional homeopathic remedy does. It enters your body through the nerves under your tongue and it "looks at" the overall functioning of every organ system in your body, including the hormones, nerves, muscles, glands, brain, etc. It does a quick scan of your entire body, much like a computer expert scans the entire hard drive on your computer. It then "knows" which parts of the hard drive are defective or, in this case, which organs and glands are not functioning optimally in your body. It then immediately and automatically goes to work at fixing the problem.

One reason you may feel a little worse when you first take your homeopathic remedy is because while it's working to optimize your overall function, it may begin by ridding your body of toxins that have been stored in your fat cells. As these toxins are released, you might feel a little worse or get a skin rash. But once you're "cleaned out," you'll feel better than ever before.

It's similar to the law firm that needs to fire a few secretaries who are not performing well but hasn't yet hired new ones. Once the new secretaries are hired a brief training period will be required to get them up to speed. During this brief transition period, the firm may notice that it's not functioning as well, but after a few weeks, it will function better than ever.

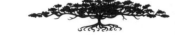

WHEN HOMEOPATHY DOESN'T WORK

I have already tried homeopathy and it didn't work. Why?

There are a lot of reasons homeopathic medicine may not have worked for you on your particular case in the past. The most common reason is that you may have not taken the remedies correctly or you may have accidentally antidoted the effects of the remedies. You may have been given the wrong remedy in the first place. You may have been given the right remedy but in the wrong potency. Or your body may not have been ready to "receive" the particular remedy you tried on a deeper level.

What do you mean that I may have antidoted the remedy?

Certain substances have the potential of stopping or antidoting the effects of the remedies. Coffee, for instance, in some cases, will ruin the effect of the remedy. Decaf coffee may do the same, but not in all cases. Some people are not sensitive to this, and some remedies are not sensitive to the effect of coffee.

Why decaf? It doesn't even contain any caffeine...

Very true and although coffee in of itself is not good for your kidneys and liver, this has nothing to do with why it is not recommended to be used when taking homeopathic remedies. It is not the caffeine which antidotes the remedies, but the chemicals in the coffee bean itself. For this reason, as far as homeopathy is concerned, drinking caffeine containing black or green tea is fine, and usually has little or no effect on most homeopathic remedies. Some remedies will even respond poorly if you are drinking a lot of tea, so ask your homeopath to be sure.

What other things will antidote a homeopathic remedy?

Mint in any form, including toothpaste, mints, gargle, gum, etc.

What else?

Raw garlic or raw onion, but cooked is fine. Also any body rubs containing camphor, eucalyptus, menthol, or any strong perfumes, etc. If you are uncertain, ask. Also, be certain not to store the remedies near perfume, makeup, kitchen or bathroom odors.

Are you telling me I may have ruined the effects of the remedies?

Yes. This is very controversial. Not all homeopaths agree on these principles. Since I am a classical homeopath, I believe these principles to be very important. If your remedies didn't work, this may have been the reason.

I have been told not to touch the remedies...

This is also very important. You should tap them into the cap and then toss them under the tongue. Also, be sure not to eat or drink anything for ten to twenty minutes before and after taking the remedies.

Is there any other reason that homeopathy may have failed to work?

The most likely reason is that you were given the wrong remedies. There are well over one thousand different remedies to choose from. A common problem such as a headache, cold, flu or back pain can have at least twenty different possible remedies to choose from. It is a science and art to match your particular set of symptoms with the right remedy. Even if you were given the right remedy, it may have been in the wrong potency. All this would make it ineffective.

How long should I wait to see if the remedy is working?

It depends on how long you have had the problem. If you have been suffering for a long time and are given a high potency remedy, it may take weeks or even a few months to feel the effect. On the other hand, in an acute case, such as a cold or flu, you should feel the effect of the correctly chosen remedy almost immediately. If you don't, then it is probably the wrong remedy. Sometimes, even in acute cases, you may need to take the remedy up to ten times or so before feeling its effect. Be sure to remain in close contact with your homeopath if you aren't sure.

What if my body or emotions are not receptive to a particular remedy?

In some cases, it may take three or four different remedies before you feel the effects. This is because each remedy subtly changes your body energy and makes it ready for the effect of the next remedy. Sometimes it's not until the fourth or fifth remedy that your body is ready to feel the effects.

I hate it when I'm given a lot of different remedies. Isn't this just a hit or miss game anyway?

No, not at all. The experienced homeopath usually knows what he or she is doing and although it may appear to you that you are a guinea pig, actually it sometimes takes a while for your body to respond to the remedies. Remember that it took you a long time to get the way you are now, and you cannot expect the damage to be undone overnight. Patience is a vital part to any natural healing approach!

> *Homeopathy could well be the medicine of the future, as it has little nor*
> *no detrimental effect on the environment, offers a holistic attitude to*
> *patient care, and has no history of animal experimentation.*
>
> —*Bernadette Vallely*
> *1001 Ways to Save the Planet*

WHAT TO DO IF YOU ANTIDOTE YOUR HOMEOPATHIC REMEDY

(or Whooops!...I Forgot and Drank a Cup of Coffee)

This is a fairly typical situation. A patient comes in for his or her monthly office visit, I open their chart, and we begin to talk. One of the things I'm always interested to know is how it went when taking their homeopathic remedy.

So after a discussion of diet and exercise, and then assessing which nutritional supplements and herbs they are running out of, I usually next ask if they have finished taking their homeopathic remedy. Many times, especially if it is a relatively new patient, they tell me that they didn't take the homeopathic remedy because they were still drinking coffee. Or they say that since they didn't obtain a new toothpaste without mint in it, they felt it would be a waste of time to take the homeopathic remedy.

I usually roll my eyes, take a deep breath and say the following: "Always, I repeat ALWAYS, take your homeopathic remedy prescribed for you, whether or not you think you may be antidoting the remedy."

If you are unsure what will antidote the remedies refer to the list of what things antidote remedies. But even if you do antidote your remedy, all you have to do is to take it again. In fact, if you drink coffee daily, you can still take your remedy. Just assure the amount of time between taking the remedy and the coffee, or the mint toothpaste, is maximized.

In other words, if all you have is mint toothpaste, go ahead and use it and wait a hour or so before taking your remedy. It is not optimal to antidote the remedies on a daily basis, but if you do it by mistake occasionally it is not a "big deal." Take the remedy anyway.

There is only one exception to this rule. If you are taking a deep-acting constitutional homeopathic remedy in a high potency (30C or 200X and above), and you are only taking this remedy one or two times, then its important not to antidote the remedy. If you antidote a high potency remedy, be sure to mention it at your next office visit so that your homeopath can decide whether to give you another dose.

GUIDELINES FOR THE USE AND STORAGE OF HOMEOPATHIC REMEDIES

The following guidelines are essential when taking homeopathic remedies:

Allow at least 20 minutes to pass *before* and *after* eating or drinking or putting anything into the mouth when taking a homeopathic remedy. This includes brushing your teeth, chewing gum, etc.

Pellets: Do not touch the homeopathic pellets. Leave the bottle uncapped for as short a time as possible. Tap your dosage of pellets (usually 3–5) into the cap and then drop them under your tongue and allow them to dissolve. Let the tablets dissolve with the mouth closed. If they do not dissolve, you may suck on or chew them after 5 minutes.

Liquid: Draw the liquid into the dropper. Do not let the dropper touch your mouth. Place the appropriate amount under your tongue and hold it there for a minute before swallowing.

Inhalants: Place the open remedy container under your nose, then breathe in deeply. Do not breathe out into the open container.

Storage and Handling: Store the remedy away from direct light or heat, microwave ovens, computers, electrical outlets, or strong odors such as perfume, incense, mothballs, etc. Do not carry the remedy on your person, such as in your pockets. At airports, do not allow the remedy to go through the X-ray. Have it hand-checked. Do not transfer the remedy to another container. Always keep it in the sterilized bottle it came in.

The following pointers will enhance the use of your remedies. I strongly urge you try to follow them to the best of your ability. If it is impossible for you to follow these rules exactly, continue to take your remedies and let me or your homeopath know which rules you are unable to follow.

These rules should be followed while taking the remedies and afterwards for two to three days. If you have taken a higher potency remedy, such as a 200X, 30C, 1M, or higher, try to follow these rules for at least a month after taking the remedy.

Refrain from drinking regular or decaffeinated coffee.

Do not eat raw garlic or raw onion.

Do not take mint. This includes most commercial toothpaste. A homeopathic drugstore or natural food store should carry a flavor of toothpaste that is mint-free. No mint flavors at all—cinnamon or licorice flavor is fine. Also be careful with chewing gum.

Do not use any products internally or externally which contain eucalyptus, camphor, mint, menthol or any other strong-smelling substances.

Do not wear perfumes or essential oils while using the remedies.

When properly stored, the remedies will be good indefinitely. Do not store them near perfumes or perfumed makeup, in your purse, near medications, foods, herbs or any other strong-smelling substances. Keep the remedies out of direct sunlight and intense heat. Avoid storing in proximity to radiation (including electrical current).

HOW TO TAKE HOMEOPATHIC REMEDIES FOR EMERGENCIES OR ACUTE CONDITIONS

The following are some simple guidelines for taking homeopathic remedies for emergencies or other acute, short term problems:

Take three to five pellets per dosage.

For an acute problem or pain, take one dose every 15 minutes until you experience relief; then stop taking it.

More is not better! Discontinue use of the remedy as soon as relief is achieved. If you get no relief after three to four doses, you have chosen the wrong remedy or wrong potency. Begin by analyzing the problem again and choosing a new remedy or potency. In some cases, however, you won't see results very quickly so if you are sure it is the right remedy, keep taking it as long as it is a low potency.

Always use 3X, 6X, or 12X potencies. For severe pain, such as an insect bite or an acute sprain, use 30X.

HOMEOPATHIC EMERGENCY MEDICINE

You are on an outing an hour or so out of town. You pack a picnic lunch and set off for a nice day's hike up the mountain. You arrive at a beautiful mountain stream, set up your picnic basket, and start eating. Seemingly out of nowhere a couple of wasps appear. One of them stings you on the back of the neck, and—*bingo!* the trip is ruined.

This has happened to me, but my trip wasn't ruined because I carried a homeopathic emergency kit. A couple doses of a remedy called *Apis mel* took the sting right out!

Homeopathic medicine is ideal as emergency medicine because it is light, easy to carry, safe, without side effects and very inexpensive. The following is an example of some of the more common homeopathic emergencies for which you can safely treat yourself.

Travel sickness

Cocculus (cocc.) for nausea with dizziness, an unsteady gait with a desire to lie down.

Nux vomica for a splitting headache with nausea, wanting warmth and craving spicy or rich foods.

Petroleum for nausea with pain in the stomach which is relieved when eating, and feeling worse from light or noise.

Sprains and strains

Arnica montana. Always start a treatment with a few doses of Arnica when you are otherwise not positive which remedy to give for a sprain. After a few doses of Arnica you may switch to *Ruta graveolens*. Ruta is used to heal the ligaments and periosteum (bone covering).

116

Rhus toxicodendron (Rhus. t.) is used when the injury feels better after you begin to move around, whereas *Bryonia alba* is used when the injured person feels better at rest without being moved or bothered in any way. If you are unsure, just stick to Arnica.

Puncture wounds

Ledum palustre (Led.) is the most common remedy for anything resembling a puncture wound. This would include side effects from injections, snake bites, stepping on a nail, and some types of insect stings. Another good remedy is *Hypericum perfolatum*, which is used whenever there is shooting pain radiating from the site of injury. Hypericum is used for any injury which involves the nerves, such as a fall on the tailbone, injury to the elbow or tooth pain from an untreated dental infection. These two remedies may also prove helpful after dental work.

Insect bites

Ledum palustre is the most common remedy.

If there is swelling then move to *Apis mellifica*.

Poison oak or stinging nettles

Rhus toxicodendron works quite well as both preventative and treatment for Poison Oak. To prevent it, take *Rhus tox.* 6X or 12X, five tablets three times per day during contact with the plant.

Use *Urtica urens (Urt. u.)* for common nettle rash or for any burning or stinging rash covering a general area of the body.

Baptisia may also be used for burning or stinging as well as *Arsenicum alb.* or *Sulfur,* depending on the person's constitution.

Food poisoning

Arsenicum album is one of the most common remedies for food poisoning if there is burning diarrhea, cramps, gas, vomiting or nausea. If after a few doses you don't feel better, switch to *Nux vomica.*

Nux vomica is great for most stomach and abdominal problems and should be carried with you on all trips across the border. Nux Vomica and Arnica are the two most indispensable emergency remedies. You should keep them both in your automobile or in your purse at all times.

Collapse and shock

Aconitum napellus (Acon.) if fear is the predominant symptom.

Arnica montana if there has been injury or bleeding.

Carbo vegetabilis if there is great hunger for air or desire to be fanned, with coldness and mental confusion.

Nosebleed

Ferrum phosphoricum is always the first remedy to try for a nosebleed.

If it does not work, go to *Phosphorus.*

To get the most benefit from your remedy it is best to avoid the following:

Foods and Beverages:

✧ Coffee, including decaffeinated coffee (it's the coffee bean, not the caffeine)

✧ Mint, including most commercial toothpaste, mints, gum, breath mints

✧ Raw onions; cooked are OK

✧ Raw garlic; cooked is fine

✧ Very spicy foods

Moderation in consuming the following is recommended:

✧ Chocolate, cola drinks, and alcohol

Miscellaneous:

Other things which may interfere with the effectiveness of your remedy are the following:

✧ Camphor oil, in any form (including Tiger Balm and other body rubs)

✧ Strong perfumes

✧ Aromatherapy

✧ Strong emotional shocks

✧ Physical trauma

✧ Dental work

✧ X-Rays

✧ Electric blankets and/or sleeping near a power line

✧ Sitting in front of a computer screen all day

✧ Acupuncture and Herbs may, in some cases; discuss this with your homeopathic doctor.

The idea of a natural healing force goes back at least to the time of Hippocrates—100 B.C.

—W. Edward Mann

HOMEOPATHIC REMEDIES & ABBREVIATIONS

REMEDY	ABBREVIATION	REMEDY	ABBREVIATION
Aconitum napellus	Acon.	*Glonoine*	Glon.
Aesulus hippocastanum	Aesc.	*Graphites*	Graph.
Allium cepa	All.c.	*Hamamelis virginica*	Ham.
Alumina	Alum.	*Hepar sulphuris calcareum*	Hep.
Anacardium	Anac.	*Hypericum perfoliatum*	Hyper.
Apis mellifica	Apis	*Ignatia amala*	Ign Ip.
Antimonium crudum	Ant.c.	*Ipecacuanha*	Ip.
Antimonium tartaricum	Ant.t.	*Kali bichromicum*	Kali.bi.
Arnica montana	Arn.	*Kali bromatum*	Kali.br.
Arsenicum album	Ars.	*Kali carbonicum*	Kali.c.
Baryta carbonica	Bar.c.	*Kali muriaticum*	Kali.m.
Belladonna	Bell.	*Kreosotum*	Kreos.
Berberis vulgaris	Berb.	*Ledum palustre*	Led.
Bryonia alba	Bry.	*Lycopodium*	Lyc.
Calcarea carbonica	Calc.	*Magnesia phosphorica*	Mag.p.
Calcarea phosphorica	Calc.p.	*Medorrhinum*	Med.
Cantharis	Canth.	*Mercurius corrosivus*	Merc.c.
Carbolicum acidum	Carb.ac.	*Mercurius vivus*	Merc.
Carbo vegetabilis	Carb.v.	*Natrum muriaticum*	Nat.m.
Caulophyllum	Caul.	*Natrum phosphoricum*	Nat.p.
Causticum	Caust.	*Nitricum acidum*	Nit.ac.
Chamomilla	Cham.	*Nux vomica*	Nux.v.
Cinchona officinalis	Chin.	*Oxalicum acidum*	Ox.ac.
Cistus canadensis	Cist.	*Phosphorus*	Phos.
Cocculus	Cocc.	*Phytolacca decandra*	Phyt.
Coffea cruda	Coff.	*Podophyllum*	Podo.
Colchicum	Colch.	*Pulsatilla nigricans*	Puls.
Collinsonia	Coll.	*Pyrogenium*	Pyrog.
Colocynthis	Coloc.	*Rhodendron*	Rhod.
Crotalus horridus	Crot.h.	*Rhus toxicodendron*	Rhus.t.
Cuprum arsenicosum	Cupr.ar.	*Ruta graveolens*	Ruta
Cuprum metallicum	Cupr.	*Sabina Sepia*	Sabin. Sep.
Dulcamara	Dulc.	*Silicea or Silica*	Sil.
Echinacea augustifolia	Echi.	*Spongia tosta*	Spong.
Equisetum	Equis.	*Sulphur Symphytum officinale*	Sulph. Symph.
Eupatorium perforliatum	Eup.per.	*Thuja occidentalis*	Thuj.
Euphrasia	Eupr.	*Tuberculinum*	Tub.
Ferrum metallicum	Ferr.m.	*Urtica urens*	Urt.u.
Ferrum phosphoricum	Ferr.p.	*Veratrum album*	Verat.a.
Gelsemium sempervirens	Gels.	*Verbascum*	Verb.

KARMA, MIASM AND HEALTH*

by Dr. Randy W. Martin

Everything in life is like a mirror of everything else.

We are only capable of perceiving that which is within our awareness parameters, that which is mirrored to us.

Our physical body is a mirror of our mental body and our thoughts.

Our physical body is also a mirror of our spiritual body and our karma.

Karma is not some metaphysical concept.

Karma is just the basic dynamic with which we enter this world.

The basic parameters, or mirrors, with which we enter the world is our karma.

Our miasm and our genetics are part of our karma, as well.

We can change our karma willfully, through "right action" and we can also get a boost or catalyze the change by the use of homeopathic remedies.

* Karma—the energy we bring into this lifetime, including physical, emotional and spiritual balance and imbalance; involves the causal relationships we have with other living things; all actions and thoughts generate karma; kind of like a pebble dropped into a pool of water; karma is the energy that radiates outwards from the drop of the pebble.

Miasm—a predisposition to illness; inherited and genetic; there are four miasms: syphillitic, sycotic, psoric and tubercular. Some homeopaths also say that cancer and AIDS are new miasms.

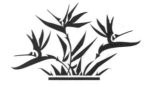

HERBAL MEDICINE

An herb is defined as any part of a plant that is used for the purpose of medical treatment, nutrition, food, seasoning, or coloring and dyeing. For medicinal use, any part of the plant may be used: root, stem, leaf, flower, or fruit.

In written history, the study of herbs dates back over 5,000 years to the Sumerians. Herbs are probably the earth's oldest and most elementary form of medical healing. For example, animals in the wild instinctively eat certain plants for health, to balance the effects of the seasons, and to alleviate disease.

Traditionally, every family had a garden or medicine cabinet of common herbal remedies. Physicians also used a variety of plant remedies to cure common ills. But as technology advanced, and with the discovery of penicillin and other patent drugs, most simple plant remedies have been gradually forgotten.

Yet many chemical drugs today have herbs as their basis. Ma Huang, for example, has been used for thousands of years. More recently, an alkaloid called *ephedrine* has been extracted from this plant and is used to relieve nasal congestion, asthma, and cough.

How do herbs work?

Specific herbs have definitive properties. Herbs can act as diuretics (clear excess water from the body), diaphoretics (cause sweating), expectorants (expel mucus), alteratives* (change bad conditions to good), or as demulcent-emollients (smooth and soften). They can also be classified as tonics, cleansers, disinfectants, etc. Most herbs actually have multiple effects.

The same herbs can also act differently on different people. In prescribing herbs, the practitioner must try to unearth the causes of the symptoms. In the case of a headache, for example, the practitioner must determine if it is caused by toothache, eyestrain, tight shoes, digestive upset, or something else entirely.

Many herbs have a tonic or strengthening effect. Some herbs tone specific organs or systems in the body. Comfrey root is a tonic for the lungs, dandelion root works on the liver, red raspberry leaves aid the uterus, and nettle tones the kidneys.

Herbs can also vary tremendously in potency, depending on their source, their storage, or drying techniques. For this reason, it is important to purchase herbs from a reliable source.

How are herbs prepared and prescribed?

For long-term effects, herbs should be taken in small doses over a period of weeks or months. Herbal formulas, or combinations of herbs, can also be used to balance certain body systems and/or to strengthen specific imbalances. Chinese herbs are almost always taken in the form of formulas.

Three of the most common methods of preparing and taking herbs are:

1. *Infusion:* $^1/_4$ teaspoon herb to 1 cup boiled water; steep
2. *Decoction:* $^1/_4$ teaspoon herb boiled in water for 20 minutes, covered, and strained
3. *Capsules*: powdered herb placed into a capsule

Other common herbal preparations are ointments, tinctures, tablets, compresses, or baths.

Herbal medicine is extremely effective, but it is not the only factor in achieving optimal health. Herbs are commonly combined with different treatments such as nutritional supplements, homeopathics, acupuncture, exercise, massage, manipulation, meditation, and other remedies.

---

*Alterative—A substance that tends to generally restore healthy bodily function

I'M SICK AND NEED ANTIBIOTICS... THINK AGAIN!!!

What do a strep throat, urinary infection, pink eye, amebic dysentery, and a bad flu all have in common? Lots!!! If you went to your medical doctor, they would all likely be treated with antibiotics. The only problem is that although the antibiotics may in fact work to get rid of your symptoms, the antibiotics may also lead to a yeast infection, indigestion, feelings of fatigue, bad taste in the mouth and an even weaker immune system.

So let's ask the same question again: What *do* a strep throat, urinary infection, pink eye, amebic dysentery and a bad cold all have in common? Well, to a Doctor of Oriental Medicine, they all fall into the classification known as Damp Heat. And I will choose different herbal formulas for each person, based not only on the name of the disease, but also on the person's basic constitution and makeup.

Some herbal treatment examples:

Strep Throat may be treated with Antiphlogistic Pills to reduce heat, swelling and redness, Coptis and Scute to get rid of the infection, or Gan Mao Ling to boost immunity if there is also a cold or flu involved;

Urinary Infection may be treated with Enterogenic, to raise the good bacteria in the system, Gentiana or Dianthus formula to rid the body of the heat and Composition A to boost immunity;

Pink Eye may be treated with Temper Fire to boost the Yin and eradicate the excess Yang, Similisan Eye Drops to homeopathically "drain" the red and inflammation out of the eye, and Euphrasia (eye bright);

Amebic Dysentery may be treated with Gentianna Formula to get rid of the Damp Heat, Aquillaria 22 to kill the amoebae and bacteria residing in the digestive tract, Enterogenic to rebuild the positive bacteria in the colon, and Condurango tincture to act as an astringent to stop the diarrhea;

Flu or Bad Cold may be treated with Gan Mao Tuire Tea to cause sweating and to break the fever, Zong Gan Ling to help the respiratory system, Dandelion Root Tea to detoxify the liver, Astragalus to boost immunity, Oscillocoxinum to boost immunity and Yin Chiao to "push" the cold out to the surface of the body.

NOTE: If you **do in fact** *need* to take antibiotics, you may also use herbs at the same time to strengthen your body so that you don't suffer side effects from the antibiotics. Never take yourself off an antibiotic prescription without first consulting your doctor. Do not assume it is always bad to take antibiotics. Sometimes they can be lifesaving and very necessary. **We need to achieve a balance in the use of Western, Oriental and Homeopathic Medicine.** This is one of my primary goals as a doctor, to open the dialogue between Western and Holistic Medicine and to work toward creating a truly holistic healing model for our future and for generations to come.

DIET, NUTRITION, AND THE WHOLE PERSON

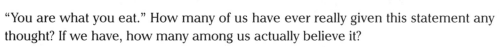

"You are what you eat." How many of us have ever really given this statement any thought? If we have, how many among us actually believe it?

The fact is that the cells which make up our bodies and minds are constantly growing and changing. It is the food we eat, the air we breathe, and the emotions we choose to entertain that affect the character and vitality of the person we are becoming, day by day, minute by minute.

Oriental medical philosophy has acknowledged this for thousands of years. For instance, in Oriental medical diagnosis, eating too much sour-flavored food is known to affect the liver and produce anger, too much spicy food affects the lungs, salty foods affect the kidneys, and sweet foods influence the stomach and pancreas. Each affected organ has a corresponding emotional effect.

Now Western medical science is recognizing how different foods can affect the organs of the body. According to recent research, eating excessive amounts of dairy products affects the pituitary gland, salt and meat stimulate the adrenals, carbohydrates and coffee affect the thyroid, and spicy foods influence the ovaries.

In short, the foods we eat *do* affect our body in the relative strength and weakness of different organs and glands, and in terms of resultant emotional states.

For each of us to consciously recognize the interconnectedness of our body, emotions, and the foods we use to nourish ourselves are the first step towards taking more responsibility for our health and well-being.

We all need to find a diet and nutritional program designed for our unique constitution. For those who want to get started now on a generic healthy diet, the following offers some guidelines. This diet is a general guideline of a healthy diet for those of you who don't have the time or inclination to do research, take tests and create an individualized metabolic diet plan for yourselves.

GENERAL DIET GUIDELINES

Most of us want a healthy body. We also want to feel healthy emotionally and spiritually. But most of us are reluctant to make the significant changes in our lifestyle that will bring about a new level of health. It is my goal to encourage and provide you with the information and emotional support necessary to make these changes. In this section, I offer you a simple eating plan, or program.

This plan is not right for everyone. Depending on your particular constitutional type, you may need to eat more or less of certain foods, whether it may be animal products, vegetables, fruits, or grains. What I provide you with is a general outline to start you on a more balanced approach to eating. You need to discuss your particular needs and possible modifications with someone like myself, who is trained to guide you in these matters within the larger context of your entire constitution and history.

The importance of eating slowly and under relaxed conditions cannot be emphasized enough. Food does not digest when you are nervous, anxious, or rushing around. Chewing your food well to begin with is also the first step toward good digestion.

According to the Chinese, you are what you eat. Food is the first step toward developing good *chi* or life force energy. Your food choices, and the way you eat them, are within your control. If you want to know what you can do today to get started on the path to better health, eat well! (Whenever possible, eat "organic"!) It is one of the simplest things to make a dramatic difference in your health and well-being.

Food Diary

Keep a record of your eating habits and your symptoms. Use these headings as an example of the type of information you should record. This is a great way to understand some of your hidden habits. I recommend that you use a looseleaf binder and put these headings at the top of each new page:

Time of Day   **What I Ate**   **Symptoms/Mood**

The Basic Plan

Breakfast

It's best to start the day with a combination of protein and a whole grain, such as a multigrain cereal, oatmeal, buckwheat, or cream of rice. There are many whole grain cereals to choose from. If you choose a cold cereal, try to use soy or almond milk instead of dairy products, if you have any allergies to milk or are lactose-intolerant. If you need to sweeten hot cereal, try using a little amasake drink or maple sugar granules, barley malt, brown rice syrup, Stevia herb, or cinnamon and ginger.

You may also want to try a coffee substitute, such as Pero, or a tea such as licorice root, ginseng, ginger, Bancha, or Pau D'arco. If you need some caffeine, try using Ponay tea, which is great for digestion and the thyroid, or a green leaf tea, which has less caffeine than coffee.

For your protein, try using tempe, an egg or two, a piece of low fat turkey or chicken, or a turkey sausage. Many people think that eggs are bad, but in actuality, if your liver is functioning properly, the eggs will never create high cholesterol. High cholesterol is a result of faulty liver metabolism and poor insulin and glucose metabolism.

Snack

Eat a piece of fruit or some vegetable sticks, or a couple of rice cakes and a piece of cheese. Herb teas and coffee substitutes are also great for between-meal snacks, and as chasers for your vitamins and herbal supplements. If you feel hypoglycemic (suffer from low blood sugar), you must be certain to add protein to your snack. If you choose to use fruit as your snack, always eat it alone, which means at least 30 minutes before or 1 hour after any other foods. This is because it's impossible for your body to digest other foods in the presence of fruit. Never combine melons with other fruit.

Lunch

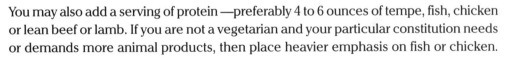

Eat a salad with lots of different vegetables and a healthy, non-hydrogenated oil dressing. Depending on your constitution, you may do better with cooked vegetables instead. If you can see "teeth marks" on the sides of your tongue, you may have what is called a Spleen Damp condition (see page 98). Most people exhibiting this condition should stay away from raw foods, as a general rule.

You may also add a serving of protein —preferably 4 to 6 ounces of tempe, fish, chicken or lean beef or lamb. If you are not a vegetarian and your particular constitution needs or demands more animal products, then place heavier emphasis on fish or chicken.

After eating protein, consider a starch such as potato, squash, or a whole grain. If you have trouble with your digestion, you may temporarily not be able to eat protein and starch at the same meal. In this case, have one or the other as your between-meal energy snack, but it's preferable to try and eat the grain and protein at the same sitting. Recent research shows that your energy uptake and assimilation is at a much higher level with you eat them together. If you are experiencing gas or bloating, you probably are deficient in digestive enzymes. A good upper and lower GI enzyme should take care of this problem. If after a few months, you have not seen an improvement in your digestion, then you need to see a holistic doctor to obtain a full workup.

An herbal or medicinal tea tops off your meal.

Always leave the table feeling not quite full.

Snack

Same as above

Dinner

Same as lunch, with additional grain ideas being brown or basmati rice, amaranth, quinoa, millet, corn, etc. Eat as much salad as you want. Your serving of grain may be a starchy vegetable, such as acorn squash or kabocha pumpkin, as well.

Evening Snacks

Same as above. If you take a calcium supplement, you may want to do so before bed in order to help you sleep.

Have fun and enjoy. Food is festive, and not the enemy. Allow your food to nurture and nourish you! As you begin to eat healthier and healthier, your cravings will shift. Try to honor your inner sense of what your body, mind, and spirit really need most.

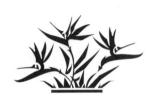

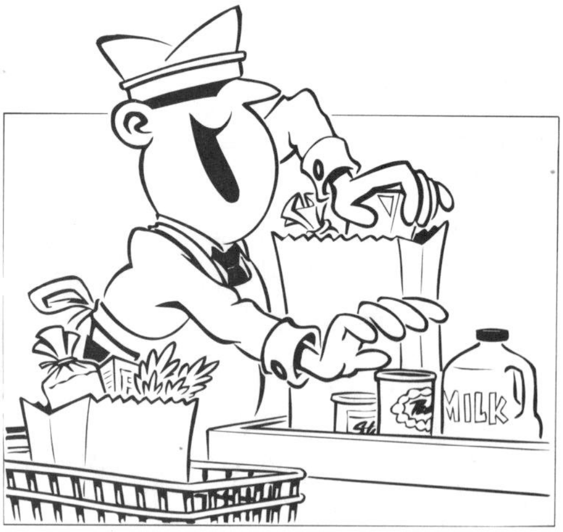

A Few Food Sources of Calcium

(beginning with the best)

Collard greens
Salmon
Blackstrap molasses
Sesame seeds
Bok Choy
Kale
Mustard greens
Broccoli
Tofu
Okra
Dandelion greens
Soybeans
Carob flour
Rutabagas

A Few Food Sources of Magnesium

(beginning with the best)

Soybeans
Beet greens
Blackeyes peas
White beans
Buckwheat
Salmon
Whole wheat flour
Tofu
Turnip greens
Collard greens
Corn meal
Wheat berries
Millet
Dandelion greens
Chicken
Lentils
Rye flour
Mustard greens
Brown Rice
Peas
Oatmeal
Sweet potatoes
Brussels sprouts
Kale
Almonds
Snap beans
Parsnips
Peanut butter
Filberts (hazelnuts)
Beets
Turnips
Corn
Broccoli
Cauliflower
Whole wheat bread
Barley
Summer squash
Onions
Asparagus
Peanuts
Carrots
Tomatoes
Walnuts
Green peppers
Mushrooms
Celery
Cabbage
Sunflower seeds
Lettuce

SEASONAL HARMONY, IMMUNITY AND DIET

Nutrition

Picture this: You're at a holiday party and the woman next to you is pigging out on your favorite chocolate cake! Your inner child says, "Go for it," yet your inner parent says, "Remember, your acupuncturist told you NO sugar or alcohol this holiday season!" What should you do?

If you are on the "healing path" described in this book, this could very well be your dilemma...WHY? Because the preventive approach to health is a superior form of medicine and there is no better way to prevent colds and flu and to increase and strengthen your immunity than to eat in a healthy way. "You are what you eat" is no joke.

According to Chinese medical principles, the food we eat is the most important factor in maintaining good health. Next most important is our assimilation of food. Many people think that colds and flu are "caught" by coming into contact with germs or bacteria. But what you may not realize is that if your immune system is strong, you will not get a cold despite being around an office or family full of "sickies."

Time and time again, my patients tell me that everyone around them is catching a cold or step throat yet they have never felt better. It is very interesting to note that according to Chinese medicine, the stomach and digestion are directly related to and affect the throat and nasal areas.

Preventing illness and boosting immunity is really as easy as eating right, strengthening digestion through acupuncture, herbs, and homeopathy, and trying your best not to worry.

What does worry have to do with digestion or colds? According to Chinese medicine, worry is said to injure and weaken the digestive organs and cause "overheating" which can cause a sore throat, diarrhea, or sinus infection.

So what to do if you don't follow your doctor's instruction and you do get sick during the winter months? Number one is to immediately find an acupuncturist and go in for an acupuncture "tune-up" treatment, massage and/or chiropractic adjustment. One or all of these together will realign your energies to more quickly fight off the "bug."

You can also take supplements such as vitamin C in a buffered or esterfied form, a dry form of vitamin E, beta carotene, CoQ_{10}, and a balanced B vitamin. Good herbs for the immune system are echinacea and goldenseal, sage, astragalus, cayenne, and garlic.

Remember to consult your homeopath or homeopathic books to determine your best homeopathic remedy. Often a well chosen homeopathic remedy will be able to cure you in literally an instant, or at least lessen the amount of time it takes for you to be "back on your feet." And remember that if you are on a homeopathic remedy, that you shouldn't be taking garlic at the same time. (See page 115).

Dietary Guidelines for Maximum Immunity

Some practical rules to follow to boost your immune system:

❋ Abstain from all fried, deep fried, and fatty foods at the first sign of a cold. These foods congest the Liver and Gall Bladder meridians, which need to be unblocked to increase immunity.

❋ Abstain from all sweeteners and sweets at the first sign of a cold, including fruits and fruit juices. Recent research indicates that sugars lower immunity.

❋ Eliminate dairy products. They are known to congest the lymph system.

❋ Generally, eat few fruits. They can create Damp Spleen conditions, which weaken digestion and immunity.

❋ In general, eat primarily good, lean, easy-to-assimilate proteins, cooked vegetables and whole grains.

Fasting and Seasonal Eating

Many of us are tempted to begin the new year with resolutions and promises to ourselves to clean up our diets—to undertake the fabled "purification diet"—especially after a holiday season of overindulgence.

In my experience this type of thinking leads to overindulgence and excuse-making in the first place—that roller coaster of up-and-down, binge-purge eating so unhealthy and degenerative to our digestive organs. The best solution is to eat in moderation at all times.

But if it's too late, and you have already overindulged, and you now want to try a purification diet, don't try to attempt an extreme one. Many people can't handle fasting. Blood sugar can drop dramatically, causing headaches and eventual boomerang bingeing.

If you were to go out to the desert and meditate for a week, then fasting might be appropriate, but it is not wise in the city under "normal" everyday stress. In normal conditions—working, going to school, running here and there—we are all under too much stress to fast. Our bodies need proper nutrients, protein and vitamins.

A more practical and effective cleansing diet is a *mono-diet.* In this diet, you chose one food at a time to "fast" on. Good mono-diet foods are brown rice, watermelon, apples, papaya, squash, pumpkin, carrots, beets, vegetable broth, or vegetable soup. You can also vary the diet and use a different single food each day. But I need to again emphasize that even this type of diet is NOT advised during normal periods of work or school.

Herbs to help in your cleansing process include dandelion for the liver, parsley or corn silk for the kidneys, and cayenne for the lungs. Lemon and lime juice in a little boiled water are always good for detoxification. A good homeopathic remedy for cleansing (if you are not being treated constitutionally) is Nux vom in a low potency (12C). Take

5 tablets once a day for about five days. This can mitigate the effects of a detoxification headache as well.

If someone expresses interest in a fast, I usually recommend simple cooked vegetables and brown rice for two weeks. This can have a tremendous cleansing and detoxing effect without straining the liver and adrenal glands like strict fasting does.

Coffee: What Evil Lurks … ?

You may have asked yourself a thousand times, "Should I give up coffee?" Or, if you have already quit as I have, the question then becomes, "Is it really worth it? Is coffee *really* that bad? Maybe I could start again."

Caffeine, one of the active constituents in coffee, increases the heart rate and is known to cause nervousness, anxiety, irritability, and mood swings. It also depletes the body of important vitamins and minerals, including Vitamin B, inositol, and potassium. It inhibits the body's ability to absorb iron.

Often people who are moody in the first place are the ones most addicted to coffee. An inability to live without coffee is a strong sign of hypoglycemia or low blood sugar. Caffeine temporarily raises blood sugar levels by stimulating the adrenal glands; it makes us feel energetic right away. Unfortunately, after this pick-me-up, it drops us down to an even lower energy level than before.

Coffee is a drug. Like any drug, it is addictive. It works just like sugar or alcohol, both of which also temporarily raise blood sugar by stimulating the adrenals.

In the long run, all of this stimulation of the adrenal glands can produce adrenal burnout. Typical signs may be tiredness between 3 and 6 P.M., black or blue circles under the eyes, and *san pa ku* (being able to see the whites of the eyes under the iris when looking straight ahead at yourself in the mirror.)

Coffee also increases breast tenderness in women who suffer from PMS. Some research also indicated increased risk of breast fibroids and ovarian cysts.

And remember—because coffee is grown in other countries, it usually contains remnants of pesticides which are illegal for use in the U.S. because of their toxicity.

More than 70 percent of the world's coffee is sprayed with synthetic chemicals including malathion and DDT.

—Utne Reader

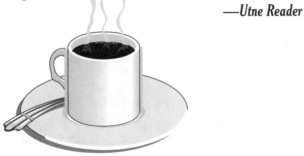

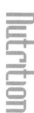

Caffeine-Containing Beverages

When examining different caffeinated beverages, it's important to read labels. Here's an example of the amount of caffeine contained in different products. The less caffeine you consume the better. Caffeine severely weakens the adrenals and your Kidney chi!

- Hot cocoa—1 oz. packet, 2 to 10 mg
- Instant coffee—5 oz., 40 to 105 mg
- Tea—5 oz. at 5-minute steep, 40 to 100 m
- Tab (soft drink)—49.4 mg
- Espresso—1 shot, 55 to 75 mg
- Percolated coffee—5 oz., 60 to 125 mg
- Anacin, Empirin, Midol—2 tabs, 64 mg
- Coke (Coca Cola)—64.7 mg
- Excedrin—65.0 mg
- Iced tea—12 oz., 67 to 76 mg
- Drip coffee—5 oz., 110 to 150 mg
- Cafergot—199.0 mg

ADRENALINE (WO)MAN
While resting, the blood contains very little adrenaline. When excited, adrenaline is released and responsible for "fight or flight."

Adrenaline:
Constricts muscles
Dilates Pupils
Increases heart rate
Stimulates breathing
Inhibits & contracts stomach
Inhibits & contracts bladder
Increases blood sugar
Stimulates metabolism

As you are probably aware, caffeine is hidden in all kinds of drinks and in many over-the-counter drugs. Most soft drinks contain caffeine too, so you have to look closely.

Decaffeinated coffee is not the best solution to the caffeine problem because it is usually processed with toxic chemicals. Even water-processed decaf is not good; it still contains the same acids and alkaloids which are thought to act as poisons and toxins in the liver. Oriental doctors think that coffee and decaf weaken the liver and the kidneys.

Black and green teas are the easiest alternatives, as they have just a little caffeine and you can regulate the amount of caffeine by the length of time you steep the tea bag. Try dipping the bag only one or two times. Among the varieties to try are China Black, Darjeeling, and Orange Pekoe. Look for organically-grown teas, preferably loose or in unbleached tea bags (no Dioxin).

Ground grains are a reasonable and very tasty alternative to coffee. They taste somewhat similar to coffees and teas. Some of the commercial grain drinks are Pero, Ovaltine, Postum, and Cafix.

Herb tea is one of the best alternatives. Drinks with ginseng can also give you an energy boost. Try peppermint tea (if you aren't taking homeopathic remedies). It is one of the best herb tea substitutes, thanks to its natural "upper" effects.

If you depend on coffee to wake you up in the morning and to help you to stay alert, substitute licorice and ginger root tea. Add 2 teaspoons of grated ginger root and 2 teaspoons of grated licorice root to 1 quart of water. Boil for 10 minutes and steep for 15 minutes.

Refreshing alternatives that shouldn't be overlooked are the flavored or plain sparkling waters such as Perrier and Crystal Geyser.

From my experience, it is best not to quit coffee "cold turkey." This can cause severe shock to the nervous system and lead to headaches, hot flashes, heart palpitations, depression, constipation, fatigue, and mood swings which can persist for a week or two. It is much gentler on the system to quit by degrees. Develop a plan of gradual abstinence which best meets your individual needs, commit to it, and then stick it out.

Daily exercise will help, because it gives the same stimulation to the brain and nervous system as coffee. Simple walking can have amazing results if done consistently.

One last suggestion: Take a close look at your diet. From an Oriental medical perspective, we often crave extreme yin substances such as coffee because of strong yang elements in our diet. Foods that contain strong yang elements include meat, fish, eggs, salt, and overcooked grains. To balance a too-yang diet, curtail yang elements and introduce more yin foods, such as salads and fresh fruits.

CAFFEINE: THE GOOD AND THE UGLY

Coffee and decaffeinated coffee are both very toxic to your liver and kidneys. Both also antidote the effects of homeopathic remedies. Most patients have a lot of trouble giving up coffee, but there is one form of caffeine that is not all bad. It comes in the form of tea. The two forms of tea I recommend to patients who have trouble giving up coffee are Ponay Tea, available exclusively through me (distributed by the Little Herb Co.) and green tea, available commercially.

Both teas come from the same type of plant, *Camellia sinensis*. Its leaves contain a substance called polyphenols, which research has shown to contain both antioxidants and anticarcinogens.

Ponay Tea also stimulates the thyroid gland, helps to detoxify the liver and helps in weight loss by burning fat on your body and in the fatty portion of the food you eat.

Green tea and Ponay both have the ability to stimulate the adrenal glands while not producing the nervous jittery reaction of coffee. The National Cancer Institute recently published a study that suggests that esophageal cancer was reduced by 57% for men and 60% for women drinking green tea. Animal studies (yuck—I don't believe in supporting them!!!) show green tea to have significant effects against all forms of cancer.

Both types of tea also have the ability to lower cholesterol. There is one form of tea that is especially great at lowering cholesterol, and that is the type found in Tuo-Cha Tea. Another safe form of tea that is used by people is twig tea, also known as Kukicha.

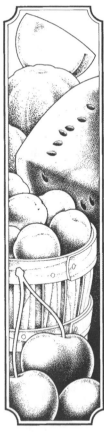

Will you teach your children what we have taught our children? That the earth is our mother? What befalls the earth, befalls all of the sons of the earth. This we know: the earth does not belong to man, man belongs to the earth. All things are connected like the blood which unites us all. Man did not weave the web of life, he is merely a strand in it. Whatever he does to the web, he does to himself.

—Chief Seattle

Deadly Pesticides

Pesticide use in California increased 31% from 1991 to 1995. Use of cancer causing pesticides increased 129%, according to Californians for Pesticide Reform, a coalition of over 70 California groups including Action Now.

Every day one million American children age 5 and under consume unsafe levels of organophosphate pesticides. Nearly one in 4 peaches and one in 8 apples have OP residues at levels that are unsafe for children, according to the *Environmental Working Group*, "Overexposed," 1/98.

Imperial Chemical Industries makes $400 million per year on the cancer-causing herbicide acetochlor and $300 million on the breast cancer drug Tamoxifen. ICI, the sole financial sponsor of Breast Cancer Awareness month, recommends mammography for "prevention," according to *Rachel's Environment and Health Weekly*.

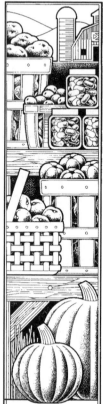

Denmark is considering a total ban on pesticide use in agriculture. By the year 2000, all pesticides considered to be hormone disrupters will be completely phased out, according to Pesticide Action Network North American.

"Can there be health of a population when we have only 'vague ideas' where our food comes from and how it gets to us?
"Our soil mineral content is now lower than any lows [in history].... Thirty cents of every consumer dollar spent for food goes for chemicals and technology. And sixty-five cents for packaging, marketing, and transportation, leaves five cents for the farmer."

—Lynn August, M.D., founder of Health Equations

Be Part of the Solution!!!
Get Involved in Your Own Health

JUMPSTART YOUR METABOLISM

How's your battery? No, not your car battery, but your internal battery, your *chi* or energy. If you don't have enough energy, it could be that your metabolism is low. (See checklist on page 136.)

Your metabolism is a direct reflection of your body heat, or the fire in your body. If it's low, you may lack energy, feel lethargy or fatigue and be unmotivated much of the time. Metabolism is related to your thyroid gland function. The thyroid gland is located in the throat at the bulge, or "Adam's Apple." Thyroid function is dependent on a wide variety of factors, including genetics, diet, daily activity and exercise level, sleep/wake cycle, emotional and physical stress, electrolytes, and the balance between your *chakras* (energy centers.)

Metabolism, or metabolic rate as it's called, is also affected by adrenal gland function, the ovaries in women or testes in men, and the pituitary gland. These glands interact to form a balancing mechanism that regulates our energy, sexual hormones and feeling of well being. These glands also affect mood through an intricate biofeedback connection to brain chemistry.

Thyroid function and metabolism tend to be determined by genetics to a large degree. If one of your parents or grandparents had a thyroid problem, you would have a susceptibility to this weakness as well. The checklist and thermometer test below will be a good start at determining if you might have this problem. If your score on the checklist test is high and your thermometer test is low, the next step is to get a complete blood workup. There are a number of different types of blood tests, so be sure you consult with a doctor knowledgeable in the area of metabolic disturbances. In addition to blood tests there are also saliva tests used to double-check sex hormone levels and adrenal hormone function. These glands will all interact with and affect the thyroid and metabolic rate, so all of them should be double-checked.

Oriental medicine also provides an avenue within which to diagnose metabolism. Here, we use the tongue, pulse and face diagnoses to determine whether there is an imbalance in the yin and yang and also to pinpoint which of the Five Elements are out of balance.

Yin refers to the Water in the body and yang refers to the Fire. If the Water is low then the Fire can flare out of control. This would correlate to hyperthyroid, or metabolism that is too fast. This also would correlate to the Fire Element being too high and the Water Element being too low. Fire correlates to the Heart and the Small Intestine. Symptoms of Fire being too high are high blood pressure, feeling "hyper," hyperactivity, ADD, palpitations, anxiety, inflammatory bowel disease, constipation, and a host of others.

Symptoms of the Fire Element being too low are fatigue, lack of motivation, low blood pressure, dislike of being with people, depression, poor circulation, brain "fog," and a host of others.

From the Chinese medical point of view, treatment for low metabolism consists of treating specific acupuncture points meant to strengthen and balance the Water/Fire (or Kidney/Heart connection.) I also give Chinese herbal combinations, some of which are thousands of years old, meant to balance and give more chi to the thyroid gland.

Typical Chinese herbal regimes might include Rehmannia Eight Formula for Kidney Yang Deficiency, Gejie Da Bu Wan and Gejie Nourishing Kidney Pills.

One important and very effective way to evaluate, diagnose and analyze metabolism is to look at the blood chemistry. This is a much different approach than simply looking at a simple thyroid blood test. Blood chemistry involves the "soil" or basis of your overall body "battery." For anyone who's done a little gardening, you might know that the basic theory is to supplement the soil with fertilizer to normalize and raise its nutrient levels. When working with body chemistry, we do the same thing by adding the missing minerals and electrolytes to balance and normalize the body's nutrient levels.

To take another analogy, we operate much as a car does, on a battery and electrical system. If the battery isn't working well, we may need a jumpstart. This jumpstart consists of giving the body various nutrients to balance its electrical system. These will be different for each person. Some people may be depleted in sodium and others in potassium. Still others may need more magnesium or calcium. Based on the blood chemistry tests, we can determine exactly what is missing in the electrical system. By supplementing with these missing minerals and electrolytes, the body will become much stronger and the metabolism will pick up substantially.

Another way of boosting metabolism is to use various vitamins, amino acids and Western herbs and glandulars. Some of the most commonly used supplements are kelp, L-tyrosine, thyroid tissue, anterior pituitary tissue, adrenal tissue, zinc, copper, iris versicolor (Blue Flag), a full-range balanced B Vitamin, ginkgo biloba and gotu-kola.

Of course, no discussion of health would be complete without addressing the issue of diet and nutrition. When the metabolism is sluggish it's a sure bet that either you aren't getting some essential nutrients in your diet, or you're getting them but not assimilating them. If you experience flatulence, bloating or burping after you eat then you probably aren't assimilating what you're eating.

If you suspect assimilation is your problem, you need to look at a number of different factors. Assimilation involves a complex process of breaking down the foods you eat into their smaller parts, so that your body can utilize them on a cellular level. You need to look at the combination of foods you are eating together. Fruit, for example, is very hard to digest with other foods. You also need to make sure you are relaxed when you eat, since it's very hard to digest when your body is in the "fight or flight" response. You might also want to consider taking digestive enzymes. Digestive enzymes will help with assimilation on a temporary basis, while we work to strengthen your digestive capabilities through acupuncture and homeopathic medicine.

It's also very important you eat enough protein, vegetables and complex carbohydrates to supply your body with the nutrients it needs to keep your metabolic "battery" running strong. Each person functions best on a particular combination of foods. If you aren't eating the right combination for you, you just won't have enough energy. This is much like putting gas in your automobile that does not have a high enough octane rating.

Let's not forget the importance of exercise in keeping your energy and metabolic rate functioning at its peak performance. There is a lot of talk these days about exercise, but dong the right kind of exercise for your metabolic type is also very important. Generally, we enjoy the type of exercise that comes the easiest for us. And although it's important to enjoy your exercise, it may be that the most enjoyable exercise is not the best for you. For example, if you are built like Ed Asner or Mary Lou Retten, you would be best with Tai Chi or ballet. On the other hand, a thin, slightly built man or woman who loves doing Yoga or Tai Chi might receive more benefit by doing weight lifting or karate. Basically, if you are of a more Yin body type and temperament, you need to balance your energy with the opposite, or Yang activity, and vice versa. This type of exercise program will also balance your metabolic rate and create an even, sustained energy.

Another way to examine this subject is via the topic of "thermogenesis," or the production of heat in the body that burns excess calories. Increasing your level of thermogenesis will not only raise your metabolic rate, but also will help in weight management. In this regard, there are some harmful herbs to avoid and some that will be helpful. If you have not checked out the health of your heart and thyroid, you shouldn't be taking herbs and supplements to increase your thermogenesis.

Some of the harmful products to avoid include caffeine in any form, including products containing the currently popular green tea additive. Gurana is also a compound closely related to caffeine and just as harmful. Ma huang, also called ephedra, should also be avoided. This is the herb that was just investigated by the FDA for the deaths of several teens at the RAVE parties. Products that are safe for increasing weight loss through thermogenesis include cayenne, malabar black pepper, ginger root, turmeric, licorice root, Vitamin B_6 and chromium.

> *We expect fruits such as bananas and oranges all year round. Many of the more exotic fruits are bought because they are on the shelf in front of us, transported thousands of miles out of season for us to eat. They are likely to have been treated with pesticides and chemicals to keep them fresher for longer. If you don't buy fruits and vegetables until they are in season, you will enjoy a better diet, too. Every item of food that is grown and consumed locally is an important addition to your diet.*
> *—Bernadette Vallely, 1001 Ways to Save the Planet*

CHECKLIST FOR LOW THYROID/LOW METABOLISM

- ❏ Decreased energy
- ❏ Depressed or low moods
- ❏ Cold hands or feet
- ❏ Dry skin
- ❏ Muscle weakness
- ❏ Low sex drive
- ❏ Thinning of head hair
- ❏ Thinning of eyebrow hair
- ❏ Nails grow slowly
- ❏ Joint stiffness in morning
- ❏ Slowed speech
- ❏ Lack of initiative
- ❏ Sleepiness during the day

- ❏ Difficulty losing weight
- ❏ Moody
- ❏ Muscle cramps or pains
- ❏ Constipation
- ❏ PMS
- ❏ Menstrual cramps
- ❏ Sleep with extra blankets
- ❏ Colder than others
- ❏ Weight gain
- ❏ Need coffee to get going
- ❏ Poor memory
- ❏ Missed periods
- ❏ Infertility

(If you checked more than 5, you may have a problem with metabolism.

If you checked more than 10, you probably have a problem.

If you checked more than 15, it is very probable that you do. You should not try to assess this entirely on your own, since you might have other problems as well.)

Learn to lead with one emotion and follow it with another. Don't let the fear lead you. Lead with the courage and follow it with the fear. You don't put down the fear and pick up the courage; you just rearrange their proximity. You don't want to suppress a God-given warning, called fear ... you just don't want it to be your opening gambit ... it's an act of will, and an act of breathing for me; it's making sure that my lower stomach is below my upper stomach, using my breath, and being really aware of the core of my body: the problem with adrenaline, which is good for all sorts of things in the work world, is that it isn't good for stamina. It's a short burst of energy, followed by a drop in the energy, so it's a short-term gain and a long-term loss...

—Anonymous

THE "UNDERARM TEMPERATURE TEST"

This is an easy test to perform on yourself to determine if you might have low metabolism.

1. At night, before retiring, shake down your thermometer and place it within arm's reach.

2. Upon waking (ideally without an alarm clock), place the thermometer so its tip is in your armpit. Hold it in place by placing your upper arm close to your side and, without moving at all, let it stay there for at least 5 minutes.

3. Read it and record the temperature. Indicate on the chart if you moved around, used an alarm clock, or were startled from your sleep.

4. For menstruating women, perform this test on days 1–5 of your period. Day 1 is the first day of your period. For men or non-menstruating women, perform this test anytime for 5 consecutive days.

NOTE: The normal underarm temperature is 97.8° to 98.2°. If you are below this reading, you may have a low thyroid and more testing is needed. You may also test your temperature in the afternoon, in which case the normal temperature is 98.6°.

Month _____ Day 1: _____

Day 2: _____

Day 3: _____

Day 4: _____

Day 5: _____

Month _____ Day 1: _____

Day 2: _____

Day 3: _____

Day 4: _____

Day 5: _____

FOOD FOR THOUGHT: MIND/BODY/SPIRIT NUTRITION AND WEIGHT LOSS

A close friend of mine was so excited by the Zone diet that she threatened to stop talking to me after I told her I felt the Zone diet was basically just another fad diet and not to be taken very seriously. A few years ago that same friend was really turned-on by the "Fit for Life" Diet, and before that it was a "high protein and no carbohydrates diet" and before that the "raw foods diet." I tried explaining to her that there simply is no one diet that's good for everybody, and that each of these "diet fads" is just that—a big fad, which will be forgotten as quickly as it came, and nothing more.

I tried explaining to my friend that I knew she had made a serious study of the human spirit-mind-body connection, and she'd have to agree that there is no single best meditation technique for everyone, no single best type of prayer or spiritual path for everyone, and no single best exercise for everyone's body, but when it came to diet, she failed to see the analogy.

As diets go, the Zone diet is actually the least harmful of the bunch. But it still doesn't allow for bioindividuality, as does my Metabolic Type Diet plan.

To complicate matters even further, there is even a different optimum diet for different seasons, to support us in different activities and that goes with different phases and cycles in our life. Combine this with the fact that many of us are very allergic to dairy products, red meat, wheat, gluten, sugar or other sweets, alcohol, chocolate, tropical fruits, and what you have is the need to create a tailor-made diet for each individual.

If there are diseases in the family such as cancer, diabetes, heart disease, hypoglycemia, fibroids or ovarian cysts, then you also must be aware enough to eliminate specific foods which will predispose you to get these diseases and instead emphasize foods which will strengthen and balance your body so that you won't be prone to illness.

Coming from a background in Chinese medicine as I do, this all makes eminent sense. In Chinese medicine, we talk about the five body types (Fire, Metal, Earth, Water, and Wood) and the specific foods that are best suited for each type (see the Five Element food charts on pages 67 and 68). But for those of us coming from a more Western way of "Black-White" thinking, it makes more sense, and obviously appears much simpler to many of us, to jump on the bandwagon of the latest diet craze for the quick fix solution to your diet and weight woes.

According to the theory of homeopathic medicine, as well as Chinese medical theory, each person craves different foods based on their particular physiologic and metabolic strengths, weaknesses and imbalances. When a person is perfectly in balance they won't crave foods that will weaken them. Instead, they will naturally crave what is good for them.

If your genetic heritage is from an area where meat was eaten, then it's likely you won't do best on the vegetarian or vegan (no animal products) diet. Generally, it best to be sensitive to your genetic heritage and the part of the world you came from.

Some of the latest fad diets, like the Fen-Phen diet are potentially the most harmful and can cause serious damage to the liver and kidneys and even be fatal in some cases. Other products that overstimulate your adrenals or thyroid gland are also potentially very dangerous.

The natural food industry has created some great weight loss and fat-burning products, but you must be very picky and read labels very carefully. Ingredients to stay away from are guarana, ephedra, kota kola, and green tea. Although these products might be safe for some people in small amounts, they all act as stimulants, just like coffee, and in doing so can create major metabolic problems for you if your body doesn't need them.

When I was a gymnast in college, my teammates and I were all very concerned with weight loss, control of fat and how to build muscle mass, so I learned firsthand what was safe and what was not. I was a strict vegetarian and needed a typical athlete's diet, high in complex carbohydrates, like potatoes, breads, rice, beans, pasta, granola, etc. I did great on this diet in college. But after college, as I stopped exercising four hours per day and my metabolism slowed with age, I required the type of diet I grew up on. This consisted of much more yang, or heavy foods, than what I ate in college. As we age, our body also needs different nutrients to stimulate various organs that slow with age and may show an imbalance.

Blood tests and hair analysis are very helpful in determining these types of imbalances, when combined with Chinese Five Element analysis and other body type diagnostic systems. According to Five Element theory, whichever of the elements you are the weakest in is the one you need to eat more foods from. If you have an overly dominant Fire element, for instance, you do not want to eat a lot from that column, but rather, you want to eat more from the Water Element, to extinguish the overactive Fire. If your Earth Element is weak, as demonstrated by an abundant craving for sweets, you want to eat more foods from the Earth Element.

When on a two-week silent meditation retreat, or even on a weekend retreat out in the desert, a vegan diet is the rule of thumb, low in fats and animal products. This lack of animal products will allow you to detoxify and realign with your natural rhythms. But if you try this type of diet while in a high stress job in L.A., most people would quickly get sick.

My advice is to stay away from fad diets and supplements which artificially increase metabolism and instead to concentrate your energetic needs on the physiological, emotional and spiritual levels and the reasons for why you eat what you eat. Developing your intuitive ability to understand food and your intimate relationship to food is one of the single most rewarding disciplines there is. What we allow into our body is a profound statement of the intimate relationship we have with ourselves and the external world. What we choose, consciously or unconsciously, to let into our body—our God-given shrine—speaks clearly to how we feel about ourselves and our world. Changing the way we eat, we automatically and simultaneously change our external world: physiologically, emotionally, spiritually and energetically.

Food for thought: the next time you crave chocolate, try taking a supplement of vitamin B_6, chromium, magnesium and calcium instead, and watch how much more relaxed you feel!

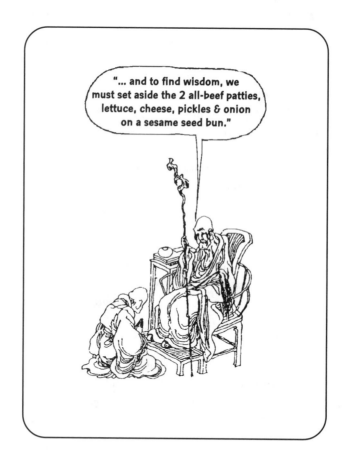

METABOLIC PROFILING: A BREAKTHROUGH IN YOUR NUTRITIONAL HEALTH

Many people are used to eating certain foods separately in their diet. This technique, called food combining, grew in popularity from the book *Diet for a Small Planet*. But now, after popularity with the Zone Diet, we are all realizing it's healthier to combine carbohydrates with your proteins and fats for optimal nutritional value. But how much of each should you eat?

The Zone Diet tells everyone to eat the same proportion of carbohydrates, fats and proteins, but this is not the optimal diet for everyone. Some people are "fast oxidizers," some are "slow oxidizers," and some fall somewhere in between.

The following questionnaire and suggested foods will give you the optimal way for you to eat given your unique metabolism. Different factors come to play when determining your metabolic type. These include your past eating habits, cultural differences, genetic inheritance, and other more subtle influences. You may also be one metabolic type and then change to another type. This is very common during pregnancy, for example.

It's also a good idea to get a blood test to confirm your metabolic type and oxidation levels and to compare these to your blood type. Although there are many different methods of analyzing which type of diet you should eat, I have found this method to be very simple and effective.

This type of eating plan will work to balance your body, if combined with nutritional supplements. If you want to really optimize your health, you can also refer to the Oriental medicine section earlier in this book, and match the foods for your particular body type according to Chinese medicine with the foods recommended there.

For most people, following the suggestions given below for your particular type and taking the recommended supplements based on your blood tests will bring you a renewed sense of health, vitality and well-being.

Some people need to do a detoxification diet before beginning this program. If you suspect you might have toxicity in the liver, kidney or lungs, then consult your health practitioner. I do not suggest that you undertake a detoxification diet without an exam and testing by your health practitioner first. In general, one shouldn't undergo any type of detoxification unless they are taking a week or two off of work and are being supervised by their health practitioner. If you are under stress, never do a detox diet. The best time to do a detox is in the fall and spring seasons, not during the summer or winter.

On the following list of characteristics, please circle the ones that most closely match you. They don't have to be perfect matches. If none of the options apply to you, then don't circle any.

Characteristic	Column 1	Column 2	Column 3
Aging	Look older than others my age	Look younger than others my age	N/A
Emotional	Loner	Very outgoing	N/A
Appetite	Small	Strong	Average
Chest Pressure	N/A	Pressure in chest	N/A
Weather	Love hot	Love cold	Doesn't matter
Cold Sores	N/A	Frequent	N/A
Coughing	N/A	Coughs daily	N/A
Skin	N/A	Frequent cracked skin	N/A
Dandruff	N/A	Frequent	N/A
Dessert	Love sweets	Prefers salty/fatty	Not particular
Digestion	Slow, poor	Fast, strong	Average
Eating at Bedtime	Worsens sleep	Improves sleep	Doesn't matter
Feelings	Hard to express	Easy to express	N/A
Eating Habits	Don't think about food much	Need to eat often to feel good	N/A
Feelings	Under control emotionally	Feelings are obvious to others around me	N/A
Eyes	Frequent dry eyes	Frequent tearing eyes	N/A
Face	Pale	Rosy, flushed	N/A
Fats	Don't like them	Love them	Take or leave it
Fats, reactions	Lowers energy	Increases energy	Average reaction
Fingernails	Thick, hard	Thin, soft	N/A
Time Between Meals	Doesn't matter	Irritable, weak, depressed if don't eat often	Feel normal
Skin	Goosebumps easily	N/A	N/A
Gums	Light, pale	Dark, pink	N/A
Hunger	Rarely get hunger pangs	Often hungry	N/A
Insect Bites	Weak reaction	Strong reaction	N/A
Itching Eyes	N/A	Tend to get	N/A
Itching Skin	N/A	Tend to get	N/A
Fasting	Can handle well	Feel terrible	N/A

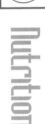

Characteristic	Column 1	Column 2	Column 3
Meal Portions	Prefer small	Prefer large	Average
Orange Juice Alone	Energizes	Bad reaction	No ill effects
Potatoes	Dislike them	Love them	Take or leave
Red Meat	Decreases energy	Increases energy	Average reaction
Saliva Amount	Dry mouth	Excessive saliva	Normal
Saliva Texture	Thick, ropy	Thin, watery	N/A
Salty Food	Dislike	Love salt	Average like
Skin Healing	Heal slowly	Heal quickly	Average
Skin Moisture	Dry	Oily or moist	Average
Skip Meals	No problem	Must eat regularly	N/A
Snacking	Rarely want them	Always snacking	N/A
Sneezing	N/A	Often and daily	N/A
Sour Foods	Dislikes them	Really like them	Sometimes like
Sweets	Agrees with me	Tastes too sweet	No effect either way
Vegetarian Meal	Is satisfying	Unsatisfying	OK either way
Wheezing	N/A	Tend to get	N/A
Meat for Breakfast	Gets tired, sleepy	Feels energetic	No reaction at all
Meat for Lunch	Feels tired after	Feels great after	No preference
If I Feel Low Energy, I Like	Fruit, pastry, candy	Meat, fats, salty	No preference
Social Setting	Introverted, shy	Extroverted, social	N/A

TOTALS   _____   _____   _____

Great. That was easy!!!

Now, add up the totals for each of the three columns.

If Column 1 and 2 are tied, or have less than 5 points difference, use profile 3.

If Column 1 and 3 are tied, or have less than 5 points difference, use profile 1.

If Column 2 and 3 are tied, or have less than 5 points difference, use profile 2.

If all 3 columns are tied or have scores with 5 points or less difference, use profile 3.

> *The most incredible thing in our world is that everybody is treated the same. In fact, not everybody is created equal.*
>
> —*Leon Hammer, M.D.*

Not only are the kinds of foods important, but also the ratio of proteins to carbohydrates are important. Think of this as your fuel mix for the engine of your metabolism. The right fuel mix will provide you with the optimum energy you need. The wrong fuel mix will result in lowered energy and fatigue.

Proteins = meat, fowl, fish, tofu, beans, legumes

Carbohydrates = fruits, vegetables, grains

Fats = butter, oils, fatty foods, seeds, cheese

Blood Type O

Dairy and grains should be eaten sparingly.

Vary your grains.

Usually Blood Type O is also the faster metabolic type, or Type 2, requiring more protein.

Try to stay away from gluten containing foods: wheat, rye, oats, barley.

Read labels for grains which may contain gluten.

Good fish are dark meat such as shark, salmon, etc.

Good meats are beef, venison, and lamb.

For vegetarian sources of protein, should eat plenty of beans, peas and lentils.

Blood Type A

Usually Blood Type A is the slower metabolic type, or Type 1, requiring less protein.

This type usually needs digestive enzymes. Consult your doctor for the enzyme best for you.

Beans can also be a bit of a problem for this type.

Focus mainly on grains, fruits, seeds and eggs.

This type can do well on the vegetarian diet, if this appeals to you.

This type may have an allergy to wheat.

Stick mainly to rice, millet, buckwheat, kamut, spelt, and quinoa and stay away from gluten.

Stay away from lima beans.

Blood Type B

This is a combination of the other types and usually corresponds to Type 3 profiles.

Moderation is the key for Type B.

You can handle a bit of everything, but should not go overboard with anything.

Stay away from chicken, buckwheat, sesame, and sunflower seeds.

Blood Type AB

These types are the most rare of all the types.

They are less than 4% of the American population.

You fall between the A and the B types.

Some of you will do well with vegetarian diets and others will need a broader range of foods.

Don't emphasize animal protein, but use vegetarian protein in larger amounts.

Finally, pay attention to what your body is asking for. Do you feel best after a huge plate of pasta, or after a piece of fish and vegetables? What gives you more energy, a steak or split pea soup? Ultimately, only you can decide on the ratio of foods that works best for your particular type.

One day you might be better on a light diet and the next on a heavier diet. Look at your background. Is your mother Italian and your father from Norway? Then you may need to mix your diet between carbohydrates and heavy protein. It takes many generations to evolve out from your genetic predisposition.

If your family ate a lot of animal protein for generations, then you probably won't do well on a macrobiotic diet. On the other hand, if your family is from Mexico and ate rice and beans for generations, then you won't do too well on steak.

Profile #1 Recommended Foods

Meat/Fowl/Fish/Legumes: chicken breast, turkey breast, eggs, cod, flounder, haddock, perch, scrod, sole, white tuna, turbot, peas, split peas, tofu products

Vegetables: bean sprouts, beets, broccoli, Brussels sprouts, cabbage, carrot, celery, cucumber, eggplant, garlic, horseradish, kale, leek, lettuce, mustard greens, onion, peppers, potato, scallion, spaghetti squash, sweet potato, tomato, yam, zucchini

Fruit: apple, apricot, berries, cherry, grape, grapefruit, lemon, lime, melon, orange, peach, pear, pineapple, plum, tangerine

Dairy: low fat only, goat cheese, tofu cheese, tofu yogurt, regular yogurt

Seeds: none

Grains: all are OK

Oils/Fats: minimize

Dessert: minimize and low fat only

Beverage: Fruit juice, vegetable juice

Miscellaneous: chicken broth, horseradish, hot sauce, catsup, mustard, tomato sauce or soup, cayenne, any spicy foods are fine

Using the recommended foods listed above, try to eat according to the following proportions (by volume):

20% Protein

70% Carbohydrate

10% Oils and Natural Fats

Profile #2 Recommended Foods

Meat/Fowl/Fish/Legumes: beef, brains, duck, goose, kidney, organ meats, lamb, liver, fowl drumsticks, fowl thigh, fowl wing, red meat, veal, venison, buffalo, heart, abalone, caviar, herring, mackerel, octopus, salmon, sardine, anchovy, squid, dark tuna, kidney beans, aduki beans, black beans, black eyed peas, lentils, lima beans

Vegetables: artichoke, asparagus, all types of beans, few carrots (cooked), cauliflower, celery (few), corn, lentil, mushroom, peas, some potato, spinach, squash

Fruit: avocado, banana, olive, some apple, some pear

Dairy: goat cheese, eggs, goat and soy milk, yogurt

Seeds: sunflower and pumpkin only

Grain: all OK

Fats/Oils: all OK

Dessert: butter-based pastries are good

Beverage: dilute fruit juices only; stay away from sweet beverages, vegetable juice

Miscellaneous: cream soups, sauces, gravies, meat stock, salt, miso, soy sauce, tamari, yeast

Using the recommended foods listed above, try to eat according to the following proportions (by volume):

50% Protein

30% Carbohydrate

20% Oils and Natural Fats

Profile #3 Recommended Foods:

All OK. Eat as much variety as possible from day to day.

Using the recommended foods listed above, try to eat according to the following proportions (by volume):

40% Protein

50% Carbohydrate

10% Oils and Natural Fats

For all types always think in terms of proportions on your plate. No matter how much food is on your plate, your food should be eaten in these proportions. You don't have to be exact, nor do I expect perfection. This is only the goal to strive for.

RAW/COOKED FOODS: QUESTIONS AND ANSWERS

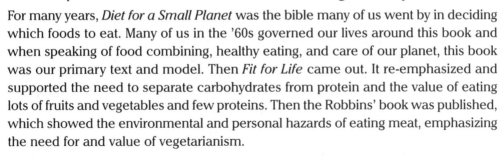

What do you think about the Zone Diet and eating a lot of protein?

For many years, *Diet for a Small Planet* was the bible many of us went by in deciding which foods to eat. Many of us in the '60s governed our lives around this book and when speaking of food combining, healthy eating, and care of our planet, this book was our primary text and model. Then *Fit for Life* came out. It re-emphasized and supported the need to separate carbohydrates from protein and the value of eating lots of fruits and vegetables and few proteins. Then the Robbins' book was published, which showed the environmental and personal hazards of eating meat, emphasizing the need for and value of vegetarianism.

Now the Zone Diet Plan is telling us the total opposite of these three "experts." The Zone is saying that because of the chemical structure of the food itself, when it interacts on a chemical level in our body, that we need to eat protein **with** carbohydrates, in order to utilize the food's potential for producing high level energy in the body.

What is the best form of usable protein?

According to the Zone Diet, the best protein comes from the demonized "dead animal parts" we were told we shouldn't eat, didn't really need, and whose production was destructive to the environment.

My experience with many patients, over a long period of time, confirms that the Zone Diet is a much more effective diet than the older, more archaic, outlook. My patients on modified Zone diet plans are experiencing much more energy then they ever have before, a reduction in chronic fatigue, less joint pains, more sex drive, less headaches and significantly better weight loss by following this modified Zone diet plan.

It seems that eggs, whey, animal protein and dairy are the most effective forms of protein and the most assimilable. I base this on my clinical experience over a 17-year period and on repeated patient blood tests where we check various indices in the blood that are reliable indicators of protein malnutrition and overall protein assimilation in the body.

What percentage of carbohydrates and proteins do I need to eat?

This differs with everyone. Some of my patients only need a little protein, and others need a lot. The important thing is to be open-minded enough to experiment on yourself. I even had one patient try a raw meat diet and found that for him, this was this best thing to do. Weird but true!

What diet do you advocate in your practice, based on your 17 years of experience in the health care field?

I personally have tried every diet there is. I was a vegan for 12 years, did a raw foods diet for years, grew up on the typical American fast food diet, got through college on candy bars and vegie burgers. I've fasted, binged, cleansed, juiced, osterized, souped, and been fairly honest with a macrobiotic diet. I'm telling you, I've done it all. What

I've found is that there is no one single diet, either cooked or raw, that is good for all people all the time. Different people need different diets for different times during their life. This is based on their individual needs and stress levels.

Are there any people who you would suggest eat a raw foods diet?

Yes, most definitely. People who have a strong Earth Element (in Five Element terminology), a good, strong, solid Yin element with an excess of Yang (Fire Element), and who have high liver enzymes on their blood chemistry panel. Also, people who have eaten meat all their lives and need to detoxify. Lastly, there are those people who have a lot of food or environmental allergies and some of these people, if their digestive tract is strong, will do very well on a raw food diet.

When on a two week silent meditation retreat or even on a weekend retreat out in the desert, a vegan or raw foods diet is the rule of thumb, low in fats and animal products. This lack of animal products will allow you to detoxify and realign with your natural rhythms. But if you try this type of diet while in a high stress job in L.A., most people would quickly get sick.

Which types of people do poorly on a raw foods diet?

People who have a history of an eating disorder, either anorexia, bulimia, chronic fasting or dieting or compulsive overeating will do very poorly on a raw foods diet plan. These people all have weak digestive tracts from years of poor eating habits and abuse of their systems, and cannot assimilate the necessary enzymes and proteins from raw foods. Also, any person who has an addictive nature and who tries to lose weight by dieting does poorly on the raw foods diet. They plug into the diet initially through their addictive personality trait, and then just yo-yo back to their old pattern. The yo-yo effect is worse than not having done anything at all.

What's wrong with using a raw foods diet for weight loss?

People who use a temporary fix or specific diet plan to lose weight are setting themselves up for failure. I have never seen a patient or friend who successfully dieted without later gaining the weight back. As the 12-Step Program of Overeaters Anonymous advises, you must develop *your relationship* with food and eat the way you need for your health and not just to lose the weight. There are very few body types who can eat a raw foods diet exclusively and sustain their energy over the long term, especially if they are living and working in a fast-paced world, such as Los Angeles.

If on a retreat or living in the desert or mountains in a retreat or slow-paced environment, it's an entirely different matter. For this reason, it's better to not fluctuate from one diet to another. One would be better off to learn to eat right for your type. This will eventually provide you with the weight loss you desire and keep it off permanently. I have seen this with many of my patients.

What should I do if I have allergies and I can't eat animal protein?

Many of us are very allergic to dairy products, red meat, wheat, gluten, sugar or other sweets, alcohol, chocolate, tropical fruits, and potatoes. Many people are allergic to almost everything and can eat only a very limited diet. What you have is the need to create a tailor-made diet for each individual. I recommend food allergy testing, and checking for exactly which foods you are allergic to.

After allergy testing, you can eliminate the foods that give you the most problems for about two months. The second step is to strengthen your digestion and immune system so that you won't have to live with the allergies any more. If you have very weak digestion, with a lot of gas, bloating or heartburn, it may take up to two years to permanently strengthen your system, but after that time, you will be able to eat whatever you want to.

What if I also have candida?

If you have *Candida albicans*, a yeast that grows in the gut, this will further weaken the digestion. I recommend we test for parasites and all types of yeasts right from the start of each client's treatment program. We can kill the yeast by using very strong yeast-fighting herbs and also supplementing with probiotics, such as L. bifidus and L. acidophilus.

What does homeopathic medicine have to say about raw vs. cooked foods?

Most Classical homeopaths won't even discuss nutrition or diet with their clients, knowing that the most important thing is to bring the body-mind-spirit into balance so that they will automatically crave what's best for their unique body type.

Homeopathic theory is based on the premise that the body-mind-spirit innately knows what's best and all you need to do is give it a little push in the right direction and we will heal ourselves. I've seen this occur hundreds of times with my patients. A prime example is a woman who had an insatiable craving for chocolate. After being given a constitutional homeopathic remedy, the craving disappeared. She's more able to give and receive love in her marriage and she craves exercise instead! Honestly! I see this happen over and over again.

Another example is a gentleman who drank 20 cups of coffee a day and after six months of homeopathic treatment, he walked into my office and proclaimed he suddenly disliked the taste of coffee! A few months latter, he also gave up eating sugar and sweets and developed a distaste for them.

Why can't I just follow my own intuition?

My experience is that if we quiet ourselves enough to listen, the spirit-mind-body and its innate inner wisdom knows exactly what it wants and needs. There is usually a dominant, "bully" voice that tries to convince us we need sugar, fries, etc., and another "still, small voice within" that knows what we really need.

One great exercise is to get quiet and give the food you crave a voice. Sit with your journal and see what comes up. Talk to the food. Ask the food what it wants from you to be your friend and ally. Keeping a food journal like this is very helpful to getting your body into balance.

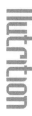

What about my parents and grandparents? Does what they ate matter?

If your genetic heritage is from an area where meat was eaten, then it's likely you won't do best on the vegetarian or vegan (no animal products) diet. Generally, it best to be sensitive to your genetic heritage and the part of the world you came from.

What's the very best way to lose weight?

Weight loss is fairly easy for most people when they take some simple, basic tests to learn what their body really needs. When combined with a moderate but daily exercise program, relaxation and stress reduction, emotional awareness techniques and simple behavioral suggestions, a sound nutritional program geared to your metabolic type is the best, safest and most effect way to lose weight, increase energy, boost stamina, increase your immunity and lift your emotional spirits.

Does my body require different foods as I age?

When I was a gymnast in college, my teammates and I were all very concerned with weight loss, control of fat and how to build muscle mass, so I learned firsthand what was safe and what was not. I was a strict vegetarian and needed a typical athlete's diet, high in complex carbohydrates, potatoes, breads, rice, beans, pasta, granola, etc. I did great on this diet in college.

But after college, as I stopped exercising four hours per day and my metabolism slowed with age, I required the type of diet I grew up on. This consisted of much more Yang, or heavy foods, than what I ate in college. As we age, our body also needs different nutrients to stimulate various organs that slow with age and may show an imbalance.

How should I eat when my body is very stressed out?

When stressed out and working hard, eating eggs, fish, turkey and buffalo burgers may provide the high quality, low fat protein necessary to keep blood sugar stable and energy high. On the other hand, many people, depending on their metabolic type and needs, do best on the vegetarian version of a high protein diet and need to eat concentrated rice- or soy-based protein powders and lots tempeh and beans at every meal.

What about macrobiotics?

Macrobiotics is based on the same Chinese Five Element and Yin-Yang theory that I believe is an effective body-type system. The only problem is that most people will not stick to their prescribed macrobiotic diet. If you can stick to the macrobiotic diet, in most cases you will eventually balance yourself out. But my experience is that you can accomplish the same goals more easily by just introducing more protein into the diet. You need to discuss these options with your health care practitioner and choose the nutritional program that will work best for you and your body type.

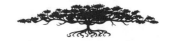

HOLISTIC WEIGHT LOSS PROGRAM

By now you may have tried many weight loss diets. Some have worked and some may not have. The difference with my philosophy towards weight loss is that it is holistic. Holistic in this sense means body, mind and spirit.

For an effective weight loss program it is important to recognize biological individuality and the use of natural means to strengthen and rebuild weak organs and glands in the body. Treatment can include acupuncture, herbal medicine, nutritional counseling, psychological counseling, and exercise.

For many of you, losing weight means simply getting rid of that extra five pounds in order to fit into the latest fashions. But for others, it is more a matter of health and good nutrition.

For everyone, the question arises: "Which diet is best for me?" Perhaps you have already tried vegetarianism, macrobiotics, the all-liquid protein diet, or an all-fruit fast. And perhaps you have wondered why your best friend is able to lose weight eating pastries and pasta, while you have only to "look at" sweets to gain an extra five pounds.

Have you noticed that not everyone craves the same foods? Have you considered the possibility that you have food allergies? Or have you wondered why weight loss has not miraculously occurred by diligently sticking to a low-caloric or low-carbohydrate diet? The truth is that not all people lose weight on the same diet. In other words, everyone needs a diet based on his or her own individual physiological and biological strengths and weaknesses.

Scientists have discovered that different people have specific weaknesses in different glands in their body. These biological differences are partly inherited and partly created through lifestyle and eating habits, and these differences account for two important factors in weight loss.

First, individual biological weaknesses are the cause for what foods we each individually crave. And second, these differences also account for what part of our body tends to accumulate extra pounds.

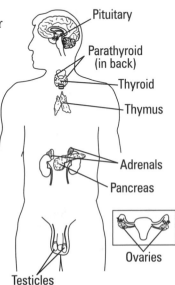

Doctors have shown that people with a weak pituitary gland, for example, tend to crave dairy products rather than sweets, and that they will more often than not accumulate "baby fat" all over their body. In contrast, people with a weak thyroid will crave sugar, caffeine and carbohydrates and gain weight mostly in the stomach, upper arms and thighs. People with weak adrenal glands crave salt, meat, potatoes and butter and tend to be stocky with big bones and a potbelly. These types of people are usually very Yang. The type of person with an imbalance in their ovaries may crave fats and spicy foods and gain most of their weight around the hips and thighs. To reverse these cravings and the accompanying weight gains, we must reverse the genetic imbalances and weaknesses.

Oriental medicine has identified these biological individualities and has a long history of effectively treating people in accordance with their differences. According to the Oriental theory of health, when our chi becomes blocked or depleted, sometimes in a particular area of the body, we experience ill health or disease. Herbs and acupuncture work to unblock the stagnant chi and allow the return of free-flowing chi, thereby allowing the body to achieve a healthy equilibrium.

The specific effect that acupuncture has on weight loss is twofold: First, it acts to relax the nervous system and lessen the anxiety and compulsiveness associated with overeating. This is accomplished by stimulation of specific acupuncture points in the ears and on the body which cause the release of endorphins, the body's own naturally-occurring opiates or relaxers. Second, acupuncture also stimulates the weak organs and glands, working to decrease the food cravings that are so hard to control. In terms of the Five Element Theory of Oriental medicine, long-term obesity or weight problems are usually a sign of weakness in the Earth or Fire Elements.

Here are seven factors that make up an effective weight loss program:

1. *A food journal*—Write down all the food you eat. Include times, day, foods, reasons, feelings, emotional and physical after-effects.

2. *Identify problems*—Foods (allergies, addictions, cravings, and aversions), situations (restaurants, social situations, etc.), time of day (biological clock).

3. *Develop strategies* to cope with Number 2.

4. *Assess your weak glands and organs*—Correct through use of nutritional supplements, acupuncture, and homeopathy.

5. *Use specific weight-loss herbal formulas* to boost metabolism, strengthen weak glands and organs in the body, work on weak energy meridians and elements, and balance the nervous system and digestive organs of assimilation.

6. *Typical acupuncture treatment schedule*—Twice a week for the first four weeks, followed by once a week for the next four weeks, followed by twice a month for the next two months, followed by once a month for the remaining time on the program, followed by periodic maintenance, usually four times a year.

7. *Exercise*—Some type of aerobic exercise will be determined with your doctor. This is important because it increases the heartbeat and burns up calories. You should exercise aerobically at least three times a week. On the other days of the week you should walk and do some simple stretching or yoga-type exercises.

There is much more to the effective loss of weight besides behavioral or physiological approaches, including emotional issues. For people serious about a holistic approach to weight loss, a thorough examination of one's reasons for overeating and the motivations for wanting to lose weight is essential. Often, overeating or undereating are old protection and defense mechanisms being revived by current stresses and emotional hurts.

In our culture, there's an overemphasis on the virtues of slenderness. *Anorexia Nervosa* (self-imposed starvation) and *Bulimia* (the binge-purge syndrome) occur in alarming proportions. In fact, many people are actually healthier—emotionally and physically—at a weight that is five to ten pounds heavier than what our popular media presents as the ideal.

On the other hand, some people are honestly confused and do not know what their optimum weight really is. For many, short-term psychological counseling may work well in conjunction with a weight loss program. Therapy helps to help clarify weight loss goals and to provide emotional support for changes in eating and exercising habits. Therapy also helps to adjust to what can be a personally and socially threatening change of self-image.

For others, the program of Overeaters Anonymous (OA) has proven very effective in providing support and helping people adjust to the psychological and social aspects of weight loss.

One very common reason that many people fail to lose weight is that they have extremes in blood sugar fluctuations. Chronic low blood sugar is called hypoglycemia and these swings in blood sugar will defeat any rational attempt at losing weight. If you study the "Dysglycemia Table" on the next page and notice you have a large number of these symptoms, then you are in danger of failure at your weight loss program. Dramatic swings up and down in blood sugar levels are called *dysglycemia*. Please study the Glycemic Index of foods (page 155) and eat the foods with the lowest glycemic index. This way, your foods will take longer to digest and not be as likely to create dramatic swings or cravings.

Weight loss *is* possible even for those who have experienced past failures. Identifying the causes of past failures, either psychological or physiological, is the first step toward insuring greater success in the future. With an honest desire to change old behaviors, weight loss can be achieved and the road to optimum health can be yours!

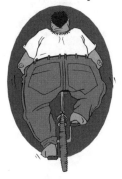

Dysglycemia: A state where blood glucose levels fluctuate sometimes radically, from a hyper- to hypoglycemic state.

Functional Symptoms:

- Allergies
- Anxiety
- Worrying
- Sweet Cravings
- Carbohydrate sensitivity
- Constant hunger
- Crying spells
- Depression
- Dizziness
- Exhaustion
- Fatigue
- Indecision

- Inner Trembling
- Insomnia
- Irritability
- Lack of Concentration
- Mental Confusion
- Nervousness
- Nightmares
- Paranoia
- Phobias
- Sinus Problems
- Weight Gain

Key Organs: Adrenals, Pancreas, and Liver

Affects: Thyroid, Ovary, Kidney, Pituitary and Brain

Wow! Now I know why nothing I tried worked! It wasn't MY fault that I craved the wrong foods—but now I understand what's going on & can do something about it! How exciting!

GLYCEMIC INDICES OF FOODS

Food	Glycemic Index	Food	Glycemic Index
Breads		**Legumes**	
Rye (Crispbread)	95	Baked Beans (canned)	70
Rye (Wholemeal)	89	Bengal gram dal	12
Rye (Whole grain)	68	Butter Beans	46
Wheat (White)	100	Chickpeas (dried)	47
Wheat (Wholemeal)	100	Chick Peas (canned)	60
Pasta		Green Peas (canned)	50
Macaroni (White, boiled 5 min.)	64	Green Peas (dried)	65
Spaghetti (brown, boiled 15 min)	61	Green Peas (frozen)	65
Spaghetti (white, boiled 15 min)	67	Haricot beans (white, dried)	54
Star pasta (white, boiled 5 min)	54	Kidney beans (dried)	43
Cereal Grains		Kidney beans (canned)	74
Barley (pearled)	36	Lentils (green, dried)	36
Buckwheat	78	Lentils (green, canned)	74
Bulgur	65	Lentils (red, dried)	38
Millet	103	Pinto beans (dried)	80
Rice (brown)	81	Pinto beans (canned)	64
Rice (instant, boiled 1 min.)	65	Peanuts	15
Rice (polished, boiled 5 min.)	58	Soya beans (dried)	20
Rice (polished, boiled 10-25)	81	Soya beans (canned)	22
Rice (parboiled, boiled 5 min.)	54	Frozen Peas	74
Rice (parboiled, boiled 15 min.)	68	**Fruit**	
Rye kernels	47	Apple (green is best)	52
Sweet Corn	80	Banana	84
Wheat Kernels	63	Orange	59
Breakfast Cereals		Orange Juice	71
"All Bran"	74	Grapes	62
Cornflakes	121	Raisins	93
Muesli	96	Pear	47
Porridge oats	89	Peach	40
Puffed rice	132	Grapefruit	38
Puffed wheat	110	Plum	34
Shredded wheat	97	**Sugars**	
"Weetebix"	108	Fructose	26
Cookies		Glucose	138
Digestive	82	Honey	126
Oatmeal	78	Lactose	57
"Rich Tea"	80	Maltose	152
Plain crackers (water biscuits)	100	Sucrose	83
Shortbread cookies	88	**Dairy Products**	
Root Vegetables		Custard	59
Potato (instant)	120	Ice Cream	69
Potato (mashed)	98	Skim milk	46
Potato (new/white, boiled)	80	Whole milk	44
Potato (russet, baked)	118	Yogurt	52
Potato (sweet)	70		

HYPOGLYCEMIC WEIGHT LOSS PLAN

There are many symptoms of *hypoglycemia* or low blood sugar. The most common ones are headaches, light-headedness, sugar cravings, weakness, and fatigue. Blood tests can be used to determine if a person is hypoglycemic.

Before you start: basic rules

❁ *Decide* before you begin each meal or snack exactly what you will eat. If you finish your meal and think you still need more food, substitute an activity instead. Substitute activities may include walking, talking on the telephone, writing in your journal, washing the dishes, doing homework, studying, reading, meditating, yoga, etc. Usually the craving will diminish after 10 to 20 minutes of activity. It takes the food you ate that long to reach the bloodstream and turn into blood sugar. If you *still* need to eat, write in your journal about how you are feeling. Try to get in touch with your emotions (i.e., guilt, anger, jealousy, resentment, lust, greed, etc.).

❁ *Rotate* all foods, including snacks, on a three- to four-day rotation. People with no known food allergies can count different strains of the same food as different foods (i.e. rice cakes made by different companies; short vs. long grain brown rice, etc.). For people who have a history of food allergies, a more strict rotation should be observed and the same food should not be eaten more often than every three to four days, but foods from the same food families may be eaten during the intervening time. For example, if you have been allergic to chicken, do not eat chicken more often than every three to four days, but you could eat turkey, duck, squab, or quail on the intervening days.

❁ *Eat* in a relaxed manner. Breathe fully while eating and try to chew each mouthful so that it is a paste by the time it is swallowed. If you rush while eating, the food will not assimilate and thus it does little good to eat it. Relax for at least five to ten minutes after eating before getting up to do anything.

❁ *Refrain* from fats, or salty or sweet foods as much as possible. Even artificial sweeteners are bad for your body; they fool the pancreas into excreting more insulin, thus driving the blood sugar even lower.

❁ *Think* of food as medicine. You would not think of taking either too much or too little medicine. So decide on your snacks and meals, and stick to your plan!

Fruits may be too sweet at first. Half a piece may be all your pancreas can handle for the time being, until your body gets stronger.

❁ *Cook* on Sunday for the whole week ahead. Cook one to two small pots of whole grains (millet, buckwheat, oats, amaranth, wheat berries, rice, corn grits, barley, etc.) and two or three portions of steamed vegetables. Each morning place snack- or meal-sized amounts in plastic containers for that day's snacks or meals. Add some raw carrots, celery, cauliflower, broccoli, jicama, avocado, or Jerusalem artichokes. Pack some rice cakes and your favorite health food cookies or cakes.

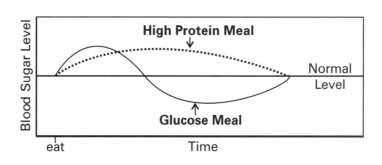

If you primarily eat in restaurants, plan your day ahead of time based on which restaurants you will be near. Decide what you will eat in each restaurant before you go in. If you are on the run and have no time to stop at a restaurant, stop at a market or minimart and pick up a tuna sandwich, banana, or other relatively healthy snack. There are no excuses for junk food any more. Even most fast food restaurants have healthy, low-, or no-fat alternatives.

When dining in a restaurant, eat half of your entree and save the rest in a doggie bag for your between-meal snack. Ask for salad dressing or sauces on the side and use them sparingly. Don't eat dessert. Instead, bring a whole grain/juice-sweetened dessert from the health food store and eat it as a between-meal snack. If you crave sweets, have a green apple an hour after your meal, or drink a cup of Ponay tea, licorice tea, or lemon juice with hot water.

❀ *Refrain* from stimulants at all costs! This includes caffeine in any form, drugs, all alcohol, and nicotine. They will only drive your blood sugar crazy and confuse your adrenal glands. In the end, they will weaken your endocrine system, making it harder to lose weight and stick to your diet plan.

❀ *Do* breathing exercises. Get plenty of outdoor exercise to oxygenate your blood cells. Sometimes exercise and breathing exercises will trick your body into making you feel full and satisfied. In this way you may be able to forgo a normally scheduled snack.

It's okay to not be perfect. A "perfect" diet will never last anyway. Progress is the goal, not perfection. Although progress can at times be slow, you need to be soft and supportive to yourself. Allow yourself the flexibility to make mistakes. Have the perseverance to bounce back and keep trying.

❀ *Keep* a record of your mistakes, slips, and what works well for you. That way you can look back in your journal and see the progress you have made, reflect on what is working and what is not.

❀ *Do* a minimum of at least *two* brisk 15- to 20-minute walks per day. A basic component to weight loss and healthy eating is keeping your metabolism running at a healthy level. Walking briskly will boost your thyroid and raise your metabolism.

It is also important for you to do some form of aerobic exercise two to three times per week. Exercise is considered aerobic when your resting pulse is approximately doubled for 10 minutes or more. If you sweat for 20 minutes straight, you are on the right track.

❋ *Drink* licorice tea, Ponay tea, a Chinese "diet" tea, or another good Chinese constitutional tea formula whenever your blood sugar begins to drop. This will keep you energized and stimulate your adrenal glands. In so doing, it will balance your blood sugar and keep you from becoming hypoglycemic.

❋ *Try* to be as honest as possible with yourself. It is also important for you to be honest with your physician about your eating and exercise. Total honesty is, in many ways, the key to the success of this entire program.

Vegetarian Hypoglycemic Weight Loss Plan

Three meals per day, with a snack every two hours.

The snack is always the same and is *not* optional: 1 rice cake plus ½ tempe burger (or a hard-boiled egg, if you eat them). In emergencies, two rice cakes and 1 whole tempe burger are okay if you are about to faint.

Breakfast: A good-sized bowl of whole grain cereal cooked (may add cinnamon for flavor) or granola with soy milk.

Lunch: Salad with cooked vegetables (steamed, with a no-fat sauce) with a whole grain or four rice cakes. For protein, add a tempe burger.

Dinner: Salad, cooked vegetables, and a protein (4 oz. fish or poultry). The only dressings allowed are: mustard, lemon, vinegar, etc. No oil-based dressings.

Total calories should be around 1,000 per day. This diet is *not* meant for long-term dieting; if it is impractical to achieve the desired weight within four weeks, this diet should be alternated with the maintenance plan.

Blood tests need to be performed before this diet and after any significant weight loss.

The Vegetarian Hypoglycemic Maintenance Plan

Here are some good snack foods for the hypoglycemic individual. Other people can use the list for healthy snack ideas as well. It's fine to make these snacks larger to psychologically experience the sensation of having a meal.

✧ 6 oz. of amasake
✧ 2 rice cakes and 6 almonds
✧ ½ rice wrap from the health food store
✧ ½ apple and 4 to 6 almonds
✧ Small can of vegetable juice with a handful of almonds
✧ Carrot and celery sticks with a couple of rice cakes and a 4 oz. piece of tofu
✧ A few slices of tempeh on a rice cake
✧ A few slices of soy cheese on a rice cake

- ✧ 2 cups hot air popcorn with a 4 oz. piece of tempe
- ✧ 2 oz. baked crackers with a 4 oz. piece of tempe
- ✧ Package of Ah Soy or Edensoy milk
- ✧ 1 cup of grain (amaranth, oats, corn, rice, quinoa, barley) with a handful of almonds
- ✧ 1 cup cooked vegetables
- ✧ ¼ cup cooked beans
- ✧ 6 oz. protein drink
- ✧ 2 tofu hot dogs
- ✧ 1 tofu or tempeh burger
- ✧ Hard-boiled egg
- ✧ ½ tuna or egg salad sandwich
- ✧ ½ small can of water-packed tuna
- ✧ Small chicken breast, wing, or leg
- ✧ ½ cup of puffed rice, millet, or corn, and ½ cup of plain yogurt
- ✧ ½ banana and 4 almonds
- ✧ Carrot with 6 almonds
- ✧ ½ carrot and a handful of pea pods
- ✧ 1 cup of lentil or other bean soup
- ✧ Miso cup of soup
- ✧ 2 oz. chicken, fish, or turkey with ½ cup cooked or raw vegetables
- ✧ Homemade muffins made from whole grains, soy milk, rice flour, grated carrots, apple juice, or other fruits or grains. Half a muffin equals a snack.

It is important for an effective weight loss program to include recognition of biological individuality and the use of natural means to strengthen and rebuild those weak organs and glands in the body. Treatment can include acupuncture, herbal medicine, nutritional counseling, psychological counseling, and exercise.

> *The changing female ideal has been documented by calculating "bust-to-waist" and "waist-to-hip" ratios of the measurements of women in popular women's magazines. You get larger ratios in eras that celebrate the big-breasted figure, and a smaller ratios in eras that endorse the boyish shape.*
>
> *Curvy, full-breasted women are in fashion during pro-maternal eras, in which motherhood and domesticity are considered women's most important roles: this was the case in the early 1900s, the 1950s, and, increasingly, today. In contrast, thin, muscular, boyish bodies are in fashion whenever women have entered the work force, specifically the traditionally male occupations: this was the case in the 1920s and again in the late 1960s and 1970s.*
>
> *—Brett Silverstein, Ph.D., and Associates*

SNACK HINTS

1. Make your snacks hard to get at. They should require preparation, like dry popped popcorn, or be hard to eat, like frozen bananas.

2. Try to avoid extremes of intake—neither fasting nor bingeing. They both lead to imbalances and stress your adrenal glands, which only creates further cravings later on. Never skip a meal. Even if you aren't very hungry, eat a snack to keep your blood sugar balanced.

3. Foods that are composed of complex carbohydrates, accompanied by a serving of protein, will decrease food cravings by maintaining blood sugar for longer periods of time.

4. Use snacks to help overcome that famished feeling. Eat animal protein following the guidelines in the section on Metabolic Profiling (page 141). Use your imagination. Take a long walk through the health food store and examine the labels to find interesting snacks.

5. Avoid tea, coffee, alcohol, and tobacco. They will artificially stimulate the adrenal glands and create cravings a few hours later. Also avoid artificially sweetened drinks and foods since they trick your body into thinking it is getting sweets and thereby weaken the associated organs and glands even further, creating even more long-term cravings for sweets.

6. Never use diet pills. They artificially stimulate the adrenal glands, causing exhaustion and poor sleep.

7. Read all labels to determine calories, fat content, sodium content and artificial ingredients.

8. If quantity is a weakness, add bulk such as raw vegetables, long grain rice, sparkling water, a natural soda before dinner, or a bowl of miso soup as an appetizer.

   Try to develop alternative responses to stresses in your life instead of snacking. Take walks, talk on the phone, read, exercise, take a bath, meditate, etc.

9. Try to always have an alternative response to snack eating: walking, talking on the phone, reading, exercise, reading, taking a bath, etc.

REALITY IS THE KEY TO WEIGHT LOSS

Many people trying to lose weight set unrealistic goals for themselves, which sets them up for failure. Other doomed-for-failure eating behaviors are the following:

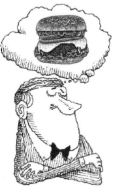

- ✧ Eat only diet and low-calorie foods
- ✧ Tell yourself you will never again be able to eat your favorite foods
- ✧ Always do the exact exercise plan you have decided on and never miss a session
- ✧ Lose the weight quickly
- ✧ Always look for a drop in weight on the scale
- ✧ Never feel threatened by a particular food or situation

These are some of the biggest obstacles to successful weight management, more so than you might expect. The cure is in developing more realistic expectations such as these:

- ✧ Change your focus to how you feel instead of how you look or how much you weigh
- ✧ Determine a logical and reasonable amount of weight to lose slowly
- ✧ Strive for improvement and not perfection
- ✧ Expect mistakes and then learn from them
- ✧ Don't set unreasonable deadlines for reaching your goals
- ✧ Forget about illegal or bad foods; you can decide for yourself which foods are best, but you can eat anything on an occasional basis
- ✧ Exercise in reasonable amounts only and don't be hard on yourself
- ✧ Some exercise is much better than none; modify your exercise to what you can handle on a regular basis.

God says: yes, no, and wait ... all you have to do is learn to listen.
—Cathy in OA

SUPPLEMENTS

Herbs

Ginger Root

Upset stomach, nausea, bloating, gas, cramps, morning sickness—what do all these problems have in common? They can all be cured with the herb Ginger Root. This herb is so versatile, you can't afford *not* to have it in your kitchen.

I keep a stick of ginger root in my freezer and it's precut into one-inch pieces. I can take a piece out and boil it for 20 minutes for ginger tea, or grate it into a vegetable sauté or soup.

It can also be combined with other teas. Boil it for 20 minutes, then turn off the heat and simmer with licorice root (for flavor), chamomile tea (for gas or cramps), or mint tea (for an energy pick-me-up).

NOTE: Never use ginger if you are taking homeopathic remedies.

For nausea or morning sickness, even gingersnaps cookies may help. Something in the ginger has a very calming effect on the stomach. If you can't keep anything at all in your stomach, try sipping ginger root tea.

Ginger is also good for a cold; it will help you increase your perspiration. Make a strong tea and then add this to bath water. This recipe is also good for sore or tired feet. Other symptoms it is used to treat include chest congestion, menstrual cramps, and children's stomach pains.

Buy ginger in the produce department of the supermarket. If you are not going to use it immediately, cut it up into small slices and freeze it. Otherwise it will go bad on you.

Ginseng: The Renowned Rejuvenator

The Chinese have been using ginseng for nearly 5,000 years. Here in the U.S. it's reputed to be a curative for impotency, low energy, failing eyesight, and just about every other problem you might have. Is it true? Is ginseng really the elixir it's cracked up to be?

Ginseng is a root, and an extremely yang root, according to Chinese medicine. It grows all over the world, but the best is said to be Korean White Ginseng. Americans also grow ginseng, and the wild version is thought to be more potent than the cultivated variety.

The ginseng root can be chewed. It can also be purchased as an extract and made into tea. It comes in a granulated tea form and in capsules. It is a great refresher for anyone with low energy, plus it strengthens weak digestion, weak adrenal glands, and the spleen. It's also used for anemia, cold hands and feet, hypoglycemia, insomnia, low blood pressure, and impotence.

Because ginseng is a very yang herb, it is good for people who are very yin. It isn't a good herb for people who have high blood pressure, high energy, those who are very strong, or those with a good sexual appetite. People built like Mary Lou Retton or a football player don't need ginseng. I rarely use it for women, as their constitutions are meant to be more yin than men's.

It is important not to take too much ginseng, because it can overstimulate the central nervous system. If you begin to use it too frequently, it will begin to weaken the body and create a dependence and long-term imbalance. In moderation, it can cure a cough, a cold, asthma, fever, lessen the effects of menopause, hay fever, sinus attacks, or glandular swelling.

A good ginseng tea is made by taking 3 cups of water and 1 shredded teaspoon each of ginseng, licorice root, and ginger. Boil for 15 minutes, steep until cool, strain, and drink.

The most innovative idea I have heard is to use it as the Chinese do—add the root to chicken soup!

Amino Acids

When a person eats enough protein and digests and assimilates that protein, they are well on their way to Optimal Health. But many people have a problem of breaking down protein into a form usable by the body where it can be used in specific metabolic pathways and to build enzymes.

Proteins in the body and the brain are formed from amino acids and the body builds over 50,000 proteins and over 15,000 known enzymes from amino acids. All enzymes, including digestive enzymes are made from amino acids, sometimes with vitamins acting as catalysts to help you utilize the amino acids.

Without amino acids, vitamins and minerals, we often become irritable, depressed, forgetful, fatigued or unmotivated. Amino acids are the basic building blocks of the foods we eat. Although vitamins and minerals are very important to life and nutrition, amino acids are the nutrients that go to make up all protein in the body.

The body cannot store amino acids for long periods of time. They must be constantly supplied in the form of foods we eat or supplements we take. There are 22 amino acids found in nature, and nine of these are essential. These nine must be supplied daily through our diet or by supplementation. Some of the most obvious functions of the amino acids are to build hair, skin, nails, hormones, muscles, and blood.

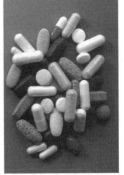

The most popular amino acid is *tryptophan*, which is used in treating insomnia. The FDA still has this one pulled from the shelves for supposed toxicity. Write your Congressman to get it back on the shelves.

The next most popular amino acid is *phenylalanine*. This is used to control pain. It works especially well with acupuncture treatments to release endorphins, the body's own naturally occurring pain relievers. DL-phenylalanine suppresses the appetite and can be used to treat addictions to sugar, compulsive overeating, and drug or alcohol dependencies.

Many psychiatrists at the forefront of pharmacology are now using certain amino acids to control depression, anxiety, and mood-related fatigue. *L-tyrosine* is an amino acid that converts to your body's own natural antidepressant, norepinephrine.

Other common uses of amino acids, when taken in various combinations that range from 8 to 15 different amino acids per formula, include treating hypoglycemia, PMS, and herpes; building muscle mass and the immune system; improving memory; and helping to sustain energy and improve athletic performance.

When taking amino acids, it is important to follow three rules. Always take the amino acids with vitamin B_6 (20 mg of pyridoxal-5-phosphate, a coenzymatic vitamin B_6 preparation). Take them in capsule form instead of tablets—they are more easily assimilated. Use the most expensive amino acids you can find. The quality of amino acids varies tremendously, and the more expensive ones are generally better than the cheaper ones.

Tryptophan scare: FDA hoax or deadly poison?

Did you have trouble getting to sleep last night? Do you remember the days when you could simply pop a couple of tryptophan capsules and, half an hour later, be in Dreamland? If so, you may be quite interested to learn the facts behind the tryptophan ban.

Tryptophan is one of the essential amino acids that must be obtained from the food we eat. It occurs naturally in high concentrations in animal and fish products and is found in especially high concentration in milk.

In the body, tryptophan triggers the release of serotonin, a neurotransmitter important to the transmission of impulses across nerve-cell connections. Serotonin is the body's natural sedative.

Tryptophan supplements have been used for nearly two decades as a natural method of relieving depression, pain, insomnia, hyperactivity, and eating disorders. So why is it suddenly supposedly making people sick?

In 1990, a rash of deaths was blamed on the rare disease *Eosinophilia Myalgia Syndrome* (EMS). This "new" disease was associated with the consumption of tryptophan products. The syndrome was first reported in New Mexico in November 1989. Symptoms included an abnormally high white blood cell count, fatigue, serious muscle pain, paralysis, and neurological damage.

According to several medical journals, the cause of EMS was not tryptophan, but a contaminant introduced during the manufacture of one particular batch. The U.S. Center for Disease Control and the FDA have known of this contamination since 1990, but refuse to retract their ban on the sale of tryptophan.

Before the ban went into effect, tryptophan was the nation's best-selling amino acid supplement, with annual sales around $150 million. One organization, the Coalition for Alternatives in Nutrition and Health Care, is suing the FDA under the Freedom of Information Act to force the agency to release what it knows.

In research published in *Advances in Therapy* in August 1990, tryptophan is reported to have been used successfully to treat EMS. Twenty EMS patients who didn't respond to steroid therapy were successfully treated with tryptophan.

Some alternatives for home treatment of insomnia, anxiety, stress, or nervousness include herbs such as Valerian Root, Passion Flower, or hops. For depression, you may want to try another amino acid called Tyrosine. Consult your health practitioner for dosage information.

There are a variety of homeopathic remedies available for treatment of like symptoms, including Coffea Cruda, Kali Phos, Mag Phos, Ignatia, Passiflora, Valeriana, Nux Vom, Lycopodium, and Gelsemium. Consult a trained homeopath before you begin using homeopathic remedies.

Vitamins

Many patients want to know whether they should take vitamins. There are many reasons for taking vitamins, but the most important ones are the following:

- Most people don't eat enough of all the right foods to meet their basic nutritional requirements.
- Most of the foods many people eat are inadequate in nutritional value. Foods are grown in soil that is depleted of vitamins and minerals due to standard agribusiness practices. Much of the food we eat is overprocessed and devoid of nutritional value.
- Due to stress, most people need extra vitamins and minerals than if they were living in a more natural, stress-free environment.
- Most people have physiological imbalances, which require extra supplementation.

Vitamins are a group of compounds that act in the body as enzymes and coenzymes, catalyzing chemical reactions within the individual cells of the body. A deficiency occurs if vitamins are not supplied by the diet in adequate amounts. Extra vitamins in varying amounts have been shown to alter body chemistry and promote better health.

Some vitamins contain herbs, amino acids, binders, fillers, coating, colorings, or flavorings. Onel difference between natural and synthetic vitamin supplements is that "natural" vitamins do not also contain preservatives, artificial colorings, or flavorings.

Another important variation to consider is whether products such as yeast or corn are used. These may cause an allergic reaction. Some vitamin supplements also use a binding process that makes chemical absorption in the body much easier. Generally, this is stated on the label.

Never take vitamins with homeopathic remedies in them. It is impossible for a vitamin to contain homeopathic remedies, as binders and fillers antidote the effects of homeopathy. Homeopathic remedies cannot be combined with any other substances.

THE OPPOSITE OF DIS-EASE IS NOT PERFECT HEALTH—IT IS WHOLENESS

Holidays can be rough for many of us. Emotional issues well up inside us. Feelings of not being good enough—not having the family we want, not having the money we want to buy gifts, not having the relationship we want. Along with these feelings of "not being enough," there sometimes arises a deep sense of longing for something more, something better, something more perfect than what we already imagine ourselves to be.

These feelings of "dis-ease" are very valuable. Although tremendously uncomfortable, they are the seeds of locating our wholeness. They point to parts of ourselves we don't like. The answers don't really belong to attaining anything "out there," and most of us already know this. Although it is hard to admit, what we long for most at the holidays is to feel whole within ourselves—to make ourselves into whole human beings. According to Chinese medicine, the winter season is a time of turning inward to plant our seeds of inner growth. If we don't take this opportunity to turn inward, to look at our dis-ease, to slow down, to integrate the lost parts of ourselves, we risk the likelihood that our emotional dis-ease will turn into physical disease.

We need to listen with our hearts and let our hearts talk to our bodies when they give us signals. The signal may be as simple as a raspy throat or a stiff neck. Learn to read these symbols of inner landscape, the inner dis-ease; slow down and take care of the inner self. Learn to express your heart to your friends, boss, and associates so that your emotional dis-ease doesn't transform into physical disease. The opposite of disease is not perfect health. It is a state of body, mind, and heart that acknowledges imperfections, accepts them, communicates them, and tries to integrate them into a greater self deep within. Trust in acceptance, the deeper wisdom of what you perceive as your imperfections is the first step toward achieving wholeness, integrity, and ridding yourself of dis-ease.

—Dr. Randy Martin

PUTTING IT TOGETHER

YOUR BODY AND YOU: QUICK FIX OR LONG HAUL?

So many of us make New Year's resolutions about wanting a healthier body for the year ahead. But we usually don't stop to think about what this really might mean on a deeper level and over the long haul of our life. Although the decision to exercise or stop eating fats or sugar or to give up coffee are good decisions in and of themselves, these simple commitments tend to be more effective if we develop a more comprehensive health strategy. When we place the individual health commitments into a long-range plan, we are taking a primary step to healing ourselves. This is very self-empowering and leads to becoming our own healer.

Many of my patients come in with specific health goals in mind, and usually these goals are shortsighted. With courage you may want to set more far-reaching goals such as the following:

- ❀ I want to be free from pain in 6 months

- ❀ I want to lose 25 pounds and keep it off the rest of my life

- ❀ I want food to nurture and nourish me instead of get in my way

- ❀ I want my brain to work more clearly so that I can be of greater service to humankind

- ❀ I want to have more energy so I can more efficiently get through my day without being tired at night

- ❀ I want to become healthier so that when I have children I don't pass my mediocre health onto them

- ❀ I want optimal health so that I can be of greater service to humankind

What I've found is that a good half of my job as holistic doctor is really as health educator. Patients need to be taught what is possible when it comes to their body-mind and its health. Many people walk around half in and half out of their body most of the time. Actually many of us are only in our body 1–2% or the time; the rest of the time we are on "automatic," in the past or future. You can't begin to heal the body until you spend more time in your body and in present time.

Much of healing the body is in learning to be present in the moment. Much of our emotional and physical pain is "old, stuck stuff" and not what is actually going on in the "now." Some physical pain is also the body's response to being worked too hard or given the wrong fuel (food) to burn. Do you know what is your optimal diet, or do you read the latest fad book and follow it instead?

Did you know that each of us has an optimal diet, and this personalized optimal diet has almost nothing to do with the latest fad books? I base an individual's optimal diet on Oriental medical principals, blood tests, hair analysis, and metabolic typing. Many of us have parasites, yeast and other digestive difficulties. According to Chinese medicine, when the digestion is working well, the rest of our body will follow suit. Have you had a test for parasites and yeast in the stool? If not, your digestive system may be operating at only one-half its potential.

When we are not feeling well, it's often only the tip of the iceberg poking its face out. If you cut off the tip, you still have the rest of the iceberg to deal with. If you had sinus problems and you cut off your nose, it wouldn't help. One of my favorite examples of how many of us relate to our physical body is my leaf blower metaphor. You know, in Santa Monica where I live, it's illegal to use leaf blowers. They are loud, noisy and inefficient. I think it should be illegal to use the kind of metaphoric leaf blowers many of us use in our bodies.

Here is the metaphor: If you had a bunch of dirt and dust in your home, would you take a leaf blower and blow it under the sofa or carpet? Then when you want to move your furniture, you'd rediscover the dirt and blow it under another piece of furniture? If you did this, then at spring cleaning time, you'd suddenly find all of the dirt! A lot of good it did. You'd just be putting off the eventual cleaning you'd have to do.

This is what we do with our bodies. We push the dirt to another location when we don't want to deal with it. If we have indigestion, we take an antacid. Headaches? We take a pain reliever; Moles or warts? We cut them off. Fibroids? We cut them out. Back pain? We ignore it. And each time we do this, we suppress the immune system and create a new problem somewhere else in our body.

Symptoms are not to be ignored or cut out or numbed out; they are our blessings in disguise. They help us to stay on track. Since we are souls temporarily inhabiting physical bodies, the physical complaints we have are often the red flags from our soul level of existence telling us where we are off and to change course.

Usually, we don't see the interconnectedness within our body any more than we see the connection between holes in the ozone layer and use of auto air conditioners. But, you see, everything in the body *is* interconnected, and I can often trace the onset of a serious disease to the suppression of a less serious disease many years earlier. Don't cut off those warts and moles. They are the body defending itself against toxicity somewhere else in the body. Don't take that pain reliever, unless absolutely necessary. Instead, wake up to a higher level of awareness to see what the headache or neck pain or cold is telling you.

I had a patient, whom we'll call Casey, who came to be treated for fibrocystic breast disease. After taking Casey's lengthy health history, I discovered not only was she a chocoholic and junk food junkie, but she also had constipation, (which she had taken laxatives for), severe menstrual cramps (which she regularly takes medications for), and had cut off several moles about three years before the onset of the breast fibroids.

Fibrocystic breast disease is, according to Chinese medical theory, usually a disease caused by an imbalance in the Liver Meridians. The Liver is involved in detoxifying the body. The moles were the body's most benign way of creating balance in a toxic environment. Due to her diet and her genetic history of having one parent an alcoholic and the other having had ovarian cancer, Casey inherited a Liver meridian problem. She was adding to this pathology by her diet high in fats and sweets and by her consistent emotional pattern of withholding and suppressing her feelings.

After a few months of cleaning up her diet and giving her homeopathic treatment, her previously cut off moles re-emerged and I told her this was a sign her body's defense mechanism was beginning to regain its health after having suppressed it for so many years. She got off all drugs and began to use herbal remedies instead. Four months into treatment, her doctor couldn't believe the breast lumps had "disappeared." She felt better, had more energy and was looking into changing careers to transfer her skills from a legal assistant to doing something more service-oriented to help her fellows.

This was a true success story, and is not uncommon when someone is willing to really look at their diet, lifestyle and how their physical symptoms are signs of an imbalance in their life on a deeper level. She could have just as easily let her doctor cut open her breasts and take out the cysts. But she was conscious enough to want to relate to herself in a truly long-range and holistic way, and as a result she can expect to have continued increasing great energy and optimal health!

LIVING WITH THE CYCLE OF THE SEASONS

Most of us live in the city. We breathe polluted air, we eat food grown under artificial conditions, and most of us have so little contact with nature that we barely notice the change in seasons. Southern California causes even more displacement because the change in seasons can be subtle indeed.

Although variations often go unnoticed, we are still animals and there are some very basic changes that take place physically and emotionally at every turn of the seasons. According to Oriental medicine, it is through seasonal changes that different organs in the body are activated and become over- or under-active.

Spring

The liver and gall bladder are the organs connected with springtime. During the spring it is appropriate to add herbs and foods to our diet that cleanse and detoxify these organs, boosting our energy and maintaining a healthier immune system—thus increasing our resistance to allergies and colds.

Foods that facilitate detoxification of the liver are green, red, and yellow vegetables such as chard, kale, beet tops, beets, carrots, dandelion greens, parsley, and string beans.

Try to avoid fats such as lard, nut butters, and red meat. Spring is the time to cleanse the body. A little lemon in warm water is a good way to start the morning or end a meal. You may also want to do a liver and gall bladder flush (see page 179).

Herbs to stimulate and cleanse the liver and gall bladder are Black Radish, Dandelion Root, Parsley Leaf, and Chelidonium. You can use these as a tea, in capsules, or in tincture form. This may also be a good time to take a nutritional supplement for liver detoxification or a Desiccated Liver tablet if you are not a vegetarian.

If you are a person who tends toward a toxic liver condition anyway, you should be especially observant of a detox diet during this time of the year. People who are the most susceptible to liver and gall bladder problems are:

❀ ACAs (Adult Children of Alcoholics or drug users, including abusers of prescription drugs)

❀ People who have uncontrollable outbursts of anger or who hold all feelings of anger inside

❀ Women with PMS or men with prostate problems

❀ Those who crave sugar, sweets, pastries, fried foods, alcohol, or recreational drugs

❀ People with hypoglycemia or diabetes in their family

❀ People prone to migraine headaches or one-sided headaches

❀ Those who belch or burp a lot or who have a lot of gas

❀ Sciatic pain sufferers

Liver toxicity worsened by spring may show up in such symptoms as allergies, muscle spasms, spinal problems, depression, headaches, digestive problems, or joint pain.

 ### Summer

The heart and small intestine are the two primary organs associated with summer, which is associated with the Fire Element. During the summer, injury to these elements is more probable, so it is wise to take appropriate steps to protect these organs and their associated meridians.

A hot climate such as Southern California is particularly apt to weaken and create problems in these meridians. The condition called *Heart Fire* is quite common in Southern California during the summer. Typical symptoms include overheating, excessive excitability, anxiety attacks, or becoming overly emotional. Depending on your constitution and imbalances in your meridians, you could experience the opposite—withdrawal, depression, lack of motivation, isolation, or feeling cold.

During the summer months, it is appropriate to add herbs and foods to your diet that will help strengthen and balance the heart and small intestines. Your energy will be more balanced and there will be more of it to sustain you through the summer and fall seasons.

Eating correctly will also boost your immunity and make you less susceptible to smog and allergies. If you eat a very yang diet—one with an excessive amount of animal proteins, salt, or other yang foods with high sodium or fat contents—you will find your cravings for sweets and cold drinks especially hard to satisfy. This is because you will need an excessive amount of yin to put out the yang Heart Fire.

Summer is the most yang of all the seasons, and it is important to offset this by adopting a diet with more yin types of foods—whole grains, beans, legumes, and lots of vegetables. Especially good for the summer diet are corn, corn meal, or popcorn. Other summer vegetables include Brussels sprouts, cucumbers, dandelions, okra, and scallions. Sunflower seeds and sunflower seed sprouts are also good at this time of year.

Red is the color associated with summer. Generally, a person with an imbalance in a particular element will have a strong opinion about the color relating to their season, whether positive or negative. A person with an imbalance in summer may not only have a red color to their face, but may prefer or dislike red clothes, red cars, red furniture, or red anything.

The direction that the summer element relates to is south, which makes sense because the summer season is hot. Southern winds are very hot winds (as compared to the northern winds associated with the cold of winter/the Water Element, or the eastern Santa Ana winds associated with the allergies of spring/the Wood Element).

Joy and laughter are the emotions associated with summer. An imbalance here may manifest itself as an inability to experience joy and laughter, or it may be manifest in a difficulty in giving and receiving warmth and love. A person may giggle or laugh too much (possibly inappropriately), or may wear a superficial smile because they are frightened.

Sometimes a person with an imbalance in the Fire Element will move very quickly and have a rounded face, broad cheeks, horizontal facial lines, and a high and cracking voice. Skin color may be red, white, or both, but it will rarely be olive, yellowish, or greenish.

The tongue is the sense organ ruled by the Fire Element and the ability to speak clearly and fluently is its associated sense. Problems with speech, such as stuttering or slurring of speech, may relate to an imbalance in the Fire Element.

Common problems include insomnia, unsettled sleep, waking too early, palpitations in the chest, sweating for no apparent reason, anxiousness or discomfort in one's environment, being "spaced out," a lack of emotional groundedness, forgetfulness, any heart problems (including tachycardia), and any assimilation problems having to do with the small intestine and duodenum (flatulence, belching, and bloating).

The time of day related to Fire is between 11 A.M. and 3 P.M., the warmest time of the 24-hour cycle. Statistically, many heart attacks occur during these hours on the *opposite* side of the clock (in the early morning), because the organs of the Fire Element, including the heart, are then at their weakest.

According to Oriental medicine, the heart is said to contain the *shen* or spirit of your being. If your shen is strong and clear, it will show up in the sparkle and clarity of your eyes. On the other hand, if a person suffers from Heart Fire or has disturbed shen from extreme anxiety, worry, or loneliness, their eyes will show this as well.

To balance the heart's shen and corresponding Heart Meridian and Fire Element, it is possible to use various meditation techniques. One such technique is to meditate on the heart chakra, located about halfway between the throat and the navel on the front center line of the body. One meditation visualizes a soothing, healing color surrounding the heart chakra. Breathe deeply into the heart, and relax the chest and shoulders. One can also use crystals set upon the heart chakra to intensify the meditation energy.

Meditation or visual imagery using the heart as your focus will help to create a stronger, better-functioning heart, and bring clarity and strength to your shen.

Fall

As we approach the fall season, trees let go of their leaves and dead wood falls. Fall is a time for letting go of our dead weight and old growth, in preparation for a winter of in energy and turning inward.

Fall and winter's inward journey is one toward our inner selves, in preparation for another springtime of outward (yang) energetic growth. The more fully we can let go in fall, the more fully we will experience the growth of spring.

It can be painful to let go of old growth. After all, it feels like it is a big part of us and who we are (old relationships, old commitments, old and inappropriate responsibilities). In times past, healers, shamans, priests, and priestesses were trained in the arts of ritual and performance. They interceded for us with the seasonal energies, acted out universal myths, and served as catalysts for change. Their ceremonies kept societies functioning in a healthy and productive way, and facilitated a natural connection with the seasons. Today we must individually and collectively recreate rituals that will make these connections meaningful.

The Jewish holiday of Rosh Hashanah includes a ritual for this time of year. Participants travel to a body of water and symbolically empty their pockets, thereby emptying the "old luggage" of the burdened soul. On Yom Kippur, participants are instructed to harvest their assets and weaknesses in the form of a personal inventory.

Tashlikh

On the afternoon of the first day of Rosh Hashanah (or that of the second if the first falls on a Saturday or is rainy), it is customary to walk to a river or spring, preferably one with fish in it, and recite special penitential prayers. The essence of these is: "You will cast all their sins into the depths of the sea, and may You cast all the sins of Your people...into a place where they shall be no more remembered or visited or ever come to mind."

This Tashlikh is accompanied by emptying one's pockets or hems or a casting of breadcrumbs into the water—symbolic of casting off one's shortcomings and starting anew.

—The First Jewish Catalog

All traditions have fall rituals enabling their participants to explore inner parts of themselves, to strengthen and balance physical and emotional bodies through the ceremonies.

According to Oriental medicine, fall relates to the large intestine, the skin, and the lungs. Theory says that the large intestine separates the pure from the impure. If you have constipation, diarrhea, colitis, abdominal pain, or rumblings, you may have a large intestine imbalance. The skin also has a role in excreting wastes. If you have eczema, psoriasis, rashes, boils, or pimples, it shows a physical difficulty in letting go of waste and of eliminating toxins from the body.

Lungs regulate the inspiration and expiration of air and propel energy throughout the body. If the lung are not healthy, you may have coughs, asthma, colds, allergies, difficulty breathing, sinus blockage, or nasal drip. You may also experience creative blocks or experience difficulties feeling "inspired."

Fall is a time when gastrointestinal and respiratory problems are likely to occur. Stomach flu, diarrhea, asthma, head colds, skin rashes, and eczema may be aggravated. If you ordinarily have any of these problems, then the fall season may make them a little worse unless you take action to strengthen your body with herbs, a cleansing diet, or acupuncture.

The color associated with autumn is white. People with a particularly pale or white complexion may be more likely to have problems with their lungs, colon, or skin at this time of year.

The emotion associated with fall is grief or sadness. Don't be surprised if you find yourself experiencing an increase in these emotions. After all, this is a time to release old attachments and feelings.

On a physical level, detoxifying herbs can facilitate the process of letting go. Chaparral, Burdock, Dandelion, or Sassafras Root bark are herbs used in detoxification. Other herbs for releasing toxins include cayenne pepper, ginger, or cinnamon taken in tea or capsule form.

Root vegetables associated with autumn such as onions, garlic, daikon radishes, and white potatoes are good to eat at this time of year to strengthen the lungs. Other fall foods include rice, navy beans, turnips, turnip greens, spirulina, and tofu.

In astrology, fall is the season of Libra, the sign of balance. It accentuates the need to balance what was attained with what needs to be released.

Winter

Have you ever wondered why some people love the winter months and others hate them? The explanation for this may be found in Oriental medicine. Winter corresponds to the Water Element, and its organs are the kidneys and urinary system or bladder. A person who has a weakness in these meridians will tend to dislike winter. These people will generally have a dislike for cold and rainy weather, display an attraction to the color black or dark blue (in clothes or cars perhaps), exhibit dark circles under their eyes and a groaning undertone in their voice. They may have dreams filled with the ocean, rivers, or ponds, feel fatigue between 3 and 7 P.M., have difficulty hearing, and crave salty foods.

On an emotional level, Water Element imbalances may manifest as a weak sense of willpower and ambition, and trouble sticking to things. Fear may also be a predominant issue. This may be a person with an unclear personal force in life, who will easily get buffeted around by other people's willpower and strengths. Other issues may be anxiety, anguish, depression, loneliness, or insomnia.

On a physical level, the Water Element may give rise to problems involving sexuality, such as sterility or impotence, loss of head hair, bone weakness such as osteoporosis, kidney stones, or low back pain. Other common problems may be fatigue, urinary infections, vaginal dryness or pain, dry or red eyes, chronic sore throats or infections, occipital headaches, low back pain, testicular pain, or yeast infections.

A person who has a weak Water Element needs to stay away from eating an excessive amount of salty foods. Salt will further weaken the kidneys.

REMEMBER YOUR SEASONAL TUNE-UP
at each seasonal change

The tune-up will help keep you in balance:

1. If you like acupuncture, I'll use those acu-points known to balance the organs related to the particular season we are going into.

2. If you prefer homeopathy, we'll take the opportunity to discuss your ongoing constitutional treatment to determine when you need your next prescription.

3. If you prefer herbs, we'll choose an herbal formula to match your constitution and the season.

4. If you want suggestions and advice on how to eat a healthy diet that is in keeping with the seasons, we can evaluate your diet and nutritional supplements as well.

The synergistic effects will be very powerful.

HOLIDAY HINTS: HOW TO HAVE A HAPPY AND HEALTHY SEASON

Winter is the season of the kidneys and urinary bladder, according to Chinese medicine. What does this mean to us, living many thousands of years after Chinese medicine originated, on the other side of the world, observing winter holiday rituals and traditions much different from those of the Chinese?

As the days get shorter, culminating with the winter solstice on December 21, many of us feel a nagging fear or confusion deep inside. Perhaps we experience it as a fear of walking in the dark to our car after work, going to a holiday party with many strangers, losing our sense of self when we visit our families, being consumed by our families, or not being understood for who we have become over the past year's growth.

Whatever the fear you may be feeling, you are on track. According to Chinese medicine, the emotion associated with the winter season and the kidneys is, in fact, fear. What can we do about it?

We can strengthen the kidney and urinary bladder meridians with acupuncture. We can access energy systems in the body associated with the emotion of fear by practicing some basic Chinese medical principles.

Make sure you get enough sleep. Make sure you eat seasonally. Strengthen your endurance by building your winter element. Eat kidney beans, pinto beans, aduki beans, miso soup, buckwheat, beets and beet greens, kale, and shiitake mushrooms. Stay away from coffee (regular *and* decaf), as it weakens the kidneys and bladder. (An alternative is Bancha Tea, which is strengthening.) Do not over-salt your food. If you must have salt, try a little tamari, Braggs aminos, or salty pickles.

Do not overeat! If you do, immediately take some herbal or homeopathic remedies to combat the negative effects you would otherwise feel the next day. Try a strong brew of Ginger Root Tea or take the capsules directly. Try Pill Curing, an herbal remedy, or a few doses of homeopathic Nux Vomica 12X or Carbo Vegetalis 6X. You can quickly relieve gas and bloating with any of these remedies.

If you're stressed and having trouble getting to sleep, you can use a variety of commercially available herbal tea formulas designed to relieve stress. Or, try a few doses of homeopathic Passiflora 6X or Avena Sativa 6X. You can also try herbal capsules of Valerian Root extract, which knock some people right out.

Take your journal out and befriend your inner child again. This is a great gift to give yourself over the holidays. Ask your inner child what s/he wants for the holidays—a walk on the beach, a drive up the coast, a relaxing video at home, that special piece of furniture, or latest electronic gizmo may go a long way toward quieting the inner feelings of anxiety or fear that many of us feel during the holidays.

Write down the dreams that come as you sleep. How often do we really take the time to honor our inner selves by taking 5 minutes in the morning to recount our dreams on paper or into a tape recorder? If you're too busy to take a major break in the form of a vacation, at least do yourself the favor of parking the car further away from your destinations and make the effort to walk and smell the flowers. Look at unique architecture; gaze at the clouds or the leaves blowing in the breeze. During the winter, the city can be quite clean and beautiful.

Life is the gift before our senses. Having the courage to go beyond our normal perspectives and enjoy the beauty of creation with all our senses, especially during the holidays, can dispel whatever fears may surface during this time of potential physical and emotional distress. Now is the time to rediscover your own inner light, to turn inward and discover the seeds of creation within your soul. Give yourself the favor of time, space, and attention—for yourself—for your own unique, desiring, and deserving inner self.

TREATING TOXICITY NATURALLY

As environmental pollution continues, the smog increases and pesticides on our foods become hard to avoid, many or us are experiencing the effects of these environmental pollutants. Homeopathic remedies, supplements, and herbs can protect us and detoxify our bodies once the pollutants have taken hold.

The best vitamin supplements to take to protect yourself are the following:
- ✧ CoQ$_{10}$
- ✧ Germanium
- ✧ Beta Carotene
- ✧ Selenium
- ✧ Vitamin E
- ✧ Vitamin C with bioflavinoids

Some of the most common and effective herbs for detoxification are:
- ✧ dandelion root for the liver
- ✧ garlic and mullein for the lungs
- ✧ corn silk and uva ursi for the kidneys
- ✧ Echinacea, burdock and red clover for blood cleansing and skin
- ✧ psyllium seed husks and betonite for the colon

You can takes capsules or purchase the bulk tea and drink the herbs.

Here are some good homeopathic remedies the detoxification:
- ✧ Chelidonium for liver and gall bladder
- ✧ Berb vulg. for the kidneys
- ✧ Kali phos for the nervous system
- ✧ Rescue Remedy upon immediate exposure to toxins or toxic sprays

Remember that environmental pollutants will effect everyone differently, depending on the individual constitution and body type. Each person will need different remedies or doses for his or her particular constitution.

DETOXIFICATION DIETS

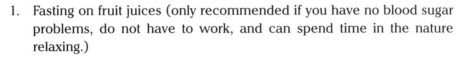

1. Fasting on fruit juices (only recommended if you have no blood sugar problems, do not have to work, and can spend time in the nature relaxing.)

2. Fasting on vegetable broth or juice (only recommended if you can relax away from all stressful situations.)

3. Single cooked vegetable diet: choose one single vegetable per day and only eat that particular vegetable, as much as desired. Suggested vegetables include string beans, squash, potatoes, carrots, beets, green leafy vegetables, celery, or any other vegetable you like.

4. Vegetable and grain diet: choose one single vegetable and one single grain per day and eat only that particular vegetable and grain on that day. Suggested grains include brown rice, millet, amaranth, quinoa, buckwheat, oats, barley or any other whole grain of your choice.

5. Vegetable, grain, legume and fruit diet: eat a variety of steamed mixed vegetables, including a lot of onions and garlic, along with a whole grain, legumes and fruits (fruits separate from other foods). Suggested legumes include tofu, tempe, split peas, black beans, lentils, pinto beans, or any other bean of your choice. Any fruit is fine but be sure to eat fruit at least one-half hour before or two hours after any other foods and never eat melon with any other fruit or food.

NOTE: If you think you may be allergic to different foods, stay away from those foods. Some of the most common allergy foods include citrus fruits, strawberries, beef, wheat, milk and all milk products, soy products, chocolate, oats, rye, barley, corn and corn products, and eggs. Of course most of these foods are not good on a detox* diet anyway.

If you should begin to experience a healing aggravation, you are detoxing too quickly. Modify your diet and go slower. A healing aggravation is any cleansing process such as a cold, skin rash, skin eruption, vaginal discharge, athlete's foot, headache or any symptom you have ever had that was suppressed by a drug, skin ointment or surgical procedure (any time in your life, back to infancy) that you are now re-experiencing.

NOTE: If you suspect you might have toxicity in the liver, kidney or lungs, then consult your health practitioner. I do not suggest that you undertake a detoxification diet without an exam and testing by your health practitioner first. In general, one shouldn't undergo any type of detoxification unless they are taking a week or two off of work and are being supervised by their health practitioner. If you are under stress, never do a detox diet.

---

*Detox—refers to the detoxification process; usually involves treatment of the liver, colon, lungs and kidneys, the primary organs which will accumulate toxins

DETOXIFICATION BROTH

(**NOTE:** This is taken from the famous "Bieler's Broth" recipe.)

Makes approximately six 1-cup servings:

3 medium	zucchini, chopped
1 medium	yellow crookneck squash, chopped
4	celery stalks, chopped
1 lb.	string beans
1 bunch	fresh parsley
2	whole garlic cloves
1 bunch	fresh dill
1	vegetable bouillon cube
1 tsp.	saltless garlic seasoner
to taste	pepper or cayenne pepper
optional	Pritikin (no fat) chicken broth
sprinkle	various seaweed powders on the soup before eating

Wash and cut all vegetables into chunks. Steam in a large soup pot, using filtered, pure water. When the vegetables are tender, place mixture in a food processor or blender. Add all seasonings and 1/2 of the remaining water used to steam vegetables. Puree contents until the soup is thick, but smooth and creamy. Add remaining liquid or additional seasonings to taste.

Broth can be eaten alone or with meals or as an in-between meal snack. It is a good way to start the day as well.

Eating Seasonably Helps You and Your Planet

Though you may love eating strawberries in January, have you considered where they come from? The strawberries you find in the supermarket in winter were probably grown in New Zealand and shipped halfway around the world. While the cost to you might only be $2.99 for a pint of berries, the cost to the planet in terms of energy and fuel wasted is immeasurable.

—Kathryn Arnol

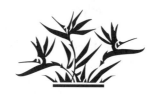

LIVER AND GALL BLADDER FLUSH
(DETOXIFICATION)

The liver and gall bladder flush is an important method to detoxify your system. The best time to do this is the beginning of spring, when the liver and gallbladder are beginning to be the most active. The method is risky, however, and patients have been known to experience severe colic and stomach pain or to get gall bladder stones caught in the bile duct. This method is not recommended for patients under twenty-five years of age or patients who know they have large stones. For these patients it is better to utilize more subtle methods, such as homeopathy and herbs.

But if you are up for a radical experience in self-healing, one that has been used for a very long time by folk healers all over the world, here it is:

1. For five or six days drink as much apple juice or apple cider as your appetite can handle in addition to regular meals and supplements you take.

2. Eat a normal lunch on the day before the flush.

3. Three hours after lunch, take two teaspoons of disodium phosphate (Standard Process brand) dissolved in one once of hot water. Follow by a little juice to kill the objectionable taste.

4. Two hours later repeat step three.

5. For your evening meal, have grapefruit juice, grapefruit or other citrus fruits or juices.

6. Before bed, drink either one-half cup of unrefined olive oil followed by a cup of grapefruit juice or one-half cup of warm, unrefined olive oil blended with one-half cup of lemon juice.

7. In bed, lie on your right side with you right knee pulled up close to your chest for thirty minutes.

8. The next morning, one hour before breakfast, take two teaspoons of disodium phosphate dissolved in two ounces of hot water.

9. That day, continue to eat your normal diet and take your supplements.

Some people experience nausea after taking the olive oil, but it usually disappears once you get into bed. If you experience vomiting, do not repeat the procedure at this time.

This flush may produce little green or yellow "stones" in your stool, so look for them. This procedure stimulates and cleans the liver and gall bladder like no other procedure.

> **NOTE:** This procedure should only be done after consulting with your health practitioner to determine whether it is safe for you to do it.

FLYING IN AIRPLANES CAUSES IMBALANCE OF YIN AND YANG

Flying in airplanes may cause an imbalance of yin and yang in most people, especially if they have a weak yin to begin with. Symptoms of yin deficiency may include headaches, nausea, dizziness, hot flashes, panic attacks, respiratory problems, and red eyes. And some people suffer for days after flying. They may also experience insomnia or constipation, two other symptoms of yang excess and yin deficiency.

Yang is associated with the sun, heat and dryness, and the primary sources of yang are the sun and sky. Yin energies are cooler and moist and the main sources of yin are the Earth, the Earth's magnetic fields and other energies of the Earth.

In a jet, high above the Earth, the air is dry and the Earth's magnetic fields are far away and weaker. The yin energies are very weak and it is very easy to finish a flight with a yang excess.

The solution is to fly as little as possible, and when you have to fly drink plenty of cold fluids, avoid alcohol, spend some time before and after the flight in meditation and walking, focusing specifically on meditation techniques to increase yin energy in the body. Utilize acupressure points to increase yin. Try to get an acupuncture treatment or massage before and after your flight. Use yin tonic herbs, homeopathic constitutional remedies or Rescue Remedy before, during and after your flight to keep your yin and yang nicely balanced.

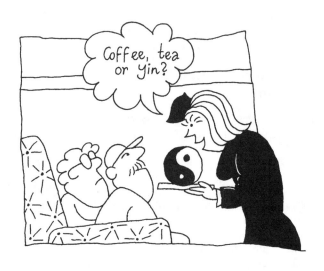

HEALTHY SEXUALITY

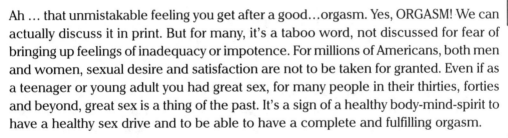

Ah … that unmistakable feeling you get after a good…orgasm. Yes, ORGASM! We can actually discuss it in print. But for many, it's a taboo word, not discussed for fear of bringing up feelings of inadequacy or impotence. For millions of Americans, both men and women, sexual desire and satisfaction are not to be taken for granted. Even if as a teenager or young adult you had great sex, for many people in their thirties, forties and beyond, great sex is a thing of the past. It's a sign of a healthy body-mind-spirit to have a healthy sex drive and to be able to have a complete and fulfilling orgasm.

So why is it that many people have trouble in the area of sex? Where did that great fulfilled sigh of pleasure go for so many people? What factors are involved? And more important, what can you do about it? If you want to have that great feeling of being sexy and horny with your partner and then be able to have sex as often as you'd like to, there *are* solutions to your problem! And for most people the solutions are neither too complex nor difficult.

First let's discuss some of the factors contributing to poor sex drive and lack of a good orgasm. For many men, fear of non-performance, commonly termed "performance anxiety" is no joke. Anticipating what the woman will think if he "can't get it up" or "can't keep it up long enough" is enough for many men to lose an erection completely. On the other end, some men simply ejaculate too soon for the satisfaction of their mates. This, too, is caused by a different type of performance anxiety.

The most common problem in many women not being fulfilled sexually is lack of experience with their partner. This is easily corrected by purchasing one of the many sex technique manuals available at your local bookstore or taking a weekend seminar and making the exercises part of your lovemaking sessions.

One of the most potent aphrodisiacs is sexual fantasy. Some people feel guilty when they find themselves slipping into sexual fantasy with their partner, but research has shown that much of our sexual attraction, desire and ultimate satisfaction is actually in our head. This is especially true for men, who tend to be turned on by visual cues more so than women. On the other hand, most women respond to touch and being caressed, spoken to, and held. So you need to educate yourself and your partner as to what turns you on and ultimately works for you. Communication is one of the most powerful aphrodisiacs.

Some of my patients come in and they already have experimented with the emotional and interactional aspects of lovemaking. For them, the issue is more physiological. What can you do to raise your man's libido? Or vice versa, what can you as a man do to get your woman to want sex more often?

In reality, there are many physiological problems that can account for a low sex drive.

The most common problem on the physical level is hormone imbalance. This can stem from either stress, lack of exercise or genetics. The solutions are usually very simple, but must be geared to each individual and the cause of their particular problem. However, it can't hurt anyone to begin by supplementing their diet with some important vitamins, minerals and herbal remedies.

For men, the most important mineral for health of the prostate and erection is zinc. I have found the most effective form of zinc to be zinc picolinate. All men should be taking zinc, especially after ejaculation. Other supplements important to male performance include vitamin E (dry form), glutamic acid, alanine, glycine and the herb uva ursi. The four indispensable supplements for men are saw palmetto extract, pygeum, ginkgo and the essential fatty acids. You can get the saw palmetto ingredient by eating pumpkin seeds, but the extract is much more potent and effective. To raise your man's sexual desire, another good herb is yohimbe bark extract. This is the herb used in a lot of the commercial products now being mass-marketed on the TV infomercials.

If you aren't a vegetarian, you can take what are called organ extracts, or glandulars. For men, the most effective is a combined extract of orchic, adrenal, thyroid and pituitary. Of course, the old standby herb is ginseng and the safest type of ginseng is Siberian ginseng. Royal jelly is also a great sexual energy stimulant.

Many doctors are also now using DHEA and pregnenolone. These are hormonal precursors to your testosterone and other endocrine hormones. These precursors are in the experimental stages here in the US, although in Europe they've been used for quite some time. I always recommend my patients take very small amounts if they are going to experiment with these hormones. A much safer way is to take wild yam extract. This is a more natural, herbal supplement and is much safer to experiment with on your own.

If these suggestions don't increase the sexual desire and performance of the man in your life, then he needs to be assessed by a holistic practitioner for deeper hormonal or emotional imbalances.

Now for you women... Is your man always bugging you for more sex, but you just aren't interested? Does your desire fluctuate throughout the month, depending on your menstrual cycle? Well, there are some very simple and easy solutions for most of you. Two of the most common herbs for regulating female hormones are vitex and damiana. Vitex can be used to regulate the menstrual cycle very effectively as well. If your period comes on either too early or too late, vitex will often do the trick.

Many woman don't realize that if they are on the pill, it is a tremendous upset to their natural hormonal balance. I always suggest my patients get off the birth control pill as soon as possible. If you are on the pill because of hormonal imbalance, this can be corrected with acupuncture and herbs just as effectively. If you're on the pill for birth control purposes, you need to learn to incorporate a barrier method of birth control into your lovemaking so that it's a "turn on" and not a "turn off." When you go off the pill, it's vital to immediately get onto a program of acupuncture and/or herbs to re-stimulate the flow of your normal hormones. Otherwise you are likely to suffer from PMS, cramps or other symptoms of imbalance for months.

Vitex, dong quai and red raspberry are the most common herbs you can use to regulate your hormones and to boost your sexual desire. If your sex drive is low, it will be increased as a result. Damiana tincture can also be used to raise sex drive. Many women are also now using DHEA and pregnenolone, but as I said with men, in my practice I usually prefer to use concentrated wild yam, in the Mannatech "Plus" formula.

Women also respond very well to acupuncture treatment used specifically to increase sexual desire. The most common acu-points used for this type of treatment are Stomach 30 and CV 3 and 4 on the lower abdomen. These stimulate and regulate the ovaries. I have had many women patients thank me for improving their sexual relationship with their husband or boyfriend after only three or four acupuncture treatments.

Homeopathic treatment can also be used and three of the most common homeo-pathic remedies are Sepia, Pulsatilla and Natrum mur. (Note that the homeopathic remedy needs to be selected by a trained Classical homeopath. This is because it's important when using homeopathy for hormonal problems to also assess and consider the emotional and spiritual aspects, along with the physical and hormonal imbalance.)

The most common characteristics in women who respond to the remedy Sepia are low sex desire or absent sex desire, liver problems (bloating, gas, acne), craving for sour-flavored foods, such as pickles, and a desire to be left alone when feeling emotionally overstimulated.

In contrast, the woman needing the homeopathic remedy Pulsatilla will crave affection and attention when stressed out, even though their desire for sex may be low. She will crave bread and butter and like the windows left open for a cool breeze. Her period may always be late, also.

The woman needing the homeopathic remedy Natrum mur may have shut down sexually after the effects of an emotional trauma or the loss of a loved one. This is a common remedy given to women who suffer from long term incapacitating grief. The Natrum mur type of woman will dislike consolation and company and prefer to be alone in their grief, in contrast to the Pulsatilla type. They may also crave fish and/or salty foods, such as chips.

I hope this brief introduction to the subject of sex and aphrodisiacs has proven helpful to you. Please remember that as people, we are incredibly complex, and the same remedy won't work for everybody. If you try some of the suggestions in this article and they don't work, then don't give up! But do get some help. Increasing your sexual desire is not that difficult, but you may need the help of a professional. Please also note that nothing in this short article is meant to replace the advice of your physician or health professional and if you are on any medications from your doctor, it is very important for you to consult with him or her before changing your medications.

APHRODISIACS

Webster's Dictionary defines an aphrodisiac as a substance which excites sexual desire. So, if you have a lover and you're lookin' to spice up your love life, than read on, because I'll give you a lot of clues for how to make that special someone even a bit more special.

If your sexual desire and interest are not up to what you'd like it to be, or if your lover's desire isn't as high as you like, the first thing to do before taking an aphrodisiac is to determine the cause From a Western medical point of view, the cause is usually related either to an endocrine gland problem or from an unresolved emotional issue.

The endocrine system is composed of a complex interaction of various glands in your body. The glands most related to sexual function include the pituitary, thyroid, adrenals, ovaries and testicles. All the endocrine glands are interconnected and it's hard to isolate which is at fault in low sexual drive. A good place to start is with a blood test to determine the condition of the thyroid gland. The thyroid regulates the heat in the body, and heat relates to Fire and sexual drive.

Other common physiological causes for either an aversion to sex or a lower than average sex drive includes frequent herpes, urinary infections, candida, painful ejaculations, painful intercourse for women, fatigue, and low back pain.

All of these problems can be easily eliminated through the use of nutritional supplements and/or Chinese herbs. To name just a few of the treatments you may want to try if you suffer from any of these problems, there are Herp-ease for herpes, Quell Fire for urinary infections, and Y-Stat for candida. Most people can be free from these annoying nuisances very quickly. Painful intercourse, painful ejaculation, fatigue and low back pain may take a few months to treat and the treatment will vary, based on the individual person.

On an emotional level, if you or your partner do not have the libido and sexual energy that you would like, you may want to also examine your emotional agenda. Many times we bring old hurts and sadness to a relationship and project it onto our current partner, thus creating "stuck" energy in the relationship. If you aren't "turned on" the way you'd like to be, first examine your "emotional agenda" or what you may be projecting onto your partner. Therapy in the form of "mind-body" therapy is a very helpful resource in this regard.

If emotionally and physically you are in good shape and just need that extra little push, then the following herbs and supplements will be of help. Women will often respond well to a Chinese herbal formula called Lycium Formula. Women who will respond particularly well to this formula will have a low libido with loss of interest in sex, general fatigue, loss of appetite and may also have low back pain and uterine fibroids or endometriosis.

Another good formula for women is Tang-kuei and Peony Formula. This one's good if you are weak in general and are having difficulty getting pregnant, have irregular menstruation with menstrual cramps, weakness and fatigue after your pregnancy, hemorrhoids or frequent urinary infections.

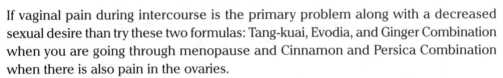

If vaginal pain during intercourse is the primary problem along with a decreased sexual desire than try these two formulas: Tang-kuai, Evodia, and Ginger Combination when you are going through menopause and Cinnamon and Persica Combination when there is also pain in the ovaries.

When fatigue is the primary cause behind low sex drive, many doctors are now using pregnenolone and DHEA, both hormones which work to strengthen libido. Vitex, dong quai, damiana and red raspberry are the most common herbs used individually to help regulate your hormones and to boost your sexual desire.

Many woman don't realize that if they are on the birth control pill, it is a tremendous upset to their natural hormonal imbalance and can affect libido. I always suggest my patients get off the pill as soon as possible. If you are on the pill because of hormonal imbalance, the imbalance can easily be corrected just as effectively with Chinese herbs, acupuncture and diet.

Traditionally, there are many more Chinese herbal formulas created to increase male sexual performance than there are for women. Here are just a few of the most commonly used: Cinnamon and Dragon Bone Combination is used when there is nervous exhaustion, generalized weakness, low back pain, impotence, insomnia and heart palpitations. Ginseng Nutritive Formula is used when there is accompanying fatigue with a poor appetite and is also a general tonic for age-related loss of sex drive. Another formula called Shou Wu is used when there is blurry vision, dizziness, dry hair, and dry throat with sexual exhaustion in men.

Some of the most well known individual herbs used to increase male sexual performance and desire include yohimbinum, ginseng and wild yam. Yohimbinum has been used for centuries all over the world. It's known to excite sexual organs and act on the central nervous system. It's a great aphrodisiac, but should not be used if there is any abdominal inflammation, such as colitis or ulcers. It will help with erections, both to strengthen and help them to last longer.

Ginseng, used before sex, enhances potency. It also helps rebuild energy following exhausting bedroom encounters. Chinese physicians prescribe ginseng as a tonic for general weakness; Russian astronauts reportedly take ginseng to improve their endurance in space. Wild yam, in either capsule or tablet form, is an excellent place to begin a holistic program of strengthening sexual interest and performance.

Any discussion of male sexual performance must also always include a discussion of prostate health. The prostate gland is located below the bladder and surrounds the urethra. The prostate is responsible for secreting a thin fluid which forms part of the semen, and also plays a large part in the muscle contractions for both urination and ejaculation. Two out of four men over the age of fifty have some symptoms of an enlarged prostate due to the typical American diet, which is high in fats and sugars and low in complex carbohydrates and roughage.

Typical symptoms of an enlarged prostate are weak urine flow, difficulty urinating, more frequent urination, low back pain for no reason, low sex drive, and painful ejaculation. Besides a poor diet being one of the causes of prostate problems, another often overlooked cause is candida and other yeast overgrowth. We often think of yeast as a woman's symptom, but actually, sexually active men and women are constantly exchanging the yeast back and forth. For men, one of the most common symptoms of an overgrowth of yeast is a prostate problem. Other than this, it may often go unnoticed in men.

The best diet for healing the prostate or for preventing a prostate problem is to stay away from caffeine and coffee products, fats, dairy products, refined carbohydrates and simple sugars, alcohol, tobacco, and drugs and to create a life where you are able to minimize stress.

Prostate health can be improved be eating pumpkin, squash and sunflower seeds and almonds, plenty of raw and cooked vegetables and fruits. Specific vitamins for both men and women's sexual health include the following:

- ✧ Vitamin E (in a dry or emulsified form)
- ✧ Vitamin F (essential fatty acids)
- ✧ Chlorophyll
- ✧ Zinc picolinate
- ✧ Vitamin C (buffered, chelated or esterfied — not ascorbic acid)
- ✧ Vitamin B_6 and a balanced B-complex as well

Foods that reduce sexual desire in both men and women include eating a diet of highly refined foods, white flour products, sugar and overly sweet foods, caffeine-containing foods and beverages, foods with additives and artificial ingredients and chemicals, and smoking, both tobacco and marijuana and other recreational drugs.

Some common medicines also interfere with sexual performance. Antihypertensives and certain tranquilizers can interfere with ejaculation and erection. Antidepressants can also decrease sexual desire in both men and women.

Note that no one herbal formula or vitamin will work for everyone. Each of us is unique and has an individual body with unique needs, so what works for one person will not work for everyone. If you have not had a complete blood test by your health professional, you should do so before self administering any herbs, especially if you have had high blood pressure or cardiac disease in your family.

Finally, the best and most effective aphrodisiac is fantasy, soft music, candlelight and romance. Try to relax and let your mind go, releasing the day's worries and using sex and foreplay as your meditation for the day. Learn to focus on the sensation of touch in your fingertips as you give your lover a massage or light spine-tingling chills. There are now many books on tantric sex. Get one and learn to use sex for your personal spiritual unfoldment. Enjoy...

(All supplements mentioned in this article should be available from your local health food store.)

CHINESE HERBAL FORMULAS FOR INCREASING LIBIDO

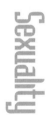

These formulas can be used to increase sexual desire and performance when the following other symptoms are also found.

Women's Formulas:

1. Women's Precious
- ✧ sallow and pale face
- ✧ dry skin
- ✧ pale lips
- ✧ tendency towards anemia
- ✧ insomnia
- ✧ dizziness
- ✧ weak vision
- ✧ heart palpitation

2. Women's Rhythm
- ✧ irregular menstrual cycles
- ✧ menstrual cramps
- ✧ breast distention at menses
- ✧ excessive blood clots during menses

3. Gather Vitality
- ✧ appetite disorders: under or over weight
- ✧ fatigue with digestive upset
- ✧ dull complexion
- ✧ tired limbs
- ✧ irregular stools
- ✧ nausea
- ✧ sleep problems

4. Dynamic Warrior
- ✧ low back pain
- ✧ cold hands or feet
- ✧ diabetes or blood sugar problems
- ✧ loose stools
- ✧ weak or cold knees

5. Woman's Treasure
- ✧ infertility
- ✧ low energy
- ✧ low back pain
- ✧ cervical dysplasia
- ✧ cold feet
- ✧ irregular menses
- ✧ anemia

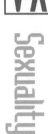

Men's Formulas:

1. Quiet Contemplative
- ✧ weak after ejaculation
- ✧ weak knees
- ✧ low back pain
- ✧ lots of wet dreams
- ✧ prostate pain
- ✧ chronic urinary infections
- ✧ hypertension
- ✧ fearful, no inner calm

2. Dynamic Warrior
- ✧ inordinately cold
- ✧ cold hands or feet
- ✧ lack of courage and will power
- ✧ asthma and shortness of breath
- ✧ lack of enough sperm, motility or fertility
- ✧ fatigue after sex
- ✧ loose stools

3. Relaxed Wanderer
- ✧ headaches
- ✧ dizziness
- ✧ fatigue
- ✧ stiffness of limbs
- ✧ digestive problems
- ✧ prostate pain or painful ejaculation
- ✧ hepatitis

4. Firm Vessel
- ✧ difficulty with erections and with maintaining erection
- ✧ low sex desire
- ✧ exhausted and dull minded
- ✧ prostatitis
- ✧ premature ejaculation
- ✧ pain on intercourse
- ✧ pale face
- ✧ lots of sexual dreams
- ✧ nervousness and anxiety

5. Quell Fire
- ✧ colitis
- ✧ prostate swelling
- ✧ indigestion with burping and gas
- ✧ painful or swollen testicles
- ✧ explosive behavior or belligerence
- ✧ genital herpes or eczema

MEN'S ISSUES

A Few Words About Birth Control and Safe Sex

There are no perfect methods for birth control. Men should take a more active role in discussing birth control methods with their partners. Women patients and friends often complain to me that their boyfriends will not use a condom. Apparently these women feel reluctant to confront their partner and force the issue. Instead, many women still take birth control pills.

If a man really cares for his partner, he will do every thing possible to keep her from taking the pill. Putting synthetically-derived hormones into the body on a daily basis is not a good idea, particularly as there are other effective and less-harmful methods of birth control.

If men were to discover that using a condom could be as vital a part of the sexual experience as intercourse, it would aid their partners quite a lot. Of course, using a condom is *pro forma* in our era of safe sex, but I am surprised by the number of couples I talk to who do not practice safe sex because one or the other of them does not want to be troubled by the use of a condom.

Sterilization for men or tubal ligation for women is not a good solution to the problem of birth control. I have seen many men and women who suffer from health problems as a result of the surgery itself. Whenever you undergo surgery you will have scar tissue, and this scar tissue will affect the flow of energy in your body. For this reason alone, you should always think twice before undergoing any surgical procedure. It is very common to develop other apparently unrelated health problems after surgery. I often see patients whose surgeries not so coincidentally preceded their current health problem.

Thank God for surgery—but only use it when necessary, and never for the sake of convenience. Get with it, men! Talk to your partner about birth control and safe sex. And women, if your man won't talk to you about pregnancy and birth control, you should seriously think about whether this is the kind of man worth your involvement.

One last point about safe sex. *Even if both you and your partner test negative for HIV, you should still practice safe sex.* Some of the latest research supports the theory that AIDS is not necessarily caused by HIV. The fact is that we still don't know a lot about AIDS. Why take needless chances?

THE PROSTATE AND SEXUAL FUNCTION IN MEN

What factors are involved in male sexual health?

There are a number of different factors involved in male sexual function and performance:

1. the relative health of the sexual organs;

2. the vital force, essential energy or what the Chinese call "chi";

3. the degree of connection within a man to other levels or centers of energy in the body; and

4. the degree to which a man is able to attain a feeling of intimacy, closeness and connectedness with his partner.

What is the prostate gland?

The prostate gland is at the root of most male sexual problems in one way or another. The prostate gland is located below the bladder and surrounds the urethra (see diagram). The prostate is responsible for secreting a thin fluid which forms part of the semen. It is also involved in controlling and maintaining muscle contractions necessary for bowel movement, urination, and ejaculation.

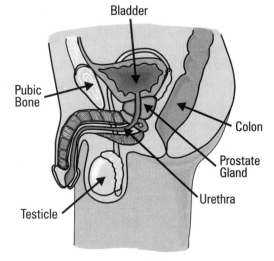

According to Western medical statistics, two out of four men over the age of fifty have at least some symptoms of an enlarged or inflamed prostate gland, i.e. prostatitis. But according to Oriental medicine, there is absolutely no need for this to occur, no matter what the age of the man.

What is prostatitis?

An enlarged prostate gland is called prostatitis. According to Western medicine, the causes are age or having a history of gonorrhea or other bacterial infections affecting the urinary tract. According to Oriental medicine, the causes are "stuck chi," or stuck energy in the area of the lower energy centers. The prostate is affected because of a weakness in this area. Oriental medicine calls prostatitis *Damp Heat in the Lower Burner.* The root of the problem is usually located in the Liver, Kidney, and Spleen meridians.

Typical signs of an enlarged or inflamed prostate can include weak urine flow, difficulty in urination, more frequent urination, low back pain for no structural reason, decreased sexual desire, painful ejaculation, pain in the perineal area (the area between the genitals and the anus), constipation, or diarrhea.

How can acupuncture help in treating prostatitis?

According to Oriental medicine, prostatitis usually originates with obstruction or blockage in the energy of the Liver and Spleen meridians, or weakness in the kidneys. Treatment is aimed at unblocking the stuck energy. Acupuncture needles are usually placed at points on the Liver, Spleen, and/or Kidney meridians (near the ankles and on the lower legs). A few needles may also be placed on the lower stomach, about two inches below the umbilicus and near the pubic bone. Acupuncture is painless and extremely relaxing.

How do diet and nutrition affect the prostate?

According to Oriental medicine, diet plays a significant role in creating prostatitis and can make a substantial contribution toward curing the disease. The best diet for this particular problem is aimed at detoxifying the liver and strengthening the kidneys. It is low in fats, oils, sweets, and sugar. Dairy products, refined carbohydrates, and simple sugars will all cause congestion in the prostate, liver, and spleen. Alcohol, tobacco, coffee, recreational drugs, and stress will also exacerbate symptoms.

The diet must be tailored to the particular constitution of each individual, but it generally should include plenty of pumpkin, squash, sunflower seeds, and almonds. A lot of raw and cooked vegetables and seasonal fruits are also beneficial. Some men need more vegetables and fruits while other men may need to eat some animal products to balance out their yin and yang.

Which vitamin supplements should be taken?

Specific vitamins and supplements often used to prevent or treat an inflamed prostate include the following:

✧ Vitamin F (essential fatty acids)
✧ Vitamin E (dry or emulsified)—400 to 800 IU per day
✧ Chlorophyll Pearls (a liver detoxifier)
✧ Zinc Picolinate—25 mg per day
✧ Vitamin C (in a buffered form)—up to 5,000 mg per day
✧ Vitamin B_6—50 mg per day

The need for various amounts of different vitamins and herbs is different for each individual. Be sensitive to your body's feedback while you experiment to find your optimal dosages.

Which herbs are good for treating prostatitis?

Ginseng, fo-ti and yohimbinum are all good for improving energy and sex drive. For the general health of the prostate and urinary tract the following herbs are good: juniper berry, damiana, kelp, echinacea, corn silk, uva ursi, birch leaf, horsetail. All herbs can be taken in capsule, tincture, or tea form. The amounts need to be determined for each individual through trial and error, or with the assistance of a health practitioner.

There are also some wonderful Chinese formulas which are very effective in the treatment and prevention of prostatitis.

Which homeopathic remedies are good for prostatitis?

❊ *Sabal serrulata* for frequency of urination and perineal pain.

❊ *Chimaphilla umbellata* for the feeling of a mass in the perineal region, the inability to pass urine except while standing with legs wide apart and body bent forward.

❊ *Clematis* for frequency of urination with weak, thin jet and dribbling afterwards; associated with epididymitis (an infection in the testicles or spermatic cords).

❊ *Conium* for older men who are sexually abstinent and who may be depressed or timid and fear being alone.

❊ *Equisetum (Equis.)* for painful urination, especially after or right at the end of urination; good for chronic urinary infections or for use as a bladder flush.

❊ *Staphysagria* for burning pains between urination, which stops during urination; occasional obsessive sexual thoughts; onset of illness can also be caused by unexpressed anger or resentment.

❊ *Causticum* for involuntary urination while coughing, laughing, sneezing, or for no reason at all; emotionally a sympathetic person. Useful for urinary retention after having had surgery.

❊ *Lycopodium (Lyc.)* is useful for urinary pain with impotence or premature ejaculation; sufferer may have low back pain or other pains which are mostly on the right side of the body; emotionally the patient may feel angry at those loved best; difficulty digesting fats; craves sweets.

NOTE: Do not take homeopathic remedies if you are unfamiliar with their use. Please refer to the section on homeopathy or see your health practitioner for directions on taking the remedies.

> *...males are not rewarded for investing in the emotional component of human relationships. In our production-oriented society, no accolades are given to men who value personalities at the expense of making one more sale, seeing one more client, or publishing one more paper... Let's face it, fame and glory do not come to men who strive to keep their lives in balance and who refuse to neglect their important relationships. The rewards in doing so can only be private ones.*
>
> —*Harriet Goldhor Lerner, Ph.D.*

SEX AND INTIMACY

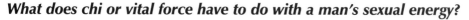

What does chi or vital force have to do with a man's sexual energy?

To a large extent, chi is dictated by heredity. But with a good diet and specific exercises, herbs, acupuncture, or homeopathy, a man can strengthen his chi to increase his vital force and sexual energy.

What exercises are good to increase sexual energy and function?

First, and most familiar to us in the West, are the Kegel exercises. These are the same exercises that women use to increase their sexual ability. The Kegel exercises for men can increase their staying power and sexual desire and help to build chi. Simply walking for an hour a day is very good, as are swimming and bicycling. Most aerobic sports are helpful, as long as they don't cause injuries.

Many yoga exercises are specifically designed to increase sexual power. Perhaps the most effective are the internal exercises of Taoist yoga. Until recently, the Taoist approach to sex was fairly unknown in the West. Now there are quite a few books available on this subject. Many of these exercises increase the connection between the lower chakras (energy centers) and the upper chakras, or between the genitals and the heart and pituitary gland. As the lower chakra (sexual energy) and the upper chakra (heart energy) are joined and integrated, a more powerful and prolonged sexual flow occurs.

What does intimacy have to do with sex?

The traditional "achievement machine" mentality programmed into men limits their ability to enjoy other aspects of sex and the sensual experience of making love. When intercourse becomes the chief goal of sex, and performance and technique dominate emotions, perceptions, spontaneity, and sensuality, there is little opportunity for intimacy. What results is eventual boredom and loss of interest in your partner.

Conversely, when sexual energy *is* tied to intimacy with your partner, different aspects are allowed to emerge. Sex becomes a microcosm of the overall health of a relationship. Various "selves" can get involved and participate more fully. The "playful child," the "romantic lover," etc.—all can have a role and thereby help to expand the overall enjoyment and fulfillment of the sexual experience.

Men's sexual health is not based on a simple formula. Emotions, the prostate and other sexual organs, diet, exercise, and attitude all play a role in sexual function. It is best to focus on a holistic approach to overall health—including mind, emotions, spirit, and body—and sexual health is sure to follow.

MEN: HOW'S YOUR PROWESS?

Webster's Dictionary defines prowess as "a brave act, superiority in ability, skill, technique, or the like. — Syn. See heroism." And I think that sometimes as men, it is in fact an act of bravery whenever we jump into bed with a woman. Whether in dating, having to overcome the fears of STDs (sexually transmitted diseases), or the performance anxiety that all men have, it takes a lot of guts to "go for it" with a woman. Let's be honest guys—it's a simple sign of masculinity to be able to perform well sexually. This article will give you many helpful suggestions and tools you can easily use to raise your prowess, your courage, bravery and performance level in bed.

To begin with, let's cut to the bottom line, and get away from the idea that performance is synonymous with ejaculation. It's not! In fact, if I might again rely on the good old Webster's Dictionary, performance is defined as "the execution of the functions required of one; effective operation, as of a motor; a deed or feat." So let's go ahead and define performance in terms of contemporary sex between a man and woman.

Sexual performance needs to be defined within the context of its being the ultimate in communion, or communication between two people. In fact, the Taoist say that sex is the ultimate way to show our love for each other and in so doing, to unite with the universal spirit, or God, or whatever you choose to call it. So the goal of our performance isn't so much the event of ejaculation as it is in the foreplay and **process** of lovemaking leading up to the ejaculation. And the best sex is actually had by both the man and the woman when the man is able to learn to control his ejaculation so that he can please the woman longer and more dynamically. When one learns to "perform" in this way, the ejaculation becomes almost anticlimactic to the entire lovemaking experience itself.

However, the first step in any lovemaking is for the guy to have a strong sexual desire to begin with. Without desire, there is no motivation to even have sex. So for those of you whose sexual desire has dwindled, here are some tips you may want to try. All of these suggestions will also help in creating better staying power, and many of these suggestions will also help in increasing potency, for those men suffering from low sperm count or low sperm motility.

❀ *Yohimbinum* in a homeopathic tincture form or in capsules is very good for most men in both increasing desire and overall potency. This herb has been used for centuries all over the world. It is known to excite sexual organs and act on the central nervous system. It's a great aphrodisiac, but should not be used if there is any abdominal inflammation, such as colitis or ulcers. It will help with erections, both to strengthen and help them to last longer. This is the primary ingredient in many of the expensive, commercially available aphrodisiacs you see advertised on late night TV infomercials.

- *Damiana* is another good herbal remedy for impotency or sexual debility from nervousness or from the nervous system being overtaxed and burned out. This is also used in homeopathic form when there are accompanying prostate problems, as in inflammation or pain in the prostate.

- *Kali phosphoricum* is a wonderful homeopathic remedy to be thought of when there is overall debility and fatigue and a disinterest not only in sex, but in life in general. It can also be used in Chronic Fatigue Syndrome and will work to perk up the entire nervous system.

- *Jin Suo Gu Jing Wan* is an incredible herbal formula from our treasure chest of Chinese herbs. This particular formula, also called Golden Lock Tea, helps to maintain erection and staying power. It's also great to take after ejaculation, to restore vitality and strength.

- *Ginseng Nutritive Formula* is a general tonic for sexual exhaustion when there is accompanying anxiety or nervousness, chronic fatigue, insomnia, heart palpitations or poor appetite.

- *Shou Wu Formula* is another general tonic for sexual exhaustion when there is accompanying graying, loss or drying of hair, dizziness, blurry vision or spots in vision, elevated cholesterol and a dry throat.

In Chinese medicine, it is common to categorize problems according to the cause, and instead of treating the symptoms alone, to treat the cause. When there is sexual debility, lack of staying power or lack of interest in sex, a Doctor of Oriental Medicine will treat the cause with much greater success and long-term effectiveness than just treating the sexual symptoms. The following four Chinese herbal formulas are to be used based on the specific cause, discussed below:

1. *Kidney Yin Deficiency:* Symptoms will be similar to those mentioned for the Shou Wu Formula and will also include dry mouth, constipation or dry stools, thirst, low back pain, possible night sweats, inability to hold the ejaculation, and irritability. One of the most common formulas used is Rehmannia Six Formula.

2. *Kidney Yang Deficiency:* Symptoms may include cold hands and feet, diabetes, chronic diarrhea, weak, painful or cold knees, weak or cold back, chronic fatigue, inability to maintain ejaculation, loss of interest in sex, fatigue, easily tires even with plenty of rest, and pale skin. A primary formula is Rehmannia Eight Formula.

3. *Stagnant Liver Chi:* Symptoms may include pain in the prostate, premature ejaculation, poor eyesight, blood in the urine, painful urination, painful ejaculation, headaches, hypoglycemia, restlessness, red eyes, hernia, gallstones, hepatitis, swollen testicles, addictions to tobacco, sugar, alcohol or drugs and muscular tension around the neck and shoulders. Two primary formulas are either Minor Bupleurum or Gentiana Formula.

4. *Damp Spleen Chi:* Symptoms of damp spleen might include a thick coating on the tongue, abdominal bloating after eating, diarrhea, flatulence, headaches, chronic prostate problems, fatigue, pain on ejaculation, indigestion in general, burping, nausea and poor appetite. Two good formulas are either Saussurea and Cardamon Formula or Ginseng and Astragalus Formula.

Any discussion of male sexual performance must also always include a discussion of prostate health. (See section on prostate health, beginning on page 190.)

Acupuncture is very effective at increasing sexual interest and performance and overall potency. The primary acupuncture points which are used include CV 4 and 5 and Spleen 4 and 6.

Exercise will increase sexual desire, help staying power and keep the prostate healthy. It's also important for men to practice the Kegel exercises, which many women practice to increase the sexual satisfaction of their male partners. The Kegel exercises can be found in many books on sex and pregnancy for women and in Mantak Chia's books on male sexuality. There are also many yoga exercises that are very effective. Yoga when combined with breathing is a very powerful healing tool.

Breathing can also be used very effectively during lovemaking to "move" energy from the lower chakras to the higher and visa versa. The ability to move energy throughout the body's chakra system at will is really the key to effective sex and sexual satisfaction. If you have too much energy in the genitals, you can learn to move it up and into the heart area. If you are too much in your head, you can learn to channel it down and into the heart and genitals.

The traditional "achievement machine" mentality that men are taught limits their ability to enjoy other aspects of the sexual and sensual experience. Certainly touch, taste, smell, breath and sound are all as arousing and fulfilling as the genital experience and can last for hours longer than a simple ejaculation. When intercourse alone becomes the chief goal of sex and performance and technique dominate over feelings, spontaneity and sensuality, there remains little opportunity for intimacy. Without intimacy, what results is eventual boredom and loss of interest in sex.

Conversely, when sexual energy is tied to intimacy with your consciously chosen partner, many different aspects of your inner world are allowed to emerge. Sex is an opportunity to become a metaphor for the overall health of the relationship, both between the man and woman and as a metaphor for the man's relationship with himself and his own inner sense of personhood and manhood.

(Please note that the suggestions in this article are not meant to be used without the advice of your health practitioner. If you are on any prescription medications or homeopathic remedies, do not change your prescription without the advice of your doctor. If you have any health conditions, you should always check with your doctor before trying any new herbs, vitamins or homeopathics.)

YEAST AND OTHER VAGINAL INFECTIONS

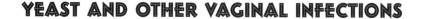

What is vaginitis?

Vaginitis refers to any inflammation of the vagina. Symptoms may include—but are not necessarily limited to—vaginal discharge, irritation, itching, odor, increased frequency of urination, reddening, burning sensation during urination, or small blisters.

What is the cause of vaginitis?

There are many possible causes. Your immune system may be run down. Vaginitis can be transmitted sexually and it can be caused by taking too many antibiotics. Other causes may include fecal contamination from wiping in the wrong direction, over-absorbent tampons, allergies to fabric softeners or synthetic underwear, the birth control pill, too frequent or too intense intercourse without sufficient lubrication, scented toilet tissue, or tight jeans.

There are different types of vaginitis, including bacterial (*gonococci* and *staphylococci*), protozoan (*trichomonas*), and fungal or yeast (*Candida albicans*). The symptoms of each type can be very similar. A vaginal culture and laboratory analysis is usually required to correctly determine the specific type.

What is the Western medical treatment?

If a culture is not taken, a physician will sometimes give the diagnosis of "nonspecific vaginitis" and treat it with sulfa drugs or topical creams. If antibiotics or antifungal creams are used, you are killing the bacteria and yeast along with some of the friendly bacteria. You're also adversely affecting your pH. The friendly bacteria and correct pH level are necessary to establish homeostasis for good health and long-term balance.

What is the holistic form of treatment?

The natural approach builds your friendly bacteria and boosts your immune system to resist unwanted or unfriendly bacteria or yeast. The long-term effect of using the holistic approach means that over time you will no longer be prone to getting yeast infections in the first place. This enables you to stop the dependence on drugs and antifungal creams that in reality *lowers* your overall resistance and immunity.

What is the treatment according to Chinese medicine?

Basically, you must have had a weakness or imbalance to be susceptible to vaginitis. The doctor of Oriental medicine takes your complete history and examines your tongue and pulses to arrive at a diagnosis. Usually, a woman who has vaginitis has what is called *Damp Heat in the Lower Burner, Cold Damp in the Spleen,* or *Liver Heat.* This is just a metaphorical way of saying that you have specific congestion in your system. Usually the tongue will have a thick coating, especially in the back. The thicker and darker yellow the coating, the more severe the condition.

Pulses will sometimes show a weakness in Fire or yang, or they may show a weakness in the Kidney meridian. If Damp Spleen is the cause, there may also be "teeth marks" or indentations along the sides of the tongue.

Because Oriental medicine tries to determine the exact cause of a problem, vaginitis can be attributed to weak Kidney Chi, Spleen dampness (immune problems, or problems assimilating cold and damp foods), or Liver stagnation (toxicity). Beyond this, Oriental medicine would say that you must have had either an inherited constitutional weakness or imbalance to begin with, a prolonged period of stress, or poor eating habits.

What is the best diet to cure vaginitis?

The best diet is one that strengthens your immune system. This is a little different for each person, depending on their constitutional imbalances.

Here are some general rules: it is usually best to stay away from dairy products, with the exception of live cultured products such as kefir and yogurt (and this unsweetened and never frozen). Fried, fatty, and oily foods also cause more congestion and weaken the immune system. Sweets and sugars provide a medium for unwanted bacteria and fungus to thrive and reproduce. Also avoid shellfish and cold or frozen foods (such as frozen yogurt), as these create dampness, congestion, and toxicity in your system.

The best diet is predominantly made up of complex carbohydrates, including vegetables and grains, and a small amount of seasonal fruits. Meat-eaters may add fish and lean poultry. Some people will do best on an all-vegetarian diet. Others will do better by adding a few animal products.

Can acupuncture help?

Yes, unless you are taking a deep-acting constitutional homeopathic remedy, which will cause interference. Besides treating the weak meridians in your body to balance yin and yang energies, acupuncture can be used to boost your immune system and build your chi to fight infection or invasion by bacteria or fungus.

What about herbs? Which ones can I use?

A combination of quince, ginger, and cloves in teas or capsule form is sometimes very effective (and also good for skin eruptions such as herpes). Black walnut and goldenseal in capsule or tincture form are also effective antibiotic and antifungal herbs. There are also many good Chinese herbal formulas, depending on the specific symptoms involved.

What is a good natural douche?

Natural douches can help to relieve discomfort and aid healing. For a yeast infection, take 2 ounces (or 6 tablespoons) crushed or rolled flaxseed. Boil the seeds in 1 quart of purified water for 10 minutes; strain. For each pint, add half a teaspoon of eucalyptus oil. Use about 4 ounces per douche. Insert using a "baby" ball syringe and retain for 20 to 30 minutes (use a tampon). Rinse with purified warm water. The mixture may be refrigerated and reheated in a double boiler for future use. The treatment is best if done one or two times daily.

Another, simpler douche mixes roughly two tablespoons of live cultured yogurt with a quarter- to a half-teaspoon of high potency acidophilus; this is inserted vaginally, followed by a tampon.

For a very simple cleansing and antiinflammatory douche on a daily basis, use one dropper of aqueous Calendula mixed with a little water.

Most pharmacies also carry vaginal homeopathic suppositories that are sometimes effective.

Should I increase my intake of vitamin and nutritional supplements?

Some women find that taking vitamins and other nutritional supplements helps amplify their immune systems. Keeping in mind that each person's vitamin needs are different, depending on diet and constitution, the following is a good general vitamin program for treatment of acute infection:

✧ Vitamin C (buffered, chelated or esterified)—1,000 to 3,000 mg per day

✧ Vitamin B (balanced, 50 mg)—1 to 2 per day

✧ Beta Carotene—25,000 IU per day

✧ Zinc Picolinate—15 to 30 mg per day

✧ Vitamin E (emulsified or dry)—400 to 800 per day

✧ High potency Acidophilus—3 times per day

Which homeopathic remedies are good for vaginitis?

Because the prescription of homeopathic remedies is based on individual symptoms, you will want to pay particular attention to the amount and type of pain and sensation (burning, bland, shooting, stabbing, pressure, hot); any discharge (white, green, yellow, reddish, clear, thick, thin, stringy, clotted); the time of occurrence (before menses, after menses, before or after intercourse, time of day); and any other unique symptoms on either a physical or emotional level that may be alternating or coinciding with the vaginitis. As the symptoms change, you may need to change homeopathic remedies unless you are being treated constitutionally.

Here are a few examples of some possible remedies with a few of their indications:

❋ *Alumina*—Thick, clear or white discharge, itching, burning, with accompanying constipation; worse after menses; menses too early, short, scanty; worse in a warm room.

❋ *Borax*—Discharge is thick and gelatinous like egg-whites; feels as if warm water is flowing; itching; menses coming too soon with profuse bleeding and severe cramps.

❋ *Graphites*—Discharge is thin and watery with burning; menses is later than normal with weakness in the back; aversion to sexual intercourse; breast tenderness.

❋ *Merc Sol*—For acute bacterial infections, including vaginitis; odorous, greenish-yellow discharge; burning; itching; worse after urination; menses are profuse; worse in damp weather.

❋ *Pulsatilla nigricans*—Discharge can vary in appearance, but usually creamy, burning, and acrid; the person is usually weepy and emotional, restless, desiring company and consolation; menses are late and scanty; person will prefer to be in open air or have windows open; rich foods will cause indigestion although they may be craved.

❋ *Sepia*—Discharge is yellow, greenish, and itching with a sensation of "bearing down" in the uterus; lower abdominal discomfort; intercourse is uncomfortable or painful with a lack of interest; the person will enjoy movement, dance, exercise, and generally want to be left alone.

❋ *Natrum phosphoricum (Nat. p.)*—Discharge is creamy or honey-colored but may be watery, sour smelling; yellow coating at the back of the tongue with a sense of a lump in the throat; excess of acidity in the digestive system; menses are earlier than normal.

❋ *Sulphur, Natrum Sulph, Medorrhinum* or *Thuja occidentalis*—These are more constitutional remedies for chronic problems and usually not used without a practitioner's assistance.

Before trying any of these homeopathic remedies, be sure to read the rules and precautions discussed in the section on homeopathic medicine.

What else can I do to prevent a yeast infection?

It is important to remember that if you are sexually active with multiple partners, or if your partner has multiple partners, you could be sharing bacterial or yeast infections.

Be sure to get plenty of rest and stay away from stressful situations as much as possible. If you are experiencing a lot of discomfort, it is best not to have intercourse. Warm baths can be soothing. Add a little aqueous solution of Calendula to the bath.

You can also microwave your cotton underwear to kill yeast. Make sure there are no synthetic fibers in the underwear, because they can damage the microwave.

BREAST AUGMENTATION*

In July 1987, a 24-year-old female expressed a desire for breast augmentation. At first I was hesitant to take the case, but after reviewing the literature and hearing her personal story, I was persuaded that acupuncture, homeopathy and herbs might help her.

She also requested help with stopping smoking and drinking alcohol. She was on birth control pills, had a diet rich in sugar, fats and animals products and expressed no desire to change her diet or stop birth control pills.

According to traditional Chinese medicine her diagnosis was Liver stagnation with Kidney Yin deficiency. Her symptoms included premenstrual syndrome, difficulty in relaxing (loves to dance/party/keep moving about), very sensitive emotionally, very

---

*This is a reprint of an article written by Dr. Martin which first appeared in *The American Journal of Acupuncture*, Vol. 17, No. 3, July–Sept. 1989.

warm emotionally, wide mood swings, warts (despite repeated surgical removal), pelvic inflammatory disease, insomnia, headaches.

She reported that due to an emotional trauma at age twelve, her breasts had significantly shrunk "almost overnight" and never grown since.

Her diagnosis according to classical homeopathic medicine was a "sycotic* miasm."

She was treated weekly at first and then every other week for the first ten months; thereafter, every two to three weeks, from July 1987 through February 1989, for a total of approximately twenty months. The following points were treated, alternating from week to week: Sp 4,6,9; Kid 3,7,25,26,27; St 36,30,29; Liv 2,3,14; CV 4,5,6,12,17,22; Hrt 1,7; Pc 6; Yintang; Zigong; UB 11,13,15,17–21,23,25,28,60.

Homeopathically, the sycotic miasm was treated with constitutional remedies, as well as consideration of the following rubrics from Kent's *Repertory*: "Chest, atrophy, mammae" and "Mind, forsaken feeling." The following homeopathic remedies were prescribed: Nat. mur., Sepia, Pulsatilla, Thuja, Sabal serr., Mammary gland, and Natrum sulph.

Herbal and nutritional supplements included the following: red raspberry, dong quai, glandular mammary, pituitary, adrenal, ovary, and thyroid, black currant seed oil, quince seed (a topical decoction on the breasts and as a tea internally).

The patient's breasts grew in size a total of three inches (measured around the chest in the traditional manner.) The treatment was an obvious success and the patient was very happy with results.

The trauma that occurred at age twelve may have altered her hormone balance. The treatment was aimed toward correcting this imbalance and the concomitant emotions.

According to the patient, the treatment was most effective when she was regular in her weekly treatments including taking and topically applying her herbs and homeo-pathic remedies. Although progress was slow, it was also very steady and, according to the patient, directly proportional to her degree of compliance.

Given the vast amount of money spent on surgical breast augmentation, it is gratifying to see these results with a non-invasive and traditional form of medicine. I have personally treated a number of women who have had surgical breast augmentation and they all were suffering symptoms of sever Liver stagnation/Fire rising, possibly at least in part resulting from the implants. (Or maybe small breasts are a symptom of a constitutional Liver stagnation condition to begin with.)

It would be interesting to conduct research on this type of treatment. There is considerable literature on this subject and given the surgical alternative, one should not hesitate to take on this type of case. On the other hand, psychotherapy may be warranted in some cases, either instead of treatment or before treatment, to clarify

*Sycotic—one of the four miasms; the sycotic miasm creates such problems as depression, sadness, moles, warts, freckles, tumors, cysts and fibroids.

the patient's goals and motives. Given the society we live in, which places so much emphasis on particular body types, it would be wise for anyone considering cosmetic surgery to consider counseling as well as non-invasive approaches well before any permanent alteration to their body.

NATURAL TREATMENT FOR PREMENSTRUAL SYNDROME

IS PMS RUINING YOUR RELATIONSHIP OR THREATENING YOUR JOB?

(The following is a selected excerpt from Dr. Martin's Doctoral dissertation on the effective holistic treatment of PMS)

"I was crying for two weeks out of the month," remembers Carol M. She had consulted with her therapist, her Western-trained physician, and tried most of the natural remedies at the health food store, and still had no success at relieving her symptoms. She ate well and exercised daily, and still nothing helped.

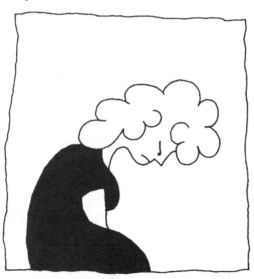

She ruled out estrogen therapy because of its links to uterine cancer and didn't want to take "the pill" because of similar risks.

After coming to my office it took only two months to relieve her symptoms by about 80%. Her treatment consisted of weekly acupuncture sessions, a change in diet based on her "body type" according to Chinese medicine, increasing her intake of specific herbs and eliminating certain foods.

In addition, I selected a constitutional homeopathic remedy based on her health history, family background and emotional and spiritual outlook on life. The homeopathic remedy immediately helped her to sleep better and feel more relaxed. It also reduced the breast tenderness, headaches and menstrual cramping.

Over seventy percent of my PMS patients see relief of most symptoms in two to three months. If there are fibroids or endometriosis then the treatment will take a bit longer since we are also working at the same time to eliminate the growths.

PMS*

What is premenstrual syndrome?

Premenstrual syndrome is one of the most common health problems facing younger women in our culture today. About one third to one half of the American adult female population between the ages of fifteen to fifty experience some sort of PMS. This translates to a lot of missed days at school and work, severe stress on relationships, as well as a lot of needless suffering.

The symptoms of PMS begin ten to fourteen days prior to the start of menstruation and end in the first few days after the onset. There are more than 150 symptoms that have been associated with PMS. Listed below are some of the most typical:**

irritability	anxiety	moodiness
anger	headaches	skin problems
vertigo	weight gain	bloating
joint pain	back pain	cramps
constipation	diarrhea	sugar craving
sore throat	vision problems	chocolate craving

It is very common for women to have many of these symptoms combined, and not unusual for there to be alternating symptoms on a month to month basis. Some months may even be symptom free.

What is the cause of PMS?

PMS is caused by both psychological and physiological imbalances. Psychologically, the primary cause is stress. Physiologically, the primary cause is an imbalance of estrogen and progesterone. Other secondary causes include poor diet, heredity, and lack of exercise.

Factors which have been shown to correlate with higher risk of having PMS include the following:**

- Being in your thirties
- Major emotional stress
- Poor eating habits
- Women who have side effects from birth control pills
- Significant weight fluctuations
- Lack of exercise
- Unmarried
- Pregnancy complicated by toxemia
- The more children, the more PMS symptoms you are likely to have.

---

*This is a condensed version of Dr. Martin's Ph.D., doctoral dissertation on the treatment of PMS using nutrition, acupuncture, homeopathy and herbal medicine, completed in 1984.

** Lark, Susan M., M.D. *Premenstrual Syndrome Self-Help Book*. Berkeley, Calif.: Celestial Arts, 1995.

From the point of view of Oriental medicine, the primary meridian systems involved in most women with PMS are the Liver, Spleen and Kidneys. The extra meridian called the Chong Mo is also often involved. (Please refer to the chapter on Oriental medicine for an explanation of PMS in these terms.)

The causes and treatments of PMS are commonly grouped together in six different types for convenience. Each type is conveniently classified according to the kinds of symptoms most commonly experienced, and each type also has its own unique causes and cures.

Type A experiences anxiety, irritability and mood swings before the period. These problems stop as soon as the menstrual flow begins. Eighty percent of women with PMS are noted to have Type A, although it is common to have more than one type at the same time. Type A is caused by a relative abundance of estrogen relative to progesterone levels.

Estrogen is a female hormone produced by the ovaries (see diagram on page 151). When there is too much estrogen circulating in the blood stream, it creates the symptoms of Type A. The cause can be either an imbalance in the endocrine loop that regulates estrogen production in the body or the liver is toxic and is not breaking down and disposing of the excess estrogen produced by the ovaries.

In Type A PMS, treatment is aimed at regulating estrogen function on the level of the endocrine glands, and in improving the function of the liver. See treatment methods discussed below.

Sixty percent of women with PMS are noted to have Type C, or an increase in craving for carbohydrates, sweets, alcohol, pastries, bread, chocolate, etc. Eating these foods creates even more craving which in turn causes mood swings, fatigue, headaches, dizziness, etc. It is a vicious, downward cycle, as those of you have experienced compulsive eating well know.

The cause of Type C is hypoglycemia, or low blood sugar. This is due to a complex chemical reaction in the body involving an endocrine gland called the pancreas (see page 151). The pancreas secretes insulin, which is meant to regulate and keep the blood sugar balanced. But for a woman who suffers with Type C PMS, the body is much more sensitive to insulin just before the period. The more sensitive your body is to insulin, the lower your blood sugar falls. The lower your blood sugar falls, the more cravings for foods to increase yur energy and oxygen to the brain and muscles.

The liver is also partially at fault in Type C. When the liver is working well, it will automatically help keep blood sugar at normal levels, but when toxic or enlarged from past overindulgence in refined carbohydrates and sweets, it is not capable of doing its job well. To some extent, Type C may also involve the adrenal and thyroid glands as well, since the complexity of endocrine gland feedback loops in the body is rather extensive.

Treatment of Type C is aimed at balancing blood sugar by changing the diet and balancing the thyroid, adrenals and pancreas.

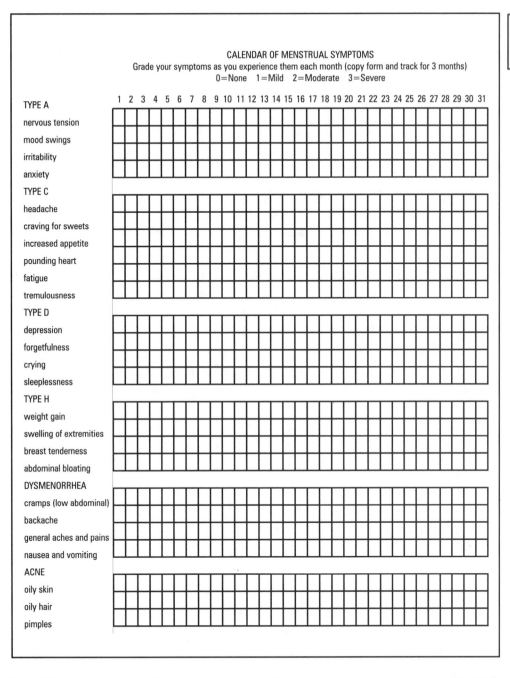

CALENDAR OF MENSTRUAL SYMPTOMS
Grade your symptoms as you experience them each month (copy form and track for 3 months)
0=None 1=Mild 2=Moderate 3=Severe

	1 2 3 4 5 6 7 8 9 10 11 12 13 14 15 16 17 18 19 20 21 22 23 24 25 26 27 28 29 30 31

TYPE A
nervous tension
mood swings
irritability
anxiety

TYPE C
headache
craving for sweets
increased appetite
pounding heart
fatigue
tremulousness

TYPE D
depression
forgetfulness
crying
sleeplessness

TYPE H
weight gain
swelling of extremities
breast tenderness
abdominal bloating

DYSMENORRHEA
cramps (low abdominal)
backache
general aches and pains
nausea and vomiting

ACNE
oily skin
oily hair
pimples

Type H, or hyper-hydration, is experienced by forty percent of women with PMS. Symptoms of Type H include bloating, swollen breasts with tenderness, weight gain, migraine headaches and vision problems. The cause is an excess output of a particular hormone from the pituitary gland called ACTH. This hormone indirectly causes the body to retain too much sodium thus causing fluid retention.

Treatment of Type H is aimed at eliminating all sodium from the diet and strengthening the kidneys and pituitary gland, thus balancing pituitary hormones.

The fourth type of PMS is called Type D, which stands for depression. Additional symptoms are confusion, insomnia, memory loss and in severe cases, suicidal thoughts. It is caused by the ovaries not producing enough estrogen. By itself Type D is seen in only five percent of women with PMS, but when combined with Type A, it is seen in twenty percent. It is potentially the most serious type.

Type D will not respond to the traditional progesterone treatment that many Western-trained medical doctors use. Instead, treatment is aimed at stimulating the secretion of female reproductive hormones, and in particular, estrogen, produced by the ovaries. This may also involve the thyroid and pituitary glands.

The fifth grouping of PMS symptoms includes acne, blackheads, cystic acne, oily skin and hair, and other skin problems. These symptoms are usually caused by lower levels of estrogen or by an increase of male hormones, called androgens, which affect the skin pH.

Skin problems are treated by eating a more alkaline diet, eliminating sugar, and taking teas and herbs to cleanse the blood. It is also important to balance the hormones, cleanse the liver, and improve overall digestion and assimilation. In terms of Oriental medicine, we look at the balance of Yin with Yang.

The sixth type of PMS is not technically PMS since it usually does not begin until after menstruation begins, but for simplicity of treatment and classification, it is ordinarily discussed along with PMS. The symptoms of this type include cramping, diarrhea, shooting pains, nausea, vomiting and low back and/or leg pains. This can last anywhere from one to four days and is due to an excess of a chemical produced in the uterus called prostaglandin F. This causes painful uterine muscle contractions.

Treatment of this last type is usually aimed at increasing prostaglandin E, which is an antagonist to prostaglandin F. Increasing dietary sources of calcium and especially magnesium also helps ease the cramping.

What are some general treatments for PMS?

Diet is the first and foremost factor that is within your control. So let us first look at your diet. Foods known to increase symptoms of PMS include the following: caffeine, milk, hard cheese, salt, chocolate, sugar, alcohol, beef, pork, lamb, and pickled foods.

Foods helpful in reducing the symptoms of PMS are the following: whole grains, brown rice, oatmeal, millet, Pritikin-type breads with no added oils, salt or sugar; all vegetables, but especially beets, carrots, collard greens, mustard greens, and beet tops; fish, and all kinds of beans are your best sources of protein (follow recommendations for your metabolic type).

Certain vitamin supplements are also helpful depending on your particular needs. The two most important are vitamin B_6 for bloating, water retention and other Type H symptoms, and magnesium for cramps and uterine pain. Vitamin C is important to combat stress, as are all the B vitamins. A good, well-rounded multiple high in vitamin B is a good preventative.

If you suffer from cramps be sure to take twice as much magnesium as you do calcium. Also take evening primrose oil or black current seed oil, which will help reduce uterine cramping by increasing the production of prostaglandin E.

Twenty to thirty minutes of exercise daily also plays a large role at balancing the hormone levels. As simple an exercise program as walking thirty minutes per day usually has a beneficial effect. Outdoor exercise has been shown to be more beneficial than indoor exercise.

Chromium is a great supplement for treatment of Type C PMS. It has a regulating effect on the blood sugar. Try this along with licorice root tea or herbal capsules to strengthen the adrenal glands. Dandelion tea will help to detoxify the liver and red raspberry leaf tea is good for tonifying the thyroid gland. Dong Quai is an herb that will help to balance the female hormones and is available in both tea or capsule form.

For skin problems use cayenne, ginger root tea to help in digestion and burdock, which has blood cleansing effects. For hypoglycemia, low energy or mood swings, add licorice toot to the dandelion root. You can also buy fresh burdock root at the health food store and use it in your stir fry, the same as you use carrots or parsnips. Burdock has a great cleansing effect on the blood, will help with acne, and also reduce bloating, due to its diuretic effects.

If you have trouble with digestion, this can lead to skin problems and/or bloating so be sure to take digestive enzymes or a good digestive tea such as Ponay. Ginger and gentian are also helpful for digestion, as is peppermint. But if you are taking homeopathic remedies, do not use peppermint.

How can homeopathy help with PMS?

Keep in mind that although it is fine to treat yourself with homeopathic remedies, a long term PMS problem may take the expertise of a trained homeopath. This will depend upon the duration and severity of your particular PMS symptoms. Either way, you can expect a significant reduction in symptoms, if not a total cure, in between two to four menstrual cycles!

For menstrual cramps there are a number of different remedies. *Colocynthis* type of cramps are relieved by doubling up, bending forward, applying pressure or warmth, as are *Magnesium phosphoricum* cramps. The pain may radiate out in all directions from the uterus. Colocynth pains are more likely to make you irritable than the woman who needs Mag. phos.

The dosage and potency for these and other suggested homeopathic remedies listed below are to take five tablets, three to five times per day in a 6X or 12X potency. If the remedy is going to work you should begin to feel an improvement either immediately or after about three doses.

Always stop taking the remedy if you feel worse or if the symptoms stop. When the symptoms decrease, also stop taking the remedy. If you keep taking the remedy after the symptoms stop, you will cause them to come back again. Note that often only one dose of the correct remedy in the correct potency is all you need. Be sure to follow all the other rules listed in the homeopathy section of this book.

For symptoms of fatigue or weakness, try *Calcium carbonate*. This remedy will be particularly helpful if you also have headaches, sweating and are cold in general. Also for fatigue is *Sepia*. For Sepia to be indicated usually you will also have low back pains, cramping in the lower abdomen, loss of interest in sex and an increase in anger and intolerance for others. Depression and moodiness is also common. Sepia is a common remedy for use in Type D PMS.

WARNING: If you have never used homeopathy, or if you are unfamiliar with the constitutional and emotional aspects of what homeopathy can do, it is best not to self medicate. This is because you could have a "healing aggravation" or "proving" and you would not know what to do or how to integrate the information that was coming to you.

For excessive weeping, sadness, or oversensitivity, a primary remedy is *Pulsatilla*. Other indications for Pulsatilla are a desire for company, a desire to be outside or to have windows open, nausea, giddiness, fainting, and unpredictable or changeable moods.

Chamomile is another remedy for excessive moodiness, with faultfinding and snapping over little things. It will also show symptoms of cramps that feel like labor pains.

The *Lachesis* personality may be angry and moody with ovarian pains that are worse on the left side. Dizziness and diarrhea, a dislike for tight clothing or anything tight around the neck are also characteristic of Lachesis.

Prognosis: How long will it take?

Usually it takes between two to four menstrual cycles to experience a significant improvement. It depends on the severity of your problems and the degree to which you are able to exercise, to change your diet, and to work on lowering your stress level.

Having suffered from severe PMS for many years, I doubted that I would ever find relief. After several months of acupuncture treatments, my menstrual cycles are practically symptom-free and I am beginning to enjoy my life again.   *—D.B., Accounting Manager*

Thank you, Randy, for the support...I can barely remember how things were before we met and I started treatment...Wow! What a change!   *—C.D., Teacher and Homemaker*

PMS DIETARY GUIDELINES

Upon Waking

✧ One cup of tea (mint, licorice, chamomile, or any caffeine-free tea); or use a coffee grain drink substitute

Breakfast

Breakfast should consist of

1. Fruit—papaya or mango is best (but an apple, pear, or banana is also okay); fruits in season are best; fruit should be eaten alone or 30 minutes before other foods

2. Grain—2 rice cakes, oatmeal, brown rice, millet, buckwheat, quinoa, amaranth, whole grain muffins, or any whole grain cereal dry or with soy milk

3. Protein—1 egg, tofu, tempeh, beans (garbanzo, lima, adzuki, black-eyed peas, kidney, pinto, etc.) or a 4 oz. piece of fish or chicken

Mid-Morning Snack (two to three hours after breakfast)

Many people have different needs for between-meal snacks. The snack food quantities are approximate and should be based on individual needs. Make certain your snacks follow the dietary guideline for your metabolic type (see page 141). You must eat some high-quality protein with your complex carbohydrates in the ratio that is best for your body type, even during your snacks.

Choose any two of these options:

✧ 1 or 2 rice cakes
✧ Handful of pumpkin seeds
✧ Soy drink
✧ Vegetable juice
✧ Carrot or celery sticks
✧ Peanut butter or tahini on rice cake
✧ 6 to 8 almonds
✧ Apple, pear, or banana
✧ ¼ avocado
✧ Small yam
✧ ½ hard-boiled egg

Lunch

✧ Raw vegetable salad
✧ Cooked vegetables (see recommended list)
✧ Whole grain or 2 rice cakes
✧ Protein (follow recommendations for your metabolic type)

Afternoon Snacks

✧ Every 2 hours until dinner, same as mid-morning snacks

Dinner

If no protein was eaten during the day, then it is necessary at dinner.

✧ Protein—fish, tempeh, tofu, lean poultry, beans, eggs, low-fat yogurt, or kefir (follow recommendations for your metabolic type)
✧ Salad
✧ Cooked vegetables (may have 2 servings)
✧ Hot tea or coffee substitute (no cold drinks!)

Late Night Snacks

Same as mid-morning, but for a sweet tooth, try

✧ Amasake
✧ Westbrae or Ah Soy
✧ Fruit kanten (see recipe below)
✧ Yam
✧ Kabocha pumpkin
✧ Fruit

Fruit Kanten Recipe

✧ 2 cups apple juice
✧ 1/3 cup agar flakes
✧ Fresh fruit of your choice

Slice fruit (try strawberries, blueberries or banana) and place into small plastic containers. Bring juice to boil and add agar flakes. Simmer on low heat for 2 to 3 minutes, until agar is dissolved. Pour this liquid over the fruit and refrigerate until hard. Then it is ready to eat. Think of it as "healthy Jello"!

This recipe can also be made with yam, amasake, soy drink, etc.

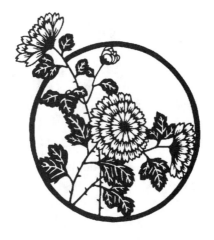

PREMENSTRUAL AWARENESS: A HOLISTIC APPROACH AND PHILOSOPHY

From a speech delivered by Dr. Martin at an international acupuncture conference in 1990

Introduction

It is important when treating PMS to remember that the doctor is treating people, not symptoms; and each person exhibits a particular energetic, intellectual, physical, and spiritual individuality. It is within this context that the treatment of PMS may play a larger role in women's lives. In addition to physical symptoms, unique emotional issues that arise during the treatment of each woman must also be addressed.

I find most women have already been run though the medical mill with progesterone therapy, the birth control pill, and referrals to psychiatrists or other therapists for antidepressants or psychotherapy. Dissatisfied, many have tried self-treatment only to be confused by various over-the-counter PMS medications, herbs, and vitamins. When combined with a toxic liver, confusion and disillusionment combine to create an irritable, skeptical, cynical, or outright angry woman.

Psychological considerations

During the time before her period, a woman may feel very sensitive, angry, sad, depressed, or experience any number of other intense emotions. In addition, many women may find they are filled with increased self-awareness and feelings of creativity. In a culture that places more emphasis on productivity than on creativity and self-expression, the creative aspects in us are that is often ignored. By ignoring this need for profound self-expression that is larger and more encompassing than the ego-self, a woman may experience even more feelings of sorrow, grief, depression, and moodiness.

Psychologist Carl Jung described this dark, repressed, cut off, or blocked part of a person as the *shadow self.* According to Jung, the shadow self has not been fully acknowledged in some way. In women, this may be a reflection of the hidden animus—the yang or male part of a woman. To the extent that the shadow remains unconscious and unexpressed, in Jungian terms a woman will be in an "animus-possessed state of judgment and emotionality."

The animus can be very difficult to contact because of its unconscious nature. It may only arise during periods of emotional turmoil such as the time just before menstruation. The animus may appear in disguise—often as a sweet, though unreal and superficial, cover for moodiness or as a very moody or very angry person afraid to get in touch with her true self.

In terms of Oriental medicine, I have found the angry animus, cloaked within the shadow, to reside in what the Chinese call the Wood Element. The other, "sweet" animus resides most often in the Fire Element.

Joyce Mills, Ph.D., points out that the time before menses provides an opportunity for women to turn inward—to examine deeper issues in their lives and portions of their psyches that may not otherwise be available for critical examination or transformational exploration. In Native American cultures, this same biological process was viewed as a source for both women's and the community's self-growth, creativity, and empowerment. By contrast, PMS is viewed negatively in our culture—women are thought of as "on the rag," and not to be taken too seriously.

In his book *The Psychobiology of Mind-Body Healing,* Dr. E. L. Rossi discusses the implications of the hormonal shift during menses and its potential to change a woman's personality. He states that when these changes are unsupported and misunderstood, they can lead to social and personal maladaptation, depression, and illness. When the changes are welcomed as an opportunity for personal growth and transformation, increased states of consciousness, awareness, and development can occur.

PMS as an opportunity for growth

Oriental medicine has the capability to catalyze and encourage women with PMS to look at it less as a problem than an opportunity to learn more about an aspect of their femininity and their personality. The process of becoming conscious of the animus and of the shadow self of the unconscious can be arduous, yet immensely worthwhile. Such changes can be profound.

Case Studies

Case 1

A 38-year-old married homemaker with two children complained of severe PMS in July 1984. Her symptoms were preceded by the birth of her second child three years before and a severe emotional trauma surrounding the critical injury of her husband.

She complained of extreme weakness, fatigue, inability to remain alert without eating frequently, muscle and joint stiffness, irritability, depression, disorientation, palpitations, a negative reaction to caffeine, and shakiness. She described herself as serious and a perfectionist. Most of these symptoms would commence a week before her period. She also suffered from cramps and backache the first two days of her period. Her diet consisted of a lot of red meat, eggs, fast foods, caffeine, and sweets.

I began treating her once a week using acupuncture points on the Stomach, Liver, Kidney, and Gallbladder meridians. She also received multivitamins and minerals for her particular symptoms. After a month the treatments were reduced to once per month, just before menses. After 4 months, she was almost free of symptoms and was instructed to return for treatment on an as-needed basis.

Case 2

A 34-year-old accountant came for treatment of PMS. Her symptoms were severe sugar cravings, irritability, moodiness, psoriasis, and left-sided sciatic pain before her period. She also had a history of abnormal uterine bleeding, pelvic inflammatory disease, and mitral valve prolapse. Her diet was high in fats, salts, dairy products, sweets, and caffeine and she rarely exercised. Her diagnosis was Damp Heat in the Lower Burner, toxic blood, depleted yin, excess yang, and blocked Liver and Gall Bladder Chi.

She began acupuncture twice a week for approximately three months, followed by treatments once a week for an additional five months. Her treatment points were primarily on the Large Intestine, Liver, Spleen, Stomach, Lung, and CV meridians. Herbal liver detoxifiers were prescribed along with a multivitamin and mineral supplement. She was also given homeopathic remedies to detoxify and balance her hormones.

Despite the fact that she did not change her diet and still got little or no exercise, her condition progressively improved. After six months of treatment she began to stop smoking and changed her diet. This was encouraging; her psoriasis also began to improve. A year after treatment she expressed a openness to counseling and discontinued acupuncture. Periodic tune-up treatments kept her symptom-free.

Case 3

A 43-year-old administrator came to my office complaining of severe menstrual cramps, constipation, and a chocolate and sugar addiction before her period. She used Advil for the pain, but expressed a desire to stop using any drug treatment.

I treated her using a homeopathic progesterone remedy and other homeopathics for hormone imbalances. She also received acupuncture on the Spleen, CV, and Stomach meridians. After one treatment, her next period was pain-free. She exercised regularly and I continued to treat her twice per month for a total of six treatments. A year later she came in for treatment of an unrelated problem and reported that she had been crampfree ever since the acupuncture.

Case 4

A 30-year-old psychotherapist complained of severe PMS with headaches, mood swings, and cramps. She was diagnosed with stagnant Liver Chi and Kidney Chi deficiency. I advised her to stop drinking coffee, increase her exercise level, take an herbal liver detoxifier and a calcium-magnesium supplement, and use homeopathic remedy for the cramps. The acupuncture points I employed in her treatment were primarily on the Stomach and Spleen Meridians. She was seen twice a month for three months and became symptom-free after two months.

Conclusions

These four cases illustrate the effectiveness of a combined approach to PMS using acupuncture, nutrition, exercise, and in some cases homeopathy and herbal

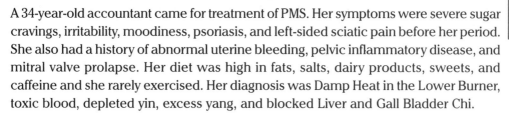

medicine. A majority of women will benefit from stress reduction; outdoor exercise is the key to success. I have also found that poor diet is a major contributing factor in cases of PMS.

There are no single answers for all women who experience PMS. Each should be encouraged to explore previously undiscovered aspects of her feminine and/or masculine side that may be denied effective creative outlets.

ENDOMETRIOSIS

Having treated endometriosis successfully for many years, the most common question women ask is: "Can you cure it?" As with most other health problems, the answer is rarely an easy yes or no.

Using a unique approach, and taking into consideration each woman's individuality, nine out of ten women will generally be symptom-free after a period of 3 to 6 months. But endometriosis is a very complex disease process and the causes are different in each woman's case. Often treatment requires active participation by the patient in the form of psychotherapy, exercise, and dietary changes. Endometriosis is a disease process that will usually require major dietary changes and a new emotional awareness for complete recovery.

Endometriosis is most often associated with imbalance in the Wood and Earth Elements. Chinese herbal formulas and acupuncture are also used to break up "congestion" in the uterine area. Homeopathic remedies are helpful; they can often facilitate the healing process and cut healing time in half. Vitamin supplements are used in some cases, depending on the eating habits and constitution of the person. The most common supplements used are the antioxidants, including vitamin C, vitamin E, beta carotene, selenium, germanium, and zinc.

Some of the herbal formulas I use to help women with endometriosis include the herbs Cinnamon, Paeonia, Bupleurum, and Dandelion Root. Other herbs are used to match the symptoms of the particular person's constitution. Fatigue, abnormal menstrual flow, and cramping are some of the most common symptoms treated with the herbal approach.

Some patients are purists and prefer to be treated with only one modality. You have your choice! After all, I believe you should take charge of your own healing process. Homeopathy is many peoples' preference. It is a good choice as a single healing modality because it so effectively treats the whole person.

There are also some specific herbs and homeopathic remedies that can be used to dissolve old scar tissue so common to this problem. Scar tissue is sometimes the major factor affecting a woman's ability to get pregnant.

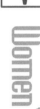

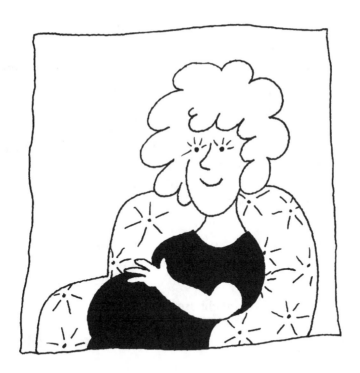

PREGNANCY AND CHILDBIRTH

The Chinese have a saying that when a baby is born, it is already nine months old. Actually, the baby is a lot older than this because it has already inherited all the genes and constitutional predispostions from both parents, its grandparents, etc. The best thing a prospective mother and father can do for their child is to undergo homeopathic and acupuncture treatment for a year or so before they conceive their baby. If both parents are in balance, the baby will be much more likely to be born healthy.

The second important factor is the women's nutritional status and emotional health, both before and during the pregnancy. It is very important for the woman to take the appropriate supplements during the pregnancy and while nursing. Especially important is the addition of easily assimilable folic acid and vitamin B_{12} during the first six months of the pregnancy. Avoiding sweets, fats, alcohol, fried foods and white flour products is also advisable. Alcohol is particularly harmful to the fetus' developing nervous system and can permanently damage it. The first six months are the most critical, but damage can occur at anytime, so alcohol should be avoided altogether if possible.

It's also important for the woman to maintain her energy during pregnancy and nursing. Many women do not get adequate exercise and this can negatively impact on her body and emotions. There are some specific Chinese formulas that can increase chi (energy) at the various stages of pregnancy.

Homeopathy and acupuncture can be used during pregnancy for such problems as headaches, morning sickness, threatened miscarriage, sore breasts, yeast infection, heartburn, emotional problems, varicose veins, colds, constipation, irritable bladder, liver toxicity, morning sickness, appetite problems and edema.

Toward the end of pregnancy, there some specific homeopathic remedies that can be given to make the birthing experience go more smoothly. The remedies can be taken without risk for the fetus or mother when a few common sense rules are followed. Recent research has shown that women receiving homeopathic remedies before labor and/or during the birth have less complications, shorter labor, less pain, and quicker recuperation time. Acupuncture is also very effective for relaxation, pain relief, or to hasten a prolonged or difficult labor.

Specific homeopathic remedies given to mother and child immediately following birth decreases the chance of complications and shortens recovery time. Postpartum depression is also treated very effectively using acupuncture and homeopathy.

Homeopathy for infant and young children is invaluable for such problems as ear infection, colic, constipation, diarrhea, skin problems, eye infection, fever, croup, colds, poor sleeping habits, allergy, teething, diaper rash or emotional upset.

MENOPAUSE

Technically, menopause is defined as the time in a woman's life after her menses has stopped. Menopause is also termed the "change of life." Although menopause is a natural process and part of human nature, because of the lifestyle most women live today, some of the symptoms most women get are anything but natural or ordinary.

Menopause usually begins between age 40 and 52 years, although in cases of surgical removal or irradiation of the ovaries, menopause may be artificially induced prematurely. The average age of menopause is 50–51 years old.

How do I know if I'm going into menopause?

Symptoms of menopause will vary greatly. Easy, symptom free menopause is possible for the average women. But most women have been used to the symptoms of severe PMS most of their lives so they assume a difficult menopausal period, as well.

Many women, by the age of 35 or 40 years, begin to experience increased PMS, menstrual irregularity and decrease in fertility. There are other women who have had no PMS symptoms and don't experience any menstrual irregularities at all until full cessation around age 50 or so.

Generally, women who have been without PMS symptoms throughout their lives can be said to have hormonal balance, and these same women's hormones will usually remain in balance throughout the menopausal transition. This will be relatively symptoms-free menopause.

It's the hormone imbalance that causes the symptoms. During the transition period of menopause there is a gradual decrease in estrogen levels. Treatment, whether natural or conventional, is aimed at correcting this imbalance in hormones.

Eighty percent of women in menopause experience hot flashes, but the degree of intensity and frequency vary tremendously. Other symptoms include changes in the vaginal and urinary tract, mood swings, anxiety, and depression.

The most common signs and symptoms of menopause are the following:

- ✧ hot flashes with sweating
- ✧ atrophy of the urogenital epithelium and skin/vaginal dryness
- ✧ osteoporosis
- ✧ high cholesterol or high triglycerides
- ✧ nervousness and irritability
- ✧ depression and insomnia
- ✧ urinary tract: frequency of urination and/or burning upon urination

Laboratory findings will usually confirm menopause by showing increased FSH hormones, decreased urinary estrogens, and a serum estrone level that is greater than that of estradiol.

Other conditions that may look a lot like, or similar to, menopause are the following:

- ✧ pregnancy
- ✧ amenorrhea

Which types of treatments are best for menopausal symptoms?

Menopause is not a fatal or even a dangerous condition, as the Western medical establishment might try to convince, although it can be extremely uncomfortable and present socially embarrassing problems. Also, the bone loss associated with menopause can lead to hip problems and difficulties later in life. Conventional treatment from your medical doctor uses hormones to replace the depletion of your naturally occurring hormones. However, estrogen replacement therapy is linked to possible cancer risk, although the data is inconclusive.

When at all possible, it's always preferable to first try some non-conventional therapies. The choices include nutritional and dietary changes, Classical homeopathic medicine, acupuncture, and herbal medicine. These four treatment modalities have always proved successful with my patients, no matter what the severity of their symptoms.

It should also be mentioned that even if a woman is symptom-free, these same treatment modalities can be utilized quite successfully to prevent or minimize any future symptoms from occurring. The sooner a woman begins a program of prevention, the more likely she will be symptom free later on down the line. A woman does not, by any means, have to be experiencing menopausal symptoms in order to begin integrating the ideas in this book into her everyday lifestyle. Dietary changes and a good vitamin/mineral supplement and herbal regimen will add energy, vitality and balance to any woman's life, whether or not she is experiencing menopausal symptoms. In addition, the correctly chosen constitutional homeopathic remedy will give further assurance of a symptom-free life.

Which homeopathic remedies do you suggest for menopause?

Well, remember that a Classical homeopath, which I am, never prescribes a homeo-pathic remedy based on the name of a disease! Rather, the remedy is chosen based on the individual and unique symptoms of the individual women. (Please refer to the homeopathy section in this book.) But the following are some of the most commonly prescribed homeopathic remedies for women who are menopausal. However, remember that there are hundreds of other good homeopathic remedies, and if you have severe symptoms you should never try to prescribe a homeopathic remedy for yourself.

Please note that the following descriptions are grossly oversimplified personality-type profiles, and to actually accurately diagnose and choose the appropriate homeopathic remedy usually takes a good homeopath about an hour.

Lachesis

This remedy, made from the venom of the Bushmaster snake, contains some of the keynotes of menopause quite strongly. The person who needs this remedy may have a fear of snakes or a fear that others are watching them or are behind them. They can't stand tight clothing, and in particular, don't like anything tight around their waist or neck.

They may have trouble getting to sleep, and will generally feel worse when they wake up. Headaches are very typical symptoms for the Lachesis individual, and they will often occur on waking and be on the left side. In fact, most symptoms will be on the left side of the body: swollen glands, ovarian cysts, sore throats, hip, back or sciatic pain, etc.

There will be the typical pulsations and hot flashes with perspiration, with a lot of excess heat in the body. There may be a lot of bruising and black and blue marks on the skin with discoloration. This individual will dislike gentle touch, but may enjoy deep massage. They are violently jealous and extremely talkative. Their symptoms will be worse in the sunlight and worse in hot weather, they may sleep on their right side and have a choking or suffocative sensation.

Finally, the Lachesis type may crave oyster and starchy foods, have severe menstrual cramps and be dealing with a chronic sense of guilt and indecision.

Sepia

Sepia is a commonly used homeopathic remedy for many types of hormonal imbalances, from PMS to menopause and uterine problems. The Sepia type will usually be cold and emotionally and physically distant, preferring to be alone and even aloof. Sepia types don't crave affection and sympathy when they don't feel well, and usually prefer to go to their room and close the door to be left alone.

Their hot flashes will be sudden, and may be accompanied by fainting or flushing headaches. There will be weakness, irritability, violent outbursts of temper, and feelings of isolation. Constipation and indigestion with hemorrhoids are very common in the Sepia type, as are a history of liver or gall bladder problems.

One outstanding feature of the woman who does well on Sepia is her strong desire for dance or active exercise of one sort or another. She may be a jogger, dancer, swimmer, or have always found solace in some active sport from early on in her life. Her symptoms, whether it be a headache or irritability, will usually be relieved with active exercise, although the sex drive in a Sepia type will usually be quite low or even absent. In fact, celibacy or spiritual abstinence is a common Sepia characteristic, although certainly doesn't pertain to all Sepia types.

A few additional points are that they may be sarcastic (even have cutting sense of humor), crave sour-flavored foods, such as vinegar or pickles, have an unusually large amount of hair on the face or body, and have had difficulty getting pregnant or have a history of miscarriage.

Sulphur

A third remedy that can often have many of the same symptoms that one finds in menopausal women is called Sulphur. The Sulphur type is known for its skin symptoms, everything from herpes to eczema, psoriasis and hives. I'll always ask a patient if they've had skin problems in the past, as a part of my normal intake questioning, and a common response is: "No, I just had the rash at age four which went away after the use of some type of ointment."

But what one must remember when treated homeopathically, is that any skin rash that was treated with ointments was actually suppressed. This suppression of the skin symptoms always creates other problems in the body/mind/spirit complex, and needs to be considered when one is choosing the constitutional homeopathic remedy. The Sulphur type will generally have had at least one instance of a suppressed eruption at some point in their life, followed later by some new symptom, like asthma, or urinary problems. (Please see the homeopathy section for more on this subject of suppression.)

Generally the Sulphur type will uncover the feet in bed during the flushes of heat. They usually will run warm, or even hot, and crave alcohol, sweets and fatty foods. They may dislike eggs, fish, and sour-tasting foods. They may have early morning diarrhea, forcing them to rush from their bed, have a history of sinusitis, and have big appetites.

The Sulphur type is more extroverted than the Sepia type, and may be a rather strong woman herself, who dislikes authority or control in others. They may also be quite the intellectual, a collector of things or ideas, and be fairly critical of others. A common sleep position will be on their left side.

Women's Issues

Arsenicum alb.

The next remedy sometimes used during menopause is homeopathic Arsenic. This type will have insomnia after midnight with many anxious dreams. They may despair their own recovery and feel it's helpless, be full of anxiety, worry, phobias, various fears, and find it impossible to quiet their mind. During their hot flashes, they may also feel chilly, and, unlike the Sulphur type, always feel better with warmth.

They may experience burning, either in the form of hot flashes, diarrhea, vaginal discharge, or elsewhere. Itching, ulcers and palpitations are also commonly found with the Arsenic type.

They are restless, "on the go" people, usually with a strong social network, who prefer the company of others, although they are quite insecure, attentive to detail, nit-picking, on the slim side, and can even be obsessive-compulsive.

Calcarea carbonica

The Calc carb type is rather opposite in many ways to the Arsenicum type. Calc carb tends to be pale, overweight, cold, easily tired, obstinate, and enjoy the company of family. They have peculiar fears, such as insects, mice, and the dark. They can be cold, clammy, and want to keep their feet covered during night sweating.

Since this remedy is made from oyster shell, and has a high degree of calcium in its composition, it may show signs of calcium deficiency, such as having a lot of cavities, weak or brittle bones and low bone density. They perspire easily, even when not having hot flushes, especially around the head.

They may crave sweets, eggs and starchy foods and have a lot of indigestion and belching. Milk may give them diarrhea. They are very responsible types, who may take the world on their shoulders and may suffer from low back pain.

Pulsatilla

The last remedy I'd like to discuss within the context of menopause is called Pulsatilla, or common windflower. This "flower-like" personality may cry easily, be very changeable, easily consoled by her friends, feel better around people who display affection towards her, and feel better in the open air. She may keep all her windows open and enjoy taking walks and hikes in the cool breeze. In fact, if kept in a closed room, she will usually feel a bit claustrophobic.

Her food preferences include a large helping of bread and butter, and other rich fatty foods. She'll always uncover her feet during hot flushes, and possibly have arthritic pains that are never in the same place. She may be heavy-hipped and be the "earth mother," care-giver type. She can be easily influenced and easily dominated by another strong type, and will usually be on the shy side.

She may also have varicose veins, headaches with red cheeks, and hay fever. Her menses will have always been changing, never the same, she may have fibrocystic breasts, and sleeps on her abdomen.

Which type of diet is the best for preventing symptoms?

It's important that the diet contain plenty of high quality, easily-assimilable protein. Following the recommendations for diet under the section "Metabolic Type Diet Plan" to assure you obtain the proper amount of protein for your body type. Emphasize fish in your diet, but stay away from shellfish. Shellfish is toxic and creates what is called "heat in the blood," which will increase your symptoms.

Also avoid sugar and white flour products, which cause toxicity in the Liver meridian. Avoiding caffeine, alcohol, and any dairy products that are high in fat is also helpful. Smoking will also cause excessive heat and make it difficult to eliminate symptoms.

Foods which are known to be helpful include yams, all soy products, peanuts, barley, oats and brown rice, all of which will stimulate and/or mimic estrogen in your body. Other estrogenic foods include all animal protein, apples, cherries, olives, plums, carrots, coconut, wheat, and the entire nightshade family (potatoes, eggplant, tomatoes, etc.)

Which types of supplements are best to take to prevent and/or treat menopausal symptoms?

Vitamin E is one of the best you can take. (You can also take Vitamin E suppositories for vaginal dryness, along with a non-alcohol-based wild yam topical ointment.) Licorice has a positive effect on the adrenal glands and so helps to balance blood sugar and stimulate/regulate the other endocrine glands.

The two most commonly used herbs used for any hormonal imbalance are Vitex (Agnus castus) and Dong Quai. Both of these herbs have a strong effect on the endocrine organs and will help to balance the estrogen. Some health practitioners claim that one should not take Dong Quai if there is a risk of fibroids, but the research on the estrogenic effects of Dong Quai are not conclusive in either direction.

For those of you who are not vegetarians, I would recommend the use of glandular supplements. These can include ovary, thyroid, uterus, pituitary and adrenal. Although available over-the-counter (OTC), glandulars are very strong and should not be experimented with unless you are under a doctor's supervision.

Two other very common supplements that are being used a lot recently are the hormones DHEA and pregnenolone. Both of these can have very important effects in the body and I would discourage any woman from experimenting with these on their own. In my practice, I always perform comprehensive blood tests before prescribing any hormones, even though these are OTC.

For anxiety, I recommend the use of tryptophan and GABA, two powerful and very effective amino acids. Remember, as mentioned in other sections, that when you take an amino acid, you always are advised to take pyridoxal-5 phosphate (a special form of vitamin B_6) to catalyze the amino acids into action.

Also of import are the essential fatty acids, including the GLAs and EPAs. You can obtain a balanced form of EFAs at the health food store, but I usually recommend fish oils and black currant seed oil. Another good form is borage oil.

What can I do to prevent osteoporosis?

Osteoporosis is occurring in frightening proportions in our culture. There are many different theories as to why it's taking place. Some researchers have connected it to the high intake of calcium in the Western diet. Others have blamed the problem on eating too much protein and meat in particular.

Women begin to lose bone minerals faster beginning at age 40. The rate of loss accelerates with the onset of menopause. Early diagnosis is difficult; that is why prevention is the best treatment. Risk factors include being Caucasian, removal of the ovaries, being underweight, a lack of calcium in the diet, lack of exercise, smoking, genetics (heredity), a small-boned and slender frame as opposed to large-boned and overweight, having poor digestion, chronic use of steroids, diuretics, or antacids containing aluminum, and a history of anorexia

The problem with most research into osteoporosis, as with most nutritional research in general, is that it's very hard to isolate nutritional factors in individuals when performing nutritional research. We are so unique and our biochemistry is so unique that it's next to impossible to isolate factors, such as calcium, in nutritional research.

To overcome this problem, I've evolved into using precise testing methods to determine osteoporosis risk and need for calcium supplementation. The two tests I always recommend for women concerned about preventing osteoporosis are the bone scan and the Health Equations analysis. There are a number of different types of bone density scans available. The important thing is to pick one and then stay with that one, year after year, carefully monitoring any changes. The Health Equations (HEq) analysis is explained on page 38. Briefly, the HEq analysis is a composite or relational blood analysis test that has the ability to show the functional utilization of the minerals in your body. Without a functional analysis, the typical static blood tests usually used are not very helpful. The functional analysis shows how your individual body is actually utilizing each of the necessary minerals in your body.

Synergistic minerals which generally need to be taken along with calcium include magnesium, silica, boron, manganese, as well as a wide array of "micro" minerals and synergistic vitamins, such as vitamin D, ovarian glandular and microcrystalline hydroxyapatite. Most of the top quality osteoporosis prevention formulas at the health food store will take a "shot gun" approach and already contain all the important elements you body needs to prevent osteoporosis, and if you don't have the time and money to get tested, then this is the direction I recommend most women take.

Which herbal treatments are best?

Common herbal treatments include dong quai, black cohosh, blue cohosh, red clover, wild yam root, and sarsaparilla. Herbs for emotional problems include oat straw, dandelion, Siberian ginseng, valerian root, passion flower, catnip, red raspberry, and chamomile.

Two of the herbal treatments I use most frequently are dandelion root and milk thistle. Both are primary herbs for use in detoxifying the liver and gall bladder and can be used in tea form, capsules or liquid tinctures.

How does Chinese medicine treat and/or prevent the symptoms of menopause?

As with other health problems and imbalances, the Chinese medical doctor uses a comprehensive variety of treatments, often including acupuncture, herbs, and nutrition, according to the five elements.

Treatment is based on imbalances in the Five Elements. In the case of menopause, the most common imbalance is between the Kidneys and the Heart. The Kidneys represent the Water element and the Heart represents the Fire element. When Fire and Water are in balance, there will be no symptoms of menopause. When Water is weak (i.e. weak kidneys), then the Fire will flare out of control and you will experience vaginal dryness, hot flashes, irritability and anxiety.

Treatment is aimed at strengthening the water and the kidneys through specific acupuncture points and Chinese herbal formulas. Nutritionally, you will want to eat foods from the Water element column of the Five Element food chart.

Specific herbal formulas will include such names as Rehmannia 6 and Quiet Contemplative. When there is Liver involvement, which is common with symptoms of hot flushes and headaches with irritability or depression, common formulas are Relaxed Wanderer; Bupleurum and Dragon Bone; and Bupleurum and Peonia.

To temper and sedate the Fire element and overactive Heart, common formulas include Compassionate Sage and Temper Fire. Finally, when there is Spleen and Earth element involvement, indicated by symptoms such as bloating, fatigue, water retention, flatulence, teeth marks on the sides of the tongue, we use formulas such as Prosperous Farmer, Gather Vitality, and Saussarea and Cardamom.

Final Thoughts

The main thing to remember is that not all women will experience menopausal symptoms. If you have been in balance hormonally during your life, the likelihood is far less that you will have any problems. Menopausal symptoms, like other health problems, are a barometer of a deeper imbalance that needs to be addressed from the holistic perspective.

If you approach your symptoms as the tip of the ice berg, and look to treat what's under the surface, rather than just to cover up the symptoms with drugs, you will be much happier and healthier in the long run. In my practice, I have many women completely overcome severe menopause symptoms within a few months using a combination of acupuncture, herbs, nutrition and homeopathy.

Women's Issues

You should also remember that if you don't have any symptoms of menopause, you can still be treated using acupuncture, homeopathy nutrition and herbs, to prevent and balance your body, and to assure you won't get symptoms later on down the line.

...The debate about hormone replacement therapy is framed against the basic assumption that the female body at menopause is deficient, primed for disease, and in need of treatment. As a result, a woman who is the least bit skeptical about the wisdom of hormone replacement therapy for herself is placed in the curious position of defending the decision not to take hormones. In truth, the burden of proof should be on her physician to show why she should take them.

—*Carol Tavris, The Mismeasure of Woman*

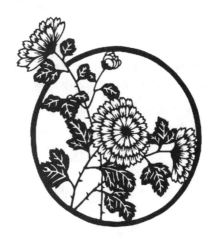

Women who stay on hormone replacement therapy for more than ten years increase their risks of developing fatal ovarian cancer by 70%.

—*American Journal of Epidemiology, 5/95*

PEDIATRICS

WHAT TO TELL YOUR DOCTOR ON YOUR CHILD'S FIRST VISIT

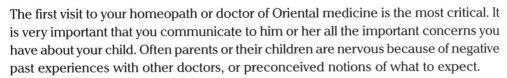

The first visit to your homeopath or doctor of Oriental medicine is the most critical. It is very important that you communicate to him or her all the important concerns you have about your child. Often parents or their children are nervous because of negative past experiences with other doctors, or preconceived notions of what to expect.

I encourage you to keep a health diary for your child (and yourself), and to bring it with you at the first and all subsequent visits. It is also most helpful if you make a list of important questions so that you don't leave without having all of your concerns addressed.

The other side of the first visit is the importance of listening to the doctor's instructions. Often, very important information on diet and remedies will be communicated. Try to stay aware of these. It is a great idea to bring a note pad and pen and to take notes. This saves both of you time in the future.

Phone calls should be reserved for emergencies. But if you discover when you get home or to the pharmacy that you forgot to ask something that might be important, always I call rather than wait for your next visit. As you explore homeopathy, you will eventually discern which questions are critical and which can wait a week or two. Here is a list of what should be discussed on your first visit to your doctor and a discussion of each:

✧ Health history of the parents and grandparents and any significant contagious diseases. This includes history of surgeries, drugs, and medications.

✧ History of the pregnancy itself.

✧ The birth.

✧ Diet.

✧ Blood work or any other laboratory work or x-rays.

✧ Complete physical health history of the child. History of vaccinations, and any adverse reactions.

✧ Complete emotional history of the child. Complete social history of the child. The child's personality characteristics, including astrology chart, if available (if you want to have your chart done, I can do it for you). The office visit itself.

✧ The treatment process and what it will entail. Your goals and expectations for the treatment of your child.

Health history of the family

The essential element is a history of any unusual diseases. Much of this may be indicated on the completed intake form. If it isn't, be sure to mention such things as cancer, diabetes, heart disease, tuberculosis, syphilis, gonorrhea, hepatitis, eczema or other skin problems, chronic headaches, depression, alcoholism, etc.

Many problems your child might be susceptible to will be genetic. The beauty of holistic treatment is that it can, in some measure, actually eradicate some of the body's cellular memory, making your child less susceptible to negative genetic influences. This may seem ridiculous to those who are more scientific in their thinking, but I encourage you to read about homeopathy and Oriental medicine before drawing your own conclusions. Much of this type of medicine acts on the cellular and molecular levels. This is why it has gained a reputation for being almost magical at times.

If either of the parents has taken a lot of recreational drugs, has a history of alcohol use, or taken over-the-counter or prescription drugs, this needs to be mentioned. Often there is a need to do some detoxification of the child before treatment begins. And, depending on the type of medications, this information can indicate a particular weakness in the child's inherited organs and glands.

It is important not to sanction any guilt you may feel for the negative physical traits you may have passed on to your child. At the same time, it is important to acknowledge and objectively report them. You will not be judged by your doctor and you shouldn't judge your past. What's done is done.

Ideally, both parents should be treated before hey conceive their child. It is important that the mother carrying the child be as strong as possible so that she can nurture and maintain a healthy child during pregnancy. Through the use of homeopathic medicine before conception takes place, it is possible to eradicate some of the negative predispositions that could otherwise be passed on to the next generation.

Homeopathy's concept of *miasm is* worthy of mention. Miasms are inherited predispositions to particular sets of diseases. It is vitally important to accurately report the parents' health history so that the doctor can determine if a miasm is involved.

Pregnancy history

This information is needed to determine if a child has undergone any trauma during gestation. Be sure to state if the mother smoked cigarettes, took any drugs, medications, alcohol, drank coffee, or ate a lot of sweets. Any trauma to the mother, whether physical or emotional, may also be of significance. The general diet of the mother and whether she was taking any nutritional supplements is also important.

The birthing process

This information determines whether there was any birth trauma, use of drugs, home birth, natural birth, etc. It's also good to note whether the birth was early, on time, or late, how long the birth took, whether the mother was under a lot of stress, if the father and other family members were lending their emotional support, or if they were absent.

Diet

The mother's diet is just as important to discuss as the infant's and child's diet, especially if the mother is currently nursing or has nursed for an extended period of time. The diet of the family in general is also notable, as the child will mimic its parents' and siblings' diets, thereby adding to or affecting genetic predisposition. The diet of the mother during the pregnancy is also to be noted.

As an infant, was the child breast-fed or bottle-fed? If bottle-fed, what type of formula was used? An especially crucial subject is whether the child is ingesting any dairy products, as they are often the primary cause of skin problems, colic, ear, and strep infections in young children. If hyperactivity is a problem, the diet in terms of sweets, additives, and artificial ingredients plays an even more important role. Skin problems or frequent infections also can be a result of poor diet.

Laboratory work

Often young children will not have previous blood or other laboratory work. If there was any significant history of health problems when lab work was performed, be sure to obtain a copy and bring it with you on your first visit. Simple problems such as anemia can easily be corrected using homeopathic constitutional remedies, but often go undiagnosed without the appropriate lab work. If any other tests have been performed, try to obtain copies and reports and bring them with you on your first visit.

It is very important for your child's healing team to include your traditional allopathic pediatrician and/or medical doctor along with your doctor of Oriental medicine and homeopathic physician. Each area or specialty should not be overlooked when the health of your child is concerned. Your pediatrician is an invaluable resource in Western diagnosis and as such can greatly enhance the achievement of optimal health.

Health history

This includes normal childhood diseases as well as any unusual problems. It is also important to discuss what form of treatment was used. If antibiotics were used, there has been a suppression of the immune system. If cortisone creams have been used on psoriasis, eczema, or chicken pox, the vital force has been suppressed—driving the disease process into a deeper and more vital level of the body. If antihistamines or inhalers are used for asthma, the same problem may arise. It i still possible to treat children who are taking prescription medications, but it may take longer to achieve the same results. If your child is taking vitamins or herbal supplements, be sure to identify these as well.

NOTE: *Never* take your child off prescription medications without the supervision of your doctor!

Vaccination history

Many parents fail to realize that many of their child's problems date back to the beginning of vaccinations. Although not all children have reactions to vaccinations, it is more common than most people realize. Think back to each vaccination and try to remember if your child suffered an adverse reaction. Common reactions include skin rashes, digestive upset or change in appetite, behavioral changes, fever, irritability, and the like.

Another approach to gathering this information is to recall when your child's problem began, then check your calendar or with your pediatrician to see if a vaccination preceded the problem. it is not at all uncommon to find a gap of a few weeks or even a month between a vaccination and when a problem began.

Emotional health history

It is important to mention any significant emotional trauma experienced by the child, even if it seems minimal to you as the parent. Remember that children are very fragile and easily affected by everything that goes on about them. If there has been a divorce or the death of a relative or pet, it may have affected the physical health of the child in some subtle way. Sleep difficulties or behavioral problems need to be assessed relative to the social dynamics of the family and siblings.

Social history

Much of this overlaps with the section on personality type. How does the child get along in preschool, school, or with siblings? If an infant, how does s/he relate to parents or siblings? Is the child outgoing or more of an intuitive or introverted type? Does s/he follow or lead in social situations? Get into fights or retreat? Play alone or prefer company? Like a shoulder to cry on or prefer to be alone to cry? How easily does s/he get upset? Does s/he repress feelings or easily express them? What do they do to get attention?

Personality characteristics

This can be the most important aspect of case-taking in homeopathic medicine. If you can read books on homeopathy it will help you define your child's personality more closely. As a tool in prescribing, I often have parents use checklists that are provided in some of the better homeopathic reference manuals. It is hard to be objective about your children—that is the main reason it's not advisable to treat them yourself for anything other than acute problems. But it is vital to report as much information on personality and social interaction as possible. Use as many examples as you can.

If you have access to the child's astrology chart it may prove helpful in discriminating the various homeopathic types. The astrology chart is especially useful in analyzing the child in terms of the Five Elements in Oriental medicine. Contact Dr. Martin and, for a minimal fee, he can create your child's astrology chart.

The office visit itself

Your child's behavior is important for the homeopath to understand, so the more you can let your child roam freely in the office, the better. (If your child is touching things that s/he shouldn't, please use a little discipline.)

Often the office receptionist will observe specific behaviors and point them out to me. This is very helpful. If your child is timid, affectionate, inquisitive, etc., the trained eye of the homeopath can use this information to evaluate the child's condition.

If your child is hyperactive, angry, or very ill, it is best to let her have free reign in the office for a few minutes. For example, if a child comes over and jumps on my lap, I immediately think of *Pulsatilla nigricans* or *Phosphorus (Phos.)* as an appropriate remedy. If the child is very scientific, asks a lot of technical questions, or wants to examine everything in the room, I may think of *Lycopodium*. If the child is destructive, I may think of *Tuberculinum* or *Medorrhinum.*

Sometimes the office visit will be very short. The homeopath may know the correct remedy right away and there will be no need to extend the visit. Other times, the visit may need to be longer than normal to collect more information. I have seen parents take offense at what they feel is a short office visit. It is best if the parent does not base an evaluation of the treatment's efficacy on the length of the office visit.

With my patients, I always include a few follow-up telephone consultations in the cost of the office visit. Often the most effective way to get some information is by the telephone. This is especially true if the child is very ill or hyperactive, when bringing him into the office would be a hardship on the child, the parent, siblings, the office staff, or the doctor.

Often a lot of homeopathic business can be conducted by telephone with only occasional office visits to monitor the child's growth and development. This is especially true for hyperactive children, small infants, and very young children. Photographs are also helpful and should be included in the child's medical chart, so that the doctor can recall the child and family when telephone consultations occur. If you have a good photo of the entire family, it will be very helpful to include it in your child's medical chart.

The treatment process and what it will entail

Be sure to discuss the treatment process with your doctor. Important points to discuss include length of treatment, frequency of office visits, costs, insurance billing, accessibility of homeopathic pharmacies, purchasing homeopathic books and remedies, and your feelings and attitudes about homeopathic treatment. It is important for the doctor to know your attitudes toward homeopathy. Often one parent will be supportive and the other antagonistic. If one parent does not live with the child, this can complicate the treatment procedure as well. Be sure to air all of your concerns during the office visits.

Goals and expectations regarding treatment

Communicate your expectations for homeopathic treatment to the doctor. Be certain that you ask the doctor what s/he thinks is the prognosis for your child's particular problem(s). Often it is not at all possible to make any predictions during the first few visits to your doctor, but after a few months s/he should be able to give you an idea of how your child will be responding to the remedies.

I always try to educate my patients that homeopathic treatment is a process that works wonders *over time.* If you can lower your expectations at first, you will be happier in the long run. With this in mind, you will be very pleased should quick, dramatic results occur. Keeping a Pediatric Homeopathic Health Journal

When using homeopathic medicines, it is important to keep a very clear journal of the person's symptoms. When the patient is your child, you can do a lot to contribute to the success of the treatment by writing a homeopathic journal.

Many parents bring their children to me for treatment and expect that the treatment will be immediately effective. This type of thinking lacks a sound understanding of what homeopathy really is and how it works. Often the treatment is immediately effective, but even in these cases there can be setbacks and complications.

With only very rare exceptions, all health problems are quite complex. A single homeopathic remedy will rarely cure your child of his or her problem(s), but don't be surprised if it happens.

I recently had a parent bring her little boy to me for a problem relating to nasal congestion. In the course of the interview it became apparent that he also had some problems with his diet. He was very particular about what he would eat. He craved frozen yogurt and other sweets but would not eat any protein foods. He disliked meat of any kind, including poultry and fish, and would not touch any legumes (another good source of protein).

His mother and I discussed his diet. I explained to the child the importance of eating either poultry or legumes. Then, in the same interview, I prescribed a homeopathic constitutional remedy for him.

His mother called me a week later to tell me her son's nasal congestion and allergies were no better and would I please consider giving him another homeopathic remedy. On further questioning, I discovered that he was suddenly eating better! He also was more amiable and easier to talk to and deal with at home and at school.

I tried pointing this out to his mother. She could only see that the symptom he came in with was no better; as far as she was concerned, the treatment had been a failure. I told her that another remedy was not yet indicated, as there had been such an obvious shift on a level deeper than that of the nasal problem. An emotional shift, one affecting his digestive organs and appetite, was occurring. Applying another remedy at this time might cut short the good process of the last remedy.

I mention this case because it's important that parents document everything that occurs with their child during homeopathic treatment. Your homeopath will use all information as clues to determine the next remedy to give your child.

This is especially true for small children and teenagers, because it is sometimes so difficult to get much information from the children themselves. The diagnosis often relies on the objective observations of parents.

If your child suddenly comes home with a pain in his or her little toe, don't ignore it. Every piece of information, no matter how apparently insignificant or small, may be vital in determining the next choice of homeopathic remedies.

The correct way to keep a homeopathic journal is to carry a small notebook with you at all times. The moment a behavior or physical symptom is observed or comes to mind, jot it down. The format is simple. Here is a suggested model:

This is just an example of a type of helpful record-keeping. If you find that your notes are becoming repetitious, summarize them before you come to the office, or talk to your homeopath on the phone. The more succinct and accurate your reporting can be, the more easily the homeopath will find the correct remedy for your child.

Date	Time	Symptom(s) or Observation(s)	Remedy
5-25-98	11:00 a.m.	Noticed that he is suddenly craving meat for the first time	None
5-25-98	9:30 p.m.	Is sleepy and not fighting me; willingly goes to bed!	None
5-29-98	3:30 p.m.	Teacher called to say he got in a fight at school	Called Dr. Martin; he says to wait
6-1-98	10:00 a.m.	He is happier and more energetic; less stuffy in nose	Dr. Martin said to wait
6-2-98	11:00 p.m.	He cannot sleep; cutting a new front tooth; irritable and wanting affection; one cheek is bright red; has low fever	Called Dr. Martin; prescribed Cham 30C, and then wait 2 weeks

Experience (Discovering Your Feelings About Your Child's Behavior)

Sit quietly in a place where you won't be bothered for five minutes or so. Have a pen and paper in hand, or have your computer's word processing program booted up. Close your eyes and begin to focus on your child. Ask yourself the following questions, and write down whatever comes up for you spontaneously, without editing any of the images, feelings or thoughts.

1. The first thing I think of when I think of my child's health is [identify thoughts or feelings].

2. I feel [describe emotion or feeling] for my child much of the time.

3. When my child says or does [describe actions], it makes me feel like [describe feelings and thoughts].

4. Sometimes I get frightened or annoyed when s/he does [describe the behavior that triggers these feelings].

Open your eyes now, if they aren't already open. The purpose of this exercise is to get you more in touch with some of your feelings toward your child. It is very hard to be objective about your child's behavior and symptoms if you have a lot of feelings about your child of which you are unaware.

Much of what is perceived as children's dysfunction can be parents' unresolved issues. To accurately report your child's behavior, preferences, likes, and dislikes, it is very important to be able to separate your feelings about yourself and your child from your observations of your child's behavior.

Again—and I can't repeat this too often—the more objectively you can help the homeopath accurately "see" your child, the easier it will be to choose the best homeopathic remedy. The more aware you are of your own emotional process as it involves your child, the easier it will be to report your child's symptoms accurately.

The homeopathic approach is a spiritual and growth-promoting path to health. As you become more familiar with various remedies, homeopathy can increase your own self-awareness. Because homeopathy works best when the whole family is being treated, you may want to consider setting up appointments for you, your spouse, and other children. The best time to get started is when you are well. You will be one step ahead of the game if and when illness strikes. You will have your remedy kit, your homeopathic doctor will already know you and be familiar with your constitution. Health will be only a phone call away.

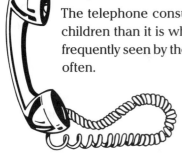

Telephone Calls

The telephone consultation is a much more valuable tool when treating children than it is when treating adults. Some children do not need to be frequently seen by the doctor, but need to be treated homeopathically more often.

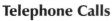

The role of the telephone call in pediatric homeopathy is a very important one. Understanding how to conduct an effective, efficient, quick telephone call can be very valuable to your child's health.

Before you call the homeopath, you should do the following:

1. Prepare a very precise list of the symptoms your child is having, along with modalities. Be sure to include the mental, emotional, and physical symptoms, including food preferences, status of the bowels, urination, fever, pains, odd behavior, etc. If you are unsure of what I am talking about, please see the homeopathy section of this book for a discussion of how to report symptoms.

2. If you have a first aid homeopathy book, do some research on your own before you call. Begin the phone conversation by telling the doctor the symptoms and then which remedies you think may be the best ones and why.

3. Have your child's homeopathic journal in front of you and be able to list the last few remedies. Be sure to include the potencies of each remedy. Most people do not realize that each potency is actually like a new remedy. If you have not seen the homeopathic doctor in a while, be ready to give a brief synopsis of the child's symptoms since you last saw the doctor. If it has been too long—more than a couple of months—you will need to visit your doctor.

Be succinct in your communication. Always remember that a busy doctor has many patients to talk to each day. While the time it takes to discuss your child's health by telephone is very important, it should be kept to a minimum. If you want to go into greater detail (more than five minutes), schedule an office appointment or a specific time for an in-depth phone consultation.

Do not call the doctor if you do not have a remedy kit at home or are unable to go to the homeopathic pharmacy to obtain a remedy—your call will be useless. If you are calling for emotional support, state so at the outset so that the doctor knows s/he doesn't need to pick your brain to make a diagnosis. Calling for emotional support or general information is a good idea, and all parents need this at times, but be clear at the outset and tell the receptionist.

If the doctor cannot take your call on the first try, leave an explicit message as to when and where you can be reached and why you are calling. Be sure to mention the degree of urgency. There is nothing more frustrating to the doctor at the end of the day than ten messages giving work numbers and no information on the degree of need. The receptionist taking your message might be new and know nothing about homeopathy!

Insist that the receptionist take a complete message and don't be intimidated if s/he is in a hurry. Your child's health is more important.

If it is an urgent matter, let the receptionist know so that s/he can immediately get the doctor, or let the doctor know to immediately return your call. If the issue isn't very urgent and can wait a day or two, please state so.

Once you have been given the name of a remedy, be sure to write down the particulars—its potency, frequency of repetition, number of pellets, when to stop the remedy, when to call back, etc.

The telephone is a very powerful tool. Often a quick conversation can lead to an incredible homeopathic remedy that changes the course of your child's life!

If you feel timid about calling and asking for help, try to express this to your doctor so that s/he can better understand your own personal process. So many people have been put off by the traditional medical profession that it takes time to realize a homeopathic doctor will actually take the time to return calls and hear the details of an illness.

Also, remember that if the doctor has a busy practice, it is often common to play "telephone tag." Keep calling back until your question is answered. If the number of calls is more than one a week, it is appropriate for the patient to be reasonably billed for time spent on the phone. This too can and should be discussed if you feel odd or uncomfortable about it.

Bring your child in for a checkup and brief office appointment every two to three months, even if s/he is well. This will ensure that the doctor has a good idea of the child's constitution, behavior, and general state of health so that if you call in an acute crisis, your child's energy will be familiar to him.

The day the child realizes that all adults are imperfect, he becomes an adolescent; the day he forgives himself, he becomes wise.

—Alder Nowlan

Experience (Identifying Issues Before Calling For Help)

Before you call, stop and close your eyes. Try to become quiet within yourself and ask yourself the following:

Am I calling for emotional support or for a homeopathic remedy?

What am I feeling relative to my child's illness?

What feelings are my child's sickness bringing up in me?

Am I prepared to run out to the homeopathic pharmacy right now to get theremedy the doctor prescribes?

Do I like working with this doctor and is s/he helpful in emergencies?

Am I happy with my child, and what does it mean that s/he is sick? What is s/he trying to tell me? How can I make him/her more comfortable?

When I was ill as a child, how was I taken care of? Did I receive the kind of love and nurturing I am giving my child? Is there healing here for me?

Stop and do some writing in your or your child's health journal. Include some of your more interesting answers.

Focus on your own "inner child" when your real child is ill. Sometimes there are very interesting connections.

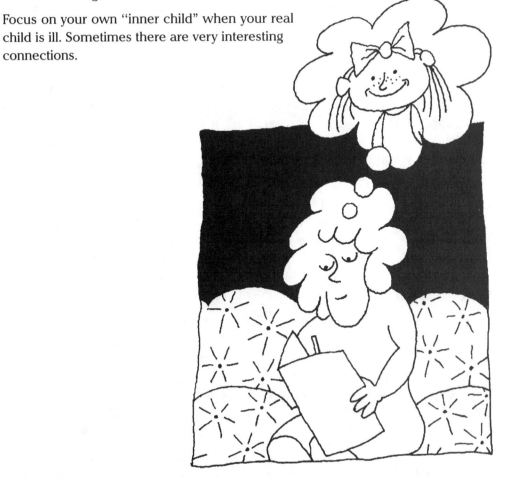

ATTENTION DEFICIT DISORDER (ADD)
"HE WON'T ACCEPT NO AS AN ANSWER"

This is the story of an eight-year-old little boy who first came to me for treatment on June 1, 1993. His mother described him as "out of control." Everything was a constant drama in the house, with the child craving constant attention. He mimicked others' behavior to spite them and was angry and demanding almost all of the time.

He had been like this for years, but over the last year he had become increasingly unmanageable. His mother said he threw frequent temper tantrums, had to be supervised 100% of the time and wouldn't "accept no as an answer."

When I saw him in my office, the first thing out of his mouth was a reaction to my computer. He came over to my desk, stood very close to me, and with a little malicious grin on his face said: "Your computer just quacked," referring to the sound effects my Macintosh computer makes.

The child would hit the mother and other children and smile while he was doing it. The mother described him as enjoying others' pain and hurt. Afterwards, he usually showed guilt or remorse and felt momentarily sad for the pain inflicted. He was described as defying his mother, and using anything as an argument.

He loves to read, but his attention and behavior was unpredictable—one moment nice, sweet or excessively affectionate and the next moment being violent and uncontrollable. He refused to go to bed at night, had a huge appetite, had frequent stomach pains, took frequent cat naps, slept on his side, was very opinionated, craved ice, beef jerky, candy, chocolate, orange juice, tomatoes, tomato juice, and fruit (especially bananas, pears, and peaches). He disliked salty foods.

He was diagnosed with Attention Deficit and Hyperactivity Disorder and had been on Prozac for three months at the time of his first visit with me. His mother reported that his behavior was a little improved on the Prozac, but not significant enough to keep him under control. They had also tried psychological counseling with little improvement. The mother decided to take him off Prozac without discussing it with the doctor (not something I would recommend!).

I prescribed a homeopathic remedy called Medorrhinum. I recommended taking the remedy only three times, at a frequency of every other day. The mother called me ten days later and reported that there was at least a 50% improvement in behavior. The mother had accidentally given the remedy daily, rather than following my instructions. I told her to wait and to not give him any more of the remedy, since improvement often will take place once the remedy is stopped. Ten days later she called again and said there was a setback. I recommended one dose of Medorrhinum in a higher potency.

Ten days later the mother called to say there was immediate improvement, but that it didn't last. I recommended one more dose of the remedy. I didn't hear back from her so I assumed she and the child were doing well. I phoned a few times to check but my calls were never returned.

I was curious about this case. Since the behavioral problem was so severe and the improvement so quick and dramatic, I wanted to know if it was holding. I finally reached the mother nine months later and she reported complete and lasting improvement without any more doses of the remedy. He just "snapped out of it" and "never snapped back," she reported.

This type of case is very gratifying for me as the doctor. This little boy's entire life will be changed thanks to the power and magic of homeopathy. Note that there are about 50 homeopathic remedies for ADD. Do not try to treat this yourself. Also, nutrition plays a large role and in my treatment program, I select a specific and individualized nutritional regimen based on either the child's blood, urine or hair lab tests.

QUESTIONS ABOUT HYPERACTIVITY AND ATTENTION DEFICIT DISORDER

What are the potential side effects of Ritalin therapy?

There are many, but the primary side effects are loss of appetite, insomnia, loss of creativity, apathy, depression, lethargy and allergic reactions.

Is there a natural way to treat hyperactivity and ADD?

Yes! Using herbs, vitamin supplements, a change in diet, homeopathic medications and amino acids has a proven track record. More and more medical literature is now available showing the positive effects of these natural therapies.

What are the causes of hyperactivity or ADD?

It can be a physiological imbalance, nutritional disorder, chemical imbalance, blood sugar disturbance, allergy to foods or artificial additives, or sensitivity to sugar or caffeine.

What are the most common foods that can cause problems?

Holistic doctors have performed a lot of research and determined that the most common foods to cause problems are the following: milk, cheese, corn, chocolate, wheat, eggs, yeast, sugar, food coloring and artificial food additives.

How do we determine if foods are a problem?

The best way is to eliminate all suspected foods for twenty-one days and then to add them back one at a time for forty-eight hours each, and see if there is any adverse reaction. If your child shows a reaction, eliminate the food. After the body chemistry is brought into balance, you may be able to add the food back to the diet.

What are typical food allergy reactions?

Typical reactions are as follows: fatigue or sleepiness, nervousness, mood swings, restlessness, irritability, inability to concentrate, nasal congestion, headaches, muscle aches, abdominal pains, bed-wetting, facial pallor or puffiness, and dark shadows under the eyes.

What vitamin supplements and amino acids are suggested for treatment?

Every child needs a slightly different formula, depending on age and the specific problems, but in general I use the following products in treating my patients for hyperactivity and ADD:

Taurine: an amino acid that has been shown to be very effective; helps in detoxification and is considered a neuromodulator.

Aminoplex: a full-range amino acid formula designed to balance blood sugar, reduce stress, provide a positive nitrogen balance, help in hormone synthesis and neurotransmitter synthesis and assist in general nutrition.

M.V.M.: a full-range multivitamin/mineral formula with adequate amounts of calcium, magnesium and the B-vitamin group.

Vitamin C: high potency vitamin C in a buffered, chelated, or esterified form.

Roboxin: coenzymatic vitamin B_2, required for maximization of electron transport.

Tryptoplex: a special tryptophan formula, helping in relaxation and insomnia, stimulates serotonin to control moods. Until the FDA reintroduces tryptophan, eating foods high in tryptophan is a good idea. These include fish, lean meat, nuts, and wheat germ.

GABA: (Gamma-aminobutyric acid), relaxes the brain and mimics Valium or Librium, but naturally.

Glycine: another amino acid, this one has a calming effect and inhibits sugar cravings.

Calcium and magnesium: for their calming and relaxing effects.

Which homeopathic medicines are used?

The following is a very brief description of some of the homeopathic remedies I use along with their various indications:

Anacardium: hyperactivity, violent behavior better by eating food.

Argenticum nit: craves sweets and sugar, but one bite of candy bar sends the child off the wall for hours.

Iodum: always hungry with a hyperactive metabolism, like a train wound up that runs and runs; may become violent without food

Medorrhinum: sexual acting out; if either parent was exposed to gonorrhea at any time in their lives; a very wild child in some cases including fits and full of wild energy; may come in waves, with a few days of calm followed by aggressive behavior or tantrums; sexually precocious; restless; worse at night; with chronic sinusitis and allergies; craves stimulation and attention.

238

Tuberculinum: don't know what they want, but always on the move; if either parent or grandparent was exposed to tuberculosis; history of ear infections or repeated colds.

Tarentula: very active all the time; talks and walks fast; constant fighting; likes to dance spontaneously when music is turned on.

Coffea cruda: similar to drinking too much coffee; mind very active and cannot sleep.

NATURAL REMEDIES FOR CHILDHOOD ILLNESS

I am delighted to see so many parents choosing homeopathy instead of antibiotics to treat their children. Whether it be a cold or flu, or something more serious like strep throat or an ear infection, parents are finally beginning to see how well homeopathy can work to strengthen the immune system and heal infants and children from the "inside out."

Some examples of common homeopathic remedies for children are the following (always be sure to consult your materia medica before using homeopathic remedies):

Ear Infection: Silica, Hepar sulph, Mercurius, Belladonna, Ferrum phos

Head Colds: Aconite, Bellodona, Gelsemium, Pulsatilla

Coughs: Drosera, Rumex, spongia, Antimonium tart, Bryonia

Asthma: Arsenicum alb, Pulsatilla, Ipecac, Lobelia

I encourage every child's family to purchase two important self-help books:

Everybody's Guide to Homeopathic Medicine by Dana Ullman

The Homeopathic Treatment of Children by Paul Herscu

Smoking may increase damage to sperm DNA and raise cancer in offspring. This study presents data suggesting that paternal smoking may increase risk of birth defects and childhood cancer in their offspring.
—*Mutation Res., 351:199-203, 1996*

HOMEOPATHIC IMMUNIZATION CHOICES

(NOTE: As your doctor, I'll help you to decide, but won't tell you what you should do with your child's immunizations. You'll need to inform yourself and decide based on your own personal values and health goals. I can refer you to books and articles that will help you to decide, but I can't make this decision for you.)

1. The most traditional approach is to get all normal immunizations that your pediatrician normally recommends and then to use homeopathy before and after each immunization to lessen the possible negative effects.

2. Another less traditional method is to take homeopathic immunizations. This is controversial and some homeopaths don't feel this really works. There is no scientific data on this subject. The way it works is to give the same immunizations you would otherwise take in allopathic form, but use them in homeopathic form instead. This requires repeated doses. There are some homeopaths who do this on all their pediatric patients.

3. Another alternative method is to have your child's health care handled by classical (constitutional) homeopathy. According to this method, your child will remain healthy and not be prone to disease because the constitutional homeopathic remedy will help to bolster the immune system. Under this approach, the sooner you begin homeopathic treatment the better. The ideal is to have the child treated before the parents even conceive, by treating the parents first. The sooner the newborn is treated the better. Note that there does not have to be anything "wrong" with your child to be treated. Constitutional treatment is *preventative*, and strengthens the overall health, vitality and immunity of your infant.

People given measles vaccine were three times as likely to develop ulcerative colitis or Crohn's disease as were those who caught measles naturally.

—The Lancet 4/29/95

QUALITY OF LIFE

ARE YOU ADDICTED????

Sugar, caffeine, cigarettes, alcohol, drugs ... these substances are the common addictions for so many of us and our most creative and sensitive friends and family members. If you, your friends, family or associates have decided to "kick" the addiction habit and begin a healthier lifestyle, a holistic approach has a lot to offer.

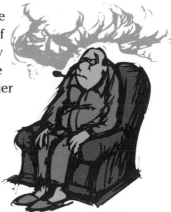

Homeopathy

Homeopathy will work in two ways. First it can be used to break the specific addiction and to release endorphins. Second, homeopathy can be used constitutionally to balance and strengthen the immune system and drastically reduce emotional anxiety.

Acupuncture

Acupuncture works to release endorphins. It's these endorphins and other similar chemical substances that are suppressed or cut off during the addictive process. Acupuncture will re-stimulate the brain to send out endorphins again, thus reducing the cravings and more quickly allowing you to feel relaxed and centered.

Chinese Herbal Medicine

Specific encapsulated herbal formulas are utilized for each type of addiction and each particular problem. Other herbs are used to detoxify the kidneys, colon, liver and lungs. Other herbal formulas are used as natural tranquilizers and for help in getting to sleep.

Nutritional Counseling

Eating right is the first and most powerful step in helping to empowering you to heal yourself. It's important that a specific, individualized nutritional program be created for you. Some of the most popular nutrition books make the big mistake of recommending the same diet for everyone. But every person's body type and metabolism is different, so there are very specific criteria to consider when creating an individualized nutritional program.

Nutritional Supplements

Each person's body has very specific requirements for nutritional supplementation. Unless you eat a nearly perfect, organic foods diet, it is important to take supplements as a part of a program tailored to meet your particular needs.

TWELVE STEP PROGRAMS AND OPTIMAL HEALTH

Introduction

Twelve-step programs (TSPs) are extremely effective for many people trying to control addictive behaviors. The reason why these programs work for some people and not for others is that they may be strong in the area of emotional, spiritual, and mental recovery, but somewhat weak in terms of physical recovery.

Keep in mind that there are four parts to any recovery program. TSP recovery tools primarily emphasize the emotional and spiritual levels, focus to a lesser degree on the mental or intellectual level, and barely touch the physical level at all.

How to pray, meditate, take a personal inventory, connect with others in the form of fellowship, community, sponsorship, inner dialogue, and ongoing assessment are certainly hallmarks of successful recovery. But on the physical level, only a few behavioral tools are discussed: "Abstain, no matter what," "Abstinence comes first," and "First things first," are common slogans. "Use the phone," or "Call before that first bite," are others.

TSPs basically offer a "white knuckle" or behavioral approach to physical recovery. One is warned of the evils of breaking abstinence. If one can diligently perform the steps and use the tools without fail, the white knuckle approach is workable. Often, however, a person is unsuccessful, especially at the beginning of the program. In fact, a very large segment of people who try to use such programs drop out. It is my feeling that while these people who fail at TSPs may be "working" their program as hard as anyone, they may be experiencing greater physical imbalance than average, which genuinely limits their ability to apply the tools and principles of the program.

It is common to judge a person's success in a program by how long the person has abstained. This is based on the assumption that if a person is working a strong program, s/he will also be successful at abstinence. Yet there are many who have achieved a great degree of spiritual balance, have a strong connection to a "higher power," or who have had a lot of therapy. Many of these individuals may work within the parameters of the TSP, yet fail miserably over the long run at abstaining from the behavior they wish to change.

Why? If people are working just as hard at the same program, why do some have an easier time of it than others? Is there is a missing link, a hidden dimension, a mysterious factor which the program does not address? I believe there is. I reiterate that this missing element is the *physical* one. TSPs assume everyone is biologically equal and the white-knuckle method will work for everyone. But some people cannot abstain; they cannot alter their behavior no matter how hard they try, because they are ignoring the physiological aspects of the addictive process.

There is a joke in Overeaters Anonymous about the mother who keeps telling her overweight child that she doesn't have an eating problem—she has an underactive thyroid. It could well be true, but unfortunately TSPs teach that the programs are complete and everything a person *should* need to achieve sobriety or abstinence is in the program. This is sad, because there are so many other excellent tools from other sources that are compatible with the program's goals and principles.

Most compulsive overeaters hope and pray that their problem is as simple as an underactive thyroid gland. In fact, most compulsive overeaters *do* have a weak thyroid, just as most alcoholics have liver problems, codependents have adrenal problems, and sexaholics have pituitary gland imbalances. There are also addictive food allergies, which cause a person to crave the food or beverage that they are allergic to. Whether the problems existed before or after the onset of the behavior is irrelevant. The fact is that there is a physical imbalance that can and needs to be treated.

I'm not trying to downplay the importance of participating in a strong TSP as a pivotal key to recovery. But for some people, the program may not be enough. People who *most* need this information are the following:

- ✧ People who, despite well-intentioned behavior and motives, fail at TSPs
- ✧ People who succeed and then slip back into their old behaviors
- ✧ People who succeed but don't get as far as they would have liked to get in the program, and ultimately achieve their goals only partway
- ✧ People who succeed at the program, achieve program goals, yet are not achieving the level of good physical health desired even after two or more years of abstinence and recovery

For these people, understanding addictions, addictive physiology, and addictive anatomy can help. Sometimes, if one is successful at working the program, physical imbalances will in fact take care of themselves over time. Through healthy diet and exercise, the liver will naturally detoxify, regenerate, and grow healthier if given the opportunity. Prayer, meditation, and visual imagery are also very helpful in this regard, but physical treatments such as acupuncture, herbal supplements, and homeopathy will facilitate the physical recovery process, as well.

It is important not to accept the addiction as the reality. Addictions are only symptoms of imbalance on a deeper level. The magic of the holistic approach, which takes into account the physical imbalance, is that often in removing the physical imbalance the emotional addiction is cured as well. Patients always have an easier time giving up alcohol, tobacco, sugar, or caffeine if they are being treated using holistic methods.

Oriental Medicine and Addictions

According to the Law of Five Elements in traditional Chinese medicine, each person is born with some weaker and stronger elements or meridians. A particular weakness may predispose a person to a particular addiction. Western medical research regards children of alcoholics as having a higher chance of becoming alcoholic themselves. Chinese medicine has known this all along.

According to Chinese medicine, if your mother, father, or grandparent was an alcoholic, you will inherit a Liver meridian (or Wood Element) that is more likely to host a precondition for substance abuse. Similarly, if a parent was obese or underweight, the child may inherit a weak Earth or Fire Element.

Depending on the particular weakness, using herbal formulas and acupuncture, a person can be successfully treated to strengthen a weak element. In strengthening a weak organ and its accompanying meridian, the predisposition to the addiction can be removed or significantly reduced. (See the section beginning on page 56 for a discussion of the Five Elements.)

Endocrinology

Another area where the holistic approach is very effective is in treating imbalanced endocrine glands and hormonal levels in the body. A weakness of each gland in the body can predispose a person to particular cravings and addictions. Using a series of blood tests and questionnaires, we can determine which weak endocrine gland is contributing to the addictive behavior. These glands can be significantly strengthened by using various minerals, glandulars, herbs, and homeopathic remedies. There are also particular exercise regimes that can strengthen each particular gland.

Amino acids

Amino acids are the building blocks of our body. Recent research has shown that a lack of specific amino acids can contribute to emotional instability and obsessive or addictive behaviors. Supplementing the diet with specific amino acids can immeasurably reduce cravings or addictions.

> *It is not heroin or cocaine that makes one an addict; it is the need to escape from a harsh reality. There are more television addicts, more baseball and football addicts, more movie addicts, and certainly more alcohol addicts in this country than there are narcotic addicts.*
>
> *—Shirley Chisholm*

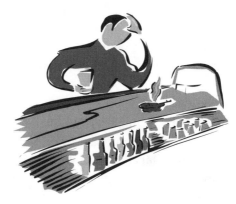

DEPRESSION, ANXIETY AND PHOBIAS

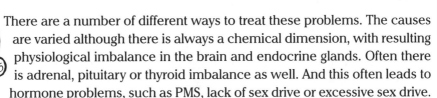

There are a number of different ways to treat these problems. The causes are varied although there is always a chemical dimension, with resulting physiological imbalance in the brain and endocrine glands. Often there is adrenal, pituitary or thyroid imbalance as well. And this often leads to hormone problems, such as PMS, lack of sex drive or excessive sex drive. Another component that is common with this type of chemical imbalance is OCD, or Obsessive Compulsive Disorder. In its extreme, this type of imbalance may lead to Bi-polar Disorder, or extreme highs and lows.

There is generally a genetic component to the disease picture, although it is often hard to trace back to a specific parent or grandparent. Sometimes there is also chemical or alcohol addiction in the family or in the person suffering from this disease.

The treatment options are many. In our culture, the most common form of treatment is the use of pharmaceutical drugs, such as Prozac, meant to correct the chemical imbalance. This approach works very well for the majority of people, but there are many who it doesn't work for or who won't take drugs. (In Europe, St. John's Wort is prescribed 25 times more often than Prozac because it provides the same benefits without any of the side effects associated with drugs.)

For these people there are alternative treatments in the form of amino acid supplements, herbs, homeopathic remedies and acupuncture. Diet almost always plays an essential role in the cause of the disease and in its cure. Exercise is also critical.

A patient with one of these problems is often in the worst possible position to make an educated decision as to which form of treatment is best suited to their particular need. Certainly, if a prospective patient is considering suicide or has attempted suicide in the recent past, they are a good candidate and should seriously consider the Western drug approach. This will bring the quickest relief and will save their life, which obviously is the most important factor.

But in less extreme cases, many people who are interested in the alternative methods lack enough information to make an educated decision. It should be said that for many people, and for many of my patients, there is no need to choose one form of treatment over the other, since they may also do a number of different methods at the same time. Some of my patients have chosen to go on Prozac for a while, while being treated with herbs and homeopathics simultaneously. This approach works for some.

Others, who are more purists, tend to want to try one thing at a time. The alternative approach to depression or anxiety can be very effective for many people. Obviously, the less severe your case and shorter you have had the problem, as with anything, the easier and quicker will be your cure. But if it is a chronic problem that you have had for many years, it will probably takes many years to achieve a complete cure.

It can also be very costly to treat using the alternative approach. Amino acid therapy can be very expensive and weekly or even monthly acupuncture can eat into your pocketbook, unless you have good health insurance.

I encourage my patients to read all they can about alternative methods before deciding. It can be a long and tedious task to cure these problems using alternative methods, although there is nothing more fulfilling to me or the patient than to look back years later and to see how far they have come—how far we have come together.

Despite the difficulties, the alternative approach is tremendously effective for those people who want a simpler, softer way, and it also opens up the road to personal and spiritual growth possibilities that were previously never thought of. And this is where the real sense of satisfaction takes place. Looking back and knowing that you chose the more difficult and longer path—AND did the personal and spiritual work to get where you are now—is very self-satisfying.

The one other component that you will need to consider regardless of which type of treatment you choose, is that you will also need to enter in-depth counseling, if you really want to see lasting results. There are many types of counseling, but at some point, most people who have been in longer-term therapy also begin to experiment with a body-mind or body-centered approach, and find it is much more effective than the type of therapy where talking is the primary modality.

THE MANY FACES OF DEPRESSION: FROM ANTIDEPRESSANT DRUGS TO HEALTH

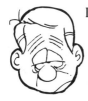 Depression is a complex, easily misunderstood and multifaceted. Most people think there is only one type of depression. In fact, depression affects over 10 million Americans annually and over 50% of the population will experience depression at least once in their life, but there are many types of depression and many different causes.

The causes of depression are often very complex, involving different psychological aspects of a person's makeup, as well as physiological, behavioral, social, environmental, energetic, and possible spiritual factors.

Unfortunately, allopathic medical doctors might easily give one of the common medications used for depression in cases of mild depression. Although these medications are very useful in cases of severe depression, it is often possible to treat mild cases of depression without the use of drugs.

As with any prescription medication, whenever an antidepressant drug is used it has a number of potential negative side effects. First, it creates more toxicity in the liver. Second, it is important to see depression as the tip of the iceberg. The weakness of the conventional drug approach is its generalized use of antidepressant drugs as a "cure-all."

Whether the problem is psychological, behavioral, environmental or spiritual, depression can be an opportunity for self-discovery and growth. The symptom of depression is an indication of an imbalance. The liver is usually toxic, or the person may have environmental allergies, food allergies, Candida or chronic fatigue syndrome.

Depression can also be caused by cofactors such as hypoglycemia, anemia, endocrine imbalances (thyroid, estrogen, progesterone, or adrenal), immune problems, toxic reactions and side effects to drugs, overdose of vitamins, electromagnetic fields, nutritional deficiencies, and more.

To determine the reason behind depression a comprehensive medical exam is required, including dietary analysis, nutritional supplementation, lifestyle and stress analysis. Possible treatments include acupuncture, acupressure, conventional drug therapy, psychotherapy, behavioral therapy, biofeedback, guided imagery, homeopathy, amino acids, herbs and dietary therapy.

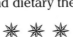

THE MANY FACES OF FATIGUE AND LETHARGY

There are many causes, or faces, that correspond to the symptoms of fatigue. Its appearance can vary tremendously, but there is one common thread. For the person who suffers from fatigue, life can be miserable, depressing, or at best difficult. But there is an answer and in the answer is found the cure. Fatigue can be cured by getting to its root cause and uprooting it!

What are the causes of fatigue?

1. *Lack of Sleep*: Without enough sleep, the body doesn't have the opportunity to rejuvenate itself and regenerate its cells. Deep sleep is also vital so that the body can achieve a deep dream state, releasing internal stress from the day's events and connecting to the collective unconscious.

2. *Incorrect Diet*: Diet must correspond to the person's activity level and their metabolic body type.

3. *Hormonal Imbalance*: This can take a number of different forms and have a few different causes. The most common imbalances involve the thyroid, adrenals and reproductive hormones, including testosterone, estrogen and progesterone.

4. *Poor Digestion*: Not assimilating one's food well can cause lots of fatigue. This can be caused by ulcers, gas, bloating, irritable bowel syndrome and Crohn's disease, parasites, and a wide variety of yeasts or Candida.

5. *Chronic Pain*: Pain can interfere with sleep and a feeling of well-being, causing chronic fatigue.

6. *Immunity Problems*: Chronic fatigue will often begin after a bad cold or flu or follow mononucleosis or other acute immune problems. Chronic sore throat or feeling "run down" will interfere with deep sleep.

7. *Emotional Stress*: Often a long-term emotional issue is the cause of fatigue. If we let an emotional issue fester and grow out of proportion for too long, it can depress our hormones and immunity and result in fatigue.

8. *Allergies*: Food and/or airborne allergies can be very exhausting, creating a kind of "false" fatigue as the body is constantly fighting to rid itself of the offending substance.

9. *Body Chemistry Imbalance*: This involves the body's "battery" running out of steam. Causes include inadequate intake of protein, lack of minerals, acid/alkaline imbalance, poor assimilation from stress, poor long-term eating habits and/or eating disorders.

The positive note is that the problem of fatigue can be completely cured, and in most cases cured fairly easily. The negative is that many people cover up their symptoms of fatigue by taking stimulants or antidepressants, and when they go off these medications they feel even worse because the cause wasn't initially addressed, located and uprooted.

How do we locate the cause of fatigue? In my practice, I ask most patients to go for complete blood testing. Blood tests can check for such things as Candida; Epstein-Barr virus; cytomegalo virus, thyroid imbalance; DHEA; testosterone, progesterone and estrogen; liver problems; immune problems; acid/alkaline imbalance; overall body chemistry, and the like.

I also perform hair analysis to check mineral levels and toxic metals in the body. Additionally, I perform various types of saliva tests to check adrenal function, hormone levels and food sensitivities/allergies to wheat and gluten. Stool tests also check for Candida, other yeasts, and parasites. Parasites are often an overlooked but leading cause of fatigue, robbing us of minerals, protein and vitamins vital to our growth and health.

Treatments vary depending on the individual and the cause of their particular type of fatigue. Some patients do very well with constitutional homeopathic medicine only. Others are more comfortable with acupuncture and herbs, or using a nutritional and dietary approach alone. I work out an individualized treatment plan with each of my patients' unique needs in mind.

> *To honor and accept one's own shadow is a profound religious discipline.*
> *It is wholemaking and thus holy and the most important experience of a*
> *lifetime.*
>
> —*Robert A. Johnson*
> *Owning Your Own Shadow*

A HEADACHE STORY WITH A HAPPY ENDING

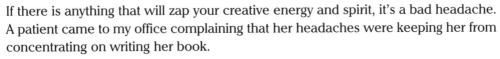

If there is anything that will zap your creative energy and spirit, it's a bad headache. A patient came to my office complaining that her headaches were keeping her from concentrating on writing her book.

What made this patient's headaches unique was that they always began when she was outdoors and in direct sunlight. I asked her more questions and discovered that the headaches were usually on her right side and began over the right eye, spreading to the back of the neck.

I asked her what made the headaches better or worse. She said they were a little better when she applied ice or a cold compress to the forehead and neck, when she took a nap, and when she laid on her right side. She said that when she ate anything salty the headaches pounded and got worse. She also said that a warm room made them worse and that they tended to begin or get worse around ten in the morning. There was one other thing, she said; after that, she became silent.

After some supportive prodding, she shared that she didn't really like talking about her headaches since talking about them or getting support from other people actually made her feel worse! She said that she was a loner and preferred to handle her problems on her own without discussing them with anyone else.

I was beginning to get an idea of which remedy would fit her symptoms, but to properly diagnose her and choose the correct remedy I needed a bit more information about the rest of her life on a physical and an emotional level. I continued to ask questions in a nonintrusive way.

"What else happens when you get your headaches?" I asked. She said that in addition to being in the sunlight when the headaches began, she also noticed she sometimes got a herpes outbreak or cold sore on her lip at the same time or a day or two later. She said she must have contracted the herpes virus from her last boyfriend. Then she shared the key piece of information: the headaches began just after the breakup of her relationship with this boyfriend.

Her complexion was oily and a bit yellow-looking, her tongue showed a crack in the center, she had a crack in the middle of her lower lip, she tended to have heartburn after greasy foods, and she craved salt.

I gave this woman a homeopathic remedy called *Natrum muriaticum* and treated her Gall Bladder and Kidney meridians with acupuncture. I also gave her a Chinese herbal formula to strengthen her Kidney yin. After eight weeks we re-evaluated her case. She had not had one headache. Previously, she had experienced headaches about once a week, particularly when it was sunny and hot.

This case illustrates how the correct diagnosis, treatment plan, and prescription can be made when the patient shares a lot about the specifics of his or her particular problem, including the emotional element. The remedy, Natrum muriaticum, fit her emotional and physical symptoms picture almost exactly, and the location of the headaches were almost always on her right-sided Gall Bladder meridian.

Mac Repertory Example Showing Homeopathic Treatment of Headaches

	Ign.	Sul-ac.	Alum.	Canth.	Arg-n.	Cann-s.	Carb-v.
Rubrics	4	3	3	3	3	2	2
% of Rubrics	80	60	60	60	60	40	40
1. HEAD PAIN; LOCALIZATION; Occiput and Forehead							
2. HEAD PAIN; LOCALIZATION; Sides; right							
3. GENERALITIES; FOOD and drinks; ice-cream; desires							
4. GENERALITIES; EXERTION; physical; amel.							
WEEPING, tearful mood; alternating with; irritability							

MIGRAINE HEADACHES

The homeopathic remedy chart above is only a small sampling of the wide variety of specific symptoms having to do with headaches. On the left side of the chart are the specific symptoms you may experience. Across the top are the abbreviations for various homeopathic remedies. The darkened areas indicate the most likely remedy for that particular symptom.

Often a combination of acupuncture and homeopathy is most effective in treating long-standing or acute headaches. To determine what may be the possible cause of your headache, refer to the Trigger Chart on the next page. Share this information with your holistic practitioner.

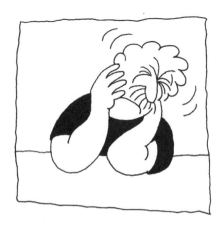

MIGRAINE HEADACHE TRIGGER CHART

Name:

Date:

Day of Week: Time of Onset:

Duration: Day of Menstrual Cycle:

Days Before Next Period:

During the 48 hours before the migraine headache:

Did you have any special worry, stress, worry, overwork or shock to your system?

❑ Yes   ❑ No

If yes, what happened?

What had you done during the day of the migraine?

Normal Work?

Unusual Activity?

Extra tired?

What foods had you eaten and when?

Breakfast: Time:

Lunch: Time:

Dinner: Time:

Snacks: Time(s):

HEADACHE DIAGNOSIS CHECKLIST

There are many different types and causes of headaches. To determine the type of headache you have, and the best type of treatment, please fill out one of these forms each time you have a headache.

Location of headache (frontal, occipital, temporal, vertex) and specify which part of the head:

Where were you when the headache began and what activity were you doing (in bed, eating, at work, in front of a computer)?

What does the headache feel like?

What is the particular sensation you feel from the headache (sharp, dull, throbbing, aching, pins and needles, numbness)?

What other sensations or things were going on in your body at the same time or before the headache occurred (back pain, stomach pain, toe pain, worry, fatigue, lack of sleep)?

What time of day did the headache begin?

Does it always begin at this time of day?

How frequently do they occur (daily, weekly, monthly)?

INSOMNIA DIAGNOSIS CHECKLIST

To better help to diagnose and treat your insomnia, please fill in this checklist as thoroughly and accurately as possible. Add any additional thoughts you have as to the possible causes of your insomnia.

Please check the applicable boxes:

❑ mind racing

❑ mind thinking about:

  ❑ grief/sadness   ❑ business/financial

  ❑ guilt/shame   ❑ other (specify):

❑ overtired

❑ nervous
  about what?

❑ body sensations keep me awake:

  ❑ restless legs   ❑ tingling

  ❑ chest   ❑ stomach pains   ❑ joint pain

❑ always get wound up at _____ A.M./P.M.

❑ always wake up at _____ A.M./P.M.

❑ wake frequently to urinate
  how many times?

❑ can't get to sleep until

❑ no trouble falling asleep, but wake up at (time):

Additional Comments:

Creating a healing space, however wide the initial chasm, is often all that therapy can do. Doing nothing but providing the space within which the body/mind/spirit can come home to, come to term with its conflicting selves, may in itself be enough.

—Dr. Randy Martin

LONGEVITY

As many as eighty percent of Americans over the age of sixty are suffering from at least one age-related disease, such as cancer, heart disease, arthritis and Alzheimer's disease. It's a fact that as we grow older and our cellular energy levels decline, our body's ability to repair and regenerate tissue drops dramatically. But correcting our nutritional deficiencies and nurturing our metabolic resources will offset this aging process and can dramatically help to prevent the numerous degenerative diseases that often plague older folks. Essentially, if we know what to do, we can "prevent" ourselves from growing older.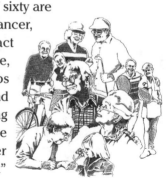

However, the difficulty arises in deciding exactly who to believe and which nutritional supplements you need to take to meet your personal goals and your specific health needs. There are many soothsayers who make all kinds of claims about being able to extend life and add bundles of energy, but who do you really believe and how do you decide for yourself?

As a Doctor of Oriental Medicine with over sixteen years experience in the health field, what I'm always recommending to my patients and what I do myself is to get tested before taking a lot of supplements. The reason I emphasize the need for testing is that, if your body doesn't really need something, then it's unwise to take it. Taking a supplement your body doesn't need will further imbalance your system, throwing your body and metabolism off even more, rather than strengthening it.

Although the particular supplement you are taking may feel good in the short run, it may actually be wearing your system down in the long run. Some supplements, such as blue green algae or ginseng can give you immediate energy, but could be depleting your kidneys and adrenals, much as caffeine does. It's a mistake to believe that just because a supplement is natural, it is healthy and a positive addition to your diet!

There a few different types of tests that can accurately determine your health and nutritional status. These tests will also be able to tell you which supplements your body needs in the long run to achieve your personal longevity goals. The types of tests which are the most accurate and commonly used for these diagnostic purposes are the following: hair, stool, and blood. I'll discuss each one in depth in just a moment.

First, it's very important to understand that in Western medicine, longevity is generally thought to be primarily of function of a healthy immune system, although other factors are also definitely involved, including the cardiovascular, endocrine and digestive systems. So with cancer and stroke being two of the leading causes of death in the US, it's vital to address immunity and cardiovascular health in any personal longevity program.

To the list of prerequisites for long life and good health, Chinese medical theory also stresses the need to counter weakness in the gastrointestinal system. This is due to the obvious but often ignored fact that we need to be efficiently *digesting* and *assimilating* the foods we eat and the supplements we take in order to maintain and improve our overall health and to give us a longer life. Chinese medicine believes that digestion is the major cornerstone to good health and increased longevity.

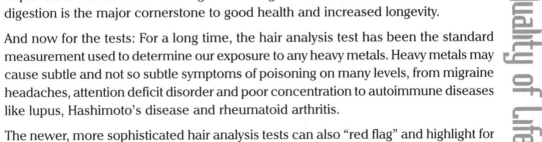

And now for the tests: For a long time, the hair analysis test has been the standard measurement used to determine our exposure to any heavy metals. Heavy metals may cause subtle and not so subtle symptoms of poisoning on many levels, from migraine headaches, attention deficit disorder and poor concentration to autoimmune diseases like lupus, Hashimoto's disease and rheumatoid arthritis.

The newer, more sophisticated hair analysis tests can also "red flag" and highlight for us problems like malabsorption, allergies, cardiac risk, stress, hypothyroidism, depression or, in children, a predisposition to violent behavior. When speaking of longevity, we're in the realm of preventive medicine, and whenever we're dealing with preventive medicine, the sooner we begin to eat the right diet and take the right supplements, the better it is for us. So it's great to have young children and teenagers tested at the earliest age possible to determine where their physiology may be "off" or where their weaknesses are.

The next test you may want to consider taking is the stool test. The stool test will reveal four very important factors that affect longevity: colon health and colon cancer risk, candida and other yeasts, parasite infestations, and digestive health. It's important when you take the stool test that you do the stool "purge" test and not the ordinary stool sample. The "purge" test evaluates contents from the entire colon, not just the last few inches.

Colon health is often ignored as a factor in longevity, but it is a reflection of digestion and assimilation. And remember what I said above—according to Chinese medical theory, if your digestion is working well, you already have the first prerequisite to longevity under your belt. If you have a large buildup of yeast, parasites, various types of worms, or a lack of beneficial bacteria in your colon, you will not be able to assimilate your food or nutritional supplements. Common symptoms of this may include gum problems, acne and other chronic skin problems, frequent gas or bloating, chronic and/or alternating diarrhea or constipation, intense stomach cramping or stabbing pains in the stomach.

But it's the blood test that is one of the most effective methods of quantifying nutritional deficiencies in your body. The most common indicators and risk factors found by the blood test are the following: dehydration, insufficient electrolytes, various types of cancer, cardiovascular health, kidney health, liver health, and digestive and assimilation problems. Modern blood tests and computer analysis will be able to tell you all this and more. If you have low energy, this can often be quickly explained by a simple blood test.

Now let's discuss some specific health recommendations for longevity and building a greater sense of well-being and energy. I want to emphasize that when you "latch onto" the correct diet and regimen for your particular body type, you can and will age more slowly, your energy will increase, you will gradually feel much younger, and you will look younger too. This is not hype. It is something I have seen in myself and my patients over many years.

Surprisingly, the first factor to consider is never which supplements to take. The right supplements should only follow after two other important aspects—lifestyle and diet. Eliminating stress from your life is by far the number one, most important factor in longevity. More and more scientific studies are confirming the stress factor in many of the common degenerative diseases in our society today. Other stress factors to meditate on are getting enough sleep and rest and reflecting on your coping mechanisms for dealing with relationship stress, work-related stress and environmental pollution and its resulting stresses.

A "new" stress factor that has only more recently been identified and acknowledged by health scientists is how we react to and cope with the increasing amount of information overload in our life. Without an effective external and internal "management" strategy for assimilating, "collating," and processing the massive amount of information that comes our way on a moment by moment basis, we will be at a higher risk of succumbing to a stress-related illness.

Once we have confronted head-on and dealt with the realities of the stress in our life by creating a realistic management strategy, it's time to confront what we put in our bodies, and the intimate relationship we have with the food we eat. Food and sex are definitely the most intimate relationships we have. Both affect us in our gut and can affect our energy and energetic system more than other factors in our life. Based on the latest scientific research, most nutritionists today are advising one of two diets: the Metabolic Type diet and the "blood type" diet. There are some differences between the two, but both tend to be higher protein then most "health-conscious" people have been eating in the past and both take into consideration our metabolic and body-type differences.

The main thing to remember is that it's very important for you to eat right for your particular metabolic or blood type, and that you don't eat the way another person has told you to eat. What's right for one person may not be right for you. Soy products may be a great source of protein and work well for one person, but a raw foods diet may work well for another and a high animal protein diet for yet another. You need to incorporate a scientific attitude when it comes to food and really learn to step back, read a few books and do some objective research to determine which "type" you are and which foods provide you with the longest, most sustained energy resources.

Another factor to consider (and one I'm finding in many of my patients) is that as we experience the relative "quickening" of time and the energy around us is apparently becoming more and more intense or compressed, many people need more protein and electrolytes in their diets then they did five, ten, or fifteen years ago, in order to remain grounded. One longevity study I read, which compared the various factors among people who lived the longest, found that one common factor was in the composition of the water in their bodies. Their water contained very high levels of electrolytes!

Many of us take calcium and magnesium supplements, but if you check your blood chemistry through blood tests, you are likely to find that you are not assimilating the supplements. Furthermore, many of us are even low on sodium, so when we drink our eight to ten glasses of water a day, we are not rehydrating our cells but just urinating the fluid right out. We need enough sodium, potassium, chloride, etc. in our body in order to catalyze all the other chemical reactions that create healthy-looking skin, good brain function and high energy.

Now we're ready to discuss the specific supplements you might want to try if your goal is to look younger, live longer, live healthier and with more mental clarity and energy. Some of these will be common ones that you have already heard of or tried and others may be more esoteric and lesser known.

The most common supplement (which has been a best seller in Europe for years but only recently has become popularized here in the States) is *Ginkgo biloba*, a species of tree that thrived 65 million years ago and continues to thrive today. It's used worldwide to treat conditions associated with aging and is sometimes referred to as a "living fossil." The tree can live for more than 1,000 years, a feat attributable to its resistance to disease, fires and other environmental hazards. In fact, it was the only tree to survive the atomic blast in Hiroshima. The Chinese also used ginkgo seeds to treat venereal disease, asthma, and impaired hearing. The most common things ginkgo can be used for today are longevity, hearing, memory, Alzheimer's, circulatory problems like cold hands and feet, and sexual potency.

While we're on the subject of circulation and memory, let's discuss a few other supplements for enhancing memory. Pregnenolone is possibly the most potent intelligence-enhancing agent ever researched. Pregnenolone is a hormone precursor that the body normally manufactures, using cholesterol as its primary raw material. In the body, it's converted into a multitude of other hormones including DHEA, estrogen, testosterone and progesterone. But pregnenolone levels generally decline with age, and some scientists are experimenting with the restoration of pregnenolone to youthful levels as an important step in dealing with symptoms of aging.

Other supplements to include in your mental fitness program include the amino acids L-phenylalanine, L-tyrosine and L-glutamine. Phenylalanine is a precursor to the neurotransmitter noradrenaline, tyrosine increases serotonin, and glutamine helps with blood sugar.

More nuts and bolts: Be sure to always take pyridoxal-5 phosphate (a form of vitamin B_6) when taking amino acids, since your body needs it to assimilate and process the amino acids. In addition to vitamin B_6, vitamin C, folic acid and copper are needed to convert phenylalanine into noradrenaline and dopamine. Your body ordinarily makes these brain chemicals all day long, but after a good night's sleep they are at a high, which is why sleep is so important.

Phosphatidylserine and phosphatidylcholine are two other important nutrients that have been shown to help with memory and brainpower. Another good one is acetyl L-carnitine, which will improve communication between the hemispheres of the brain, improve memory, relieve fatigue, enhance energy metabolism, improve eye-hand coordination, enhance mood and increase immune function. These, as well as the amino acids discussed above, always need to be taken on an empty stomach. This is because the proteins in the food you eat will interfere with and lessen the overall action and effectiveness of these supplements.

Now, for the heart: I recommend taking Coenzyme Q_{10} to help improve energy production on the cellular level, enhance heart muscle function, lower cholesterol, and restore immune functions. Folic acid and L-carnitine have also been shown to protect the heart from disease. Any program for cardiovascular health needs to also include natural stable fish oil in the diet. Marine fish oil supplementation has been shown to protect against many cardiovascular and inflammatory disorders (including arthritis and migraines) and to lower risk factors associated with these diseases.

In particular, fish oils have been shown to significantly improve and normalize parameters associated with HDLs (the good cholesterol) and LDLs (the bad cholesterol), total cholesterol and homocysteine. There is a lot of very recent research that shows that homocysteine levels in the blood have a lot to do with cardiovascular risk. Fish oils are beneficial because they are a plentiful source of omega-3 fatty acids, which have been shown to lower homocysteine levels and raise the good HDLs, so they can help to prevent heart attack, atherosclerosis, hypertension, and arrhythmias. In his Zone program, Barry Sears cautions that one should emphasize the omega-6 fatty acids over the omega-3 fatty acids, to tip the balance toward the "good eicosanoids" that promote good health. Omega-6 fatty acids are found in raw nuts, seeds, and legumes; borage oil, grape seed oil, and primrose oil are also good sources and are available as dietary supplements.

For the heart, I generally recommend my patients also take one of the many Chinese herbal formulas containing an herb called Salvia. This herb has been shown to match and in some studies even outperform the effectiveness of some of the common heart and cholesterol-lowering pharmaceutical medications. Salvia works by dilating the vessels and increasing cardiac output. And also always remember that vitamin E is a natural blood thinner and also increases the oxygen flow to the heart muscle.

Speaking of vitamin E, it's generally recognized that E and the other antioxidants are the foundation of any longevity program due to the wide array of functions they stimulate and support. Antioxidants are the major protectors against disease and premature aging. We've all seen butter or oil become rancid when left out, or metal become rusty from exposure to oxygen. In the body, these same oxidative reactions can also take place, deep down at the cellular level, and if these reactions overwhelm your body's natural ability to control or "quench" them, your risk of illness is accelerated.

To assure you are getting everything you need, it's a good idea to take a multiple antioxidant formula. Make certain it has all the basics in it. They should include the following: beta carotene, vitamin C (buffered, chelated or Ester C), vitamin B_1, B_2, B_3, vitamin E (in a non-oily, water-soluble form), folic acid, zinc and selenium.

Additional antioxidants, which are sometimes more expensive, but have been shown to help with immunity and protect from a broad range of aging diseases, include the following: grape seed pycnogenols, Boswellia (an ancient Ayurvedic herb), Bilberry extract (a medicinal herb used for centuries in the West), Coenzyme Q_{10}, garlic, NADH, (the first nutritional supplement tested by the FDA), and reduced glutathione. Reduced glutathione is one of the "newer" antioxidant discoveries that have now been shown to "spare" or "recycle" your other antioxidants, so that you are actually getting maximum benefit, or recycling from whichever other antioxidants you're taking.

Although the antioxidants are your easiest and best protection against any and all immune problems, you may also want to consider other specific supplements that strengthen the thymus gland. It's a well-accepted fact that the thymus gland function declines with age and in many individuals it is barely functioning by age forty. The thymus gland is the primary gland in the body that controls T-cell production, and our T-cells are our body's protection and first line of defense from disease.

There are many different types of T-cells, including T-4 helper white blood cells and T-8 killer (or lymphocyte) white blood cells. Cancer, AIDS, colds, flu, herpes and every other type of virus are only able to get a foothold in the body because these T-cells, which are our first line of defense, are not responding strongly enough or not "programmed" properly. Products that help directly with T-cell production include herbs such as astragalus and echinacea and glandular supplements made from the thymus gland.

Of the many different types of ginseng, Siberian ginseng is known to stimulate mental clarity and give physical energy while not depleting the body. Siberian ginseng is generally the only one I recommend for women, since the other types may be too yang in nature. Korean ginseng and American ginseng are also used for energy and vitality, but it's important that these only be used for a quick "pick-me-up" or to recover from an acute illness; they should not be used on a regular basis

The Chinese have a long tradition of preserving youth and have a host of herbal formulas with a proven track record of mitigating the aging process, but these Chinese herbal formulas need to be selected based on which individual weakness a person has. Some examples are the following:

❖ *Dynamic Warrior* is used to tonify Kidney Yang and build Jing (essence)

❖ *Women's Precious* is used to nourish and tonify Liver and Heart blood and support the Spleen

✧ *Rehmannia 6* is used to tonify Kidney Yin and protect from sexual weakness, poor eyesight, and to nourish the tendons and ligaments

✧ *Central Chi Pills* are used to tonify and help digestion and Spleen chi

✧ *Shou Wu* is used as a general tonic against aging.

Generally, each Chinese herbal company has its own specific line of formulas to combat the aging process, but each needs to be prescribed based on your own individual constitution. If you take a formula that is not indicated for your particular weakness, you may cause an imbalance in your meridians and organs. I consider the well-selected Chinese formula to be an essential part in any anti-aging strategy.

Finally, you may also want to consider consulting a classical homeopath. In conjunction with the right diet and supplements, a well-selected constitutional homeopathic remedy will work on a cellular level to strengthen all your body's physical and mental functions.

Here are three very important general guidelines you need to always remember when taking any and all supplements: Begin by taking the smallest potency you can find. You can even cut a tablet in half or take only a few drops, if it's in liquid form. Reactions are always possible, as are allergies to substances, so you should always begin with the smallest amount possible and slowly work your way up.

Second, never take any supplement, whether it is an herb, vitamin or mineral, on an ongoing basis. In my medical practice, I generally tell my patients never to take anything more than three months. This is because of a little-known law, or rule, of natural healing: Any substance you take can and will eventually cause a "proving" in your system. A proving is when your body becomes saturated, either energetically or physiologically, with the substance. When this happens, the substance itself will begin to create in you the exact symptoms you were taking it to eradicate!

For example, if ginkgo was initially raising your libido and you were to continue taking it, eventually it will decrease your libido. To prevent this, rotate your supplements, so that you are not "addicted to" any one single product. In the case of vitamins and minerals, always rotate the product by changing the company or the chemical composition of the product. For example, don't always take colloidal calcium, or blue green algae, but change to something else which has the same benefits, but acts in a slightly different way.

Lastly, please remember that none of the advice in this or any article should be taken as gospel. Everyone writes from his or her own point of view and experience. You should always check with your own health practitioner or doctor before embarking on a new program or supplement. And never discontinue any prescription medication or combine a prescription medication with a natural supplement without sitting down and discussing it with your doctor.

Over the past year, I have recently been invited to lecture on vitamins, herbs and homeopathy to various groups of medical doctors. This says to me that there is finally an increased openness and acceptance, even from traditional medical doctors, about integrating different health care approaches.

STRESS AND THE GLOBAL VILLAGE

In our modern culture, we are increasingly subjected to the "global village" concept first coined by Marshall McLuhan in the 1960s. Everything going on in the world is intricately interconnected and within our daily grasp. We are immediately made aware of styles and fashions in Europe, fighting in Eastern Europe, upheaval in Africa, crime across the country, and all the other disasters occurring everywhere else in the world.

The problem with this is that when it comes to our emotions we still function on a basic, animal level. Intellectually, we might think that all of this data bombarding us is wonderful; emotionally, however, it creates a lot of stress. It *deeply* affects many of us, particularly if we are at all sensitive.

Our adrenal glands that trigger action and response—"fight or flight"—are designed to be stimulated when faced with danger. The adrenals go into survival mode regardless of whether the stimulation is real or on the TV. For the individual, the global village concept implies only the ability to receive a vast amount of incoming information. There is little or no opportunity for appropriate "global" reactions to such information. In a practical sense, appropriate reactions are limited to slow-paced, rational, or political plans that offer little immediate relief or satisfaction on the animal level. This immense intake of information with a relatively small opportunity for action creates a disparity—a major source of internal stress.

Here are some suggestions for sensitive individuals who are faced with this type of stress:

❁ Learn to set appropriate goals and boundaries. Ignore—or at least be selective— about what you allow into your frame of awareness. Healthy censorship is an important way to keep your stress levels to a minimum and will keep your adrenal glands from being in constant overdrive.

❁ Develop a rational plan of action—personally or within your community— to address larger issues of most concern to you; that way, at least intellectually you can feel plugged into the "larger picture."

❁ Get into the habit of doing enough physical stress-reduction exercise to keep your adrenals balanced. Many people in our culture turn to addictive substances or behaviors and avoid calming down and relaxing. This keeps the body from getting rid of stress and adds to more muscle tension and other stress-related symptoms

Stress busters

Here are some practical exercises you can do each day:

- Breathe.
- Take a walk.
- Eat well. Eliminate, or at least minimize, your intake of salt, sugar, alcohol, caffeine, and fats.
- Reduce your intake of stimulation and stress-related data {such as news).
- Get a massage.
- Receive an acupuncture treatment.
- Reduce negative internal messages by learning self-acceptance and embark on a program to increase your self-esteem.
- Get emotional support wherever you can; concentrate on creating solid friendships.
- Journal; learn to express your feelings on paper.
- Meditate or at least spend quiet time alone.
- Take naps. Some people do better on less sleep and a few small naps during the day.
- Read things that you find entertaining.
- Rent an entertaining video or see a mindless movie.
- Play with children (unless you are already a parent—then play with adults).
- Play with an animal.
- Walk in nature. Go to the beach and listen to the waves, or listen to the trees in a forest.
- Change your lifestyle to allow for more of all of the above.
- Take a bath and get some bath toys to play with.
- Create a hobby that brings no income, only enjoyment.
- Pray and get in touch with your gratitude.

MEDITATION-BASED STRESS REDUCTION

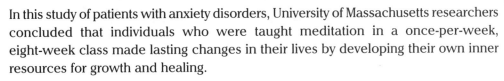

In this study of patients with anxiety disorders, University of Massachusetts researchers concluded that individuals who were taught meditation in a once-per-week, eight-week class made lasting changes in their lives by developing their own inner resources for growth and healing.

Participants learned a technique known as "mindfulness meditation," which they were required to practice at home. Specific improvements included reduction in depression and anxiety, fewer panic attacks and more mobility for agoraphobics. Most participants were still practicing the technique at a three-year follow-up and were able to decrease or eliminate medications they had been taking.

—Gen. Hosp. Psychiatry 1995; 17:192-200

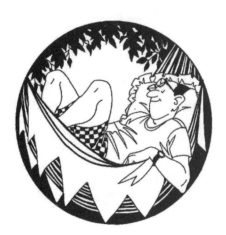

The question is not whether we can help the patients who come to our offices with complaints, but whether we can help them cope long-term with the changing environment in which they live.

—Roy Martina, M.D.

SPECIFIC CONDITIONS

COMMON NATURAL TREATMENTS

Accident/Injury/Trauma:

Immediately take a dose of homeopathic *Arnica* if you don't have any other remedies available or don't know what else to give. Keep Arnica handy in the car or anywhere else you go. If you don't have Arnica, then you can use the Bach flower remedy called *Rescue Remedy*.

Headache:

Frontal Headache: Massage below the occiput (at Gall Bladder 20).

Sinus Headache: Use Tiger Balm on Yin Tang (between the eyebrows).

Migraine: Use peppermint oil rubbed into the temples and forehead; place your feet and hands in hot water and place ice on your forehead and back of the neck.

Use these teas for headache (mix or use separately): catnip; peppermint; sage leaves.

Abdominal Gas and Bloating or Pain:

Charcoal tablets or capsules for gas and diarrhea

Pill curing, a Chinese herbal formula

Slippery elm bark tea: one teaspoon powdered bark to two cups of water, simmered for twenty minutes; strain and drink as needed.

Nausea:

Use either peppermint tea or clove tea.

Ginger root tea, made from the fresh root or ginger capsules

Vomiting:

Slippery elm bark tea (same recipe as above)

Same herbs as for nausea

Fever:

Peppermint and elder flower tea: take one tablespoon of each of the leaves to two cups boiled water; steep for fifteen minutes and strain; sip as needed.

Sage tea also helps to break a fever; one tablespoon to one cup of boiled water.

Herpes:

Two great herbal formulas are combinations of 1) Echinacea, burdock, and capsicum or 2) quince, ginger, and clove. Take one capsule of each every two to three hours.

Use no stimulating foods, sweets, alcohol, caffeine, or spices.

Use goldenseal or calendula ointment, mixed with a little lysine, topically on blisters or sores.

Lysine, 1000 mg. three or four times per day during an acute outbreak

Quell Fire and Rehmannia 6

Bladder Infection:

Cranberry juice

Vitamin C, beta carotene, vitamin E, zinc picolinate

Corn silk tea

Berb. vulg. tincture, ten drops, three to four times per day

Menstrual Cramps:

Ten days before the period, increase your intake of magnesium to 1,000 mg. per day.

Raspberry leaf tea used throughout the menstrual cycle

Diarrhea:

Acidophilus capsules

Peppermint tea

Charcoal capsules if accompanied by gas

To prevent traveler's diarrhea, use digestive enzymes, garlic capsules and homeopathic *Nux vom.*

Sore Throat:

Sage Tea: drink it and also make a large portion in the bathroom sink and inhale the vapors to clear out the nose. You can also gargle with it.

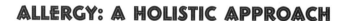

ALLERGY: A HOLISTIC APPROACH

Allergies can be divided into two general groups: food allergies and environmental allergies. Environmental allergies can be further divided into airborne and household. Airborne allergies consist of pollens, dust, exhaust fumes, etc., and household allergies include animal hair, mites, molds, detergents, cleansers, bedding, synthetic fibers in clothing, etc.

The approach to curing allergies from the holistic perspective is twofold. First is to eliminate the allergen (i.e. the irritating substance). Second is to strengthen your body so that the allergen no longer bothers you. In my practice, I have seen many people cured of all types of allergies using natural methods without the use of drugs.

Symptoms of allergy are highly individual. The most common symptoms are nasal congestion, sore throat, coughing, red and itching eyes, headaches, depression, fatigue, muscle cramps, indigestion, acne, runny nose, skin rash and hives, mental fog, irritability and anxiety. But there are many other symptoms experienced by different individuals.

There are many ways to "test" for allergies. These include blood tests, skin scratch tests, pulse tests, dowsing and muscle testing. Depending on the person and their financial constraints, I use any variety of these tests in my practice. Each has certain strengths and weaknesses.

Food allergies are treated by eliminating the suspected foods while at the same time strengthening the digestive system. The most common foods that people are allergic to are dairy, wheat, chocolate, citrus fruits, sugar, red meat, and barley. Other common food allergens are eggs, shellfish, tomatoes and potatoes.

The reason a particular food manifests as an allergen in your body is because your digestive system is sensitive to that food and cannot break it down into its basic parts. As a result, whole food "particles," so to speak, enter the blood stream as poisons and then circulate throughout the body to produce allergy symptoms in the weakest area of your body. (Note that this theory is very controversial and is generally not accepted as fact by Western-trained doctors.)

The treatment used to cure food allergies is to strengthen the digestive tract, breakdown of foods and their assimilation. This is done by treating the weak meridians using acupuncture and Chinese herbal formulas. Digestive teas, specific enzyme formulas and homeopathics are also used. Some of the most common herbs used include mint, gentian and ginger root.

Depending on the individual symptoms, the following homeopathic remedies may also be used:

1. *Pulsatilla:* when fats are the major problem, in a person who craves fats, and is emotionally rather soft, needy, or desiring a lot of support;

2. *Nux vomica:* for toxicity in the liver with a craving for spicy foods and stimulants; constipation; rather angry and irritable emotionally and tends to be a workaholic type;

3. *Lycopodium:* for a lot of flatulence, right sided pains, sciatica, shoulder pain, irritability, craving for sweets and an explosive temper, but only around those he or she is close to; can be emotionally very sweet around work and social situations;

4. *Carbo veg:* for flatulence and general indigestion with bloating and a slow metabolism.

You can also use homeopathic remedies that are made from the foods you are allergic to, in much the same way as allergy shots work.

Allergies to pollens are also treated very effectively with acupuncture and homeopathy. Specific remedies may include the following:

1. *Pollintinum:* composed of a variety of the most common pollens;

2. *Histaminum:* to suppress the histamine reaction of watery and itchy eyes, asthma or runny nose;

3. *Euphrasia:* for red, burning or itching eyes;

4. *Allium cepa:* for a runny and burning nose with much mucus;

5. *Sabadilla:* for uncontrollable sneezing;

6. *Baptisia:* for a skin rash and hives with itching;

7. *Cat Hair:* to desensitize you to an allergy to cats.

Depending on the individual symptoms, Chinese herbal formulas are often used. Usually a person with allergies has toxicity in the liver meridian and herbs to detoxify the liver are very helpful.

When you are allergic to household products, the treatment approach is to try to eliminate all the offending products while at the same time working to boost your immune system in general. The basic treatment consists of herbs, nutritional supplements, and counseling. Acupuncture is sometimes used at well.

Nutritionally, foods to avoid when trying to build your immune system include sugar, red meat, coffee, dairy products and fats, but this list varies tremendously from person to person.

Specific vitamins and herbs that may be used to boost immunity include vitamin C (buffered, chelated, or esterified), vitamin E (dry), beta carotene, zinc and selenium. Bee pollen, barley greens, sun chlorella, acidophilus, ginseng, codenopsis and astragalus are also commonly used as tonics.

If you think you are experiencing allergies, please talk to me or another trained medical practitioner who has experience diagnosing and treating allergies. It is often difficult to differentiate allergic reactions from Candidiasis (a yeast infection), dysglycemia (blood sugar swings), Epstein-Barr virus, and Chronic Fatigue Syndrome.

FOOD ALLERGY CHECKLIST

1. Insomnia
2. Foggy thinking
3. Crying Spells
4. Withdrawal
5. Mood swing(s)
6. Fatigue
7. Irritability
8. Gas
9. Bloating
10. Diarrhea
11. Tremors
12. Nausea
13. Anxiety
14. Headache
15. Skin rash
16. Stomach pain
17. Sweating
18. Chills
19. Itching
20. Muscle spasms
21. Sugar craving
22. Chocolate craving
23. Craving for bread or other starches
24. Pain behind the eyes
25. Sleepy within ½ to 1 hour after eating

EARTHQUAKE PREPAREDNESS: YOUR PERSONAL HOMEOPATHIC FIRST AID KIT

When we think of preparing for earthquakes and other natural disasters, we usually think in terms of flashlights, a battery-operated radio, sturdy shoes, and other traditional first aid equipment. Of course it's important to have all the traditional items contained in a first aid kit, but in addition you may want to prepare a homeopathic first aid kit.

1. Include Traumeel lotion, or some other topical lotion containing *Arnica montana*, which can be applied to the skin for swelling, sprains, bruising, muscle spasm and stiffness, and internal injuries of any kind, including bleeding. There are other companies producing Arnica ointments, but I like Traumeel© because the particular combination of remedies it contains in addition to Arnica make it effective for many first aid emergencies.

2. *Calendula Cerate* for an open wound; a gentle, healing formula of calendula in cerate form in a Vaseline base. Besides being very soothing, it will help to heal and disinfect even the worst open wound. If you suspect infection or want to keep infection away, apply this formula and keep the wound covered. Do not apply to mucus membranes or very sensitive parts of the body.

3. Lysine Plus ointment. This topical ointment is generally used for herpes on the skin, but it contains a large portion of Hydrastis (Goldenseal) which makes it a gentle, soothing, and healing ointment for use on sensitive body parts (nose, mouth, genitals, ears, etc.) It will help to keep infection away, remove pus, and promote healing.

4. *Echinacea augustifolia* tincture. Use this as a disinfectant to scrub open wounds before applying a topical ointment. Use about ten drops per quarter cup of water.

5. *Hydrastis* tincture. Use this the same way you use the Echinacea tincture; it is particularly helpful cleaning any wound where there is pus. It is also a useful gargle for throat infections, strep, or sore throat.

6. *Arnica montana 12X.* This is the first remedy to use for any trauma to your body.

7. Rescue Remedy. A combination Bach Flower Remedy which is very useful for the emotional or physical effects of trauma, jet lag, and disorientation. If you don't know which remedy to use and you have access to Rescue Remedy, use it first. Put 2 drops under the tongue every 15 to 30 minutes in an acute stage.

8. *Nux vomica 12X.* Probably the next most-useful *polycrest* (remedy of many uses) to have on hand. One survey of homeopaths stated that when asked which *one* remedy each would take to a desert island (if s/he only could only take one) the majority said *Nux vomica.* Of course, if you know your particular constitutional remedy, it would probably benefit you more to take it instead of *Nux vomica.*

   Nux vomica is good for any type of digestive problem including constipation, diarrhea, or indigestion. It may also be helpful in dizziness if you don't have another remedy on hand.

9. *Belladonna* for fever and inflammation.

10. *Hypericum perfoliatum* for nerve injury.

11. *Ipecac* for vomiting and nausea.

12. *Conium* and *Cocculus* for dizziness and disorientation.

13. *Ledum palustre* for contusions and bruising.

14. *Ruta graveolens (Ruta)* for injury to ligaments and tendons, such as sprains and tears (after using *Arnica*).

In general, I recommend purchasing a homeopathic first aid remedy kit and keeping it near your traditional first aid kit. Also, make a smaller version, using a fishing tackle box or camera case, and keep it in your car for emergencies.

TUMORS, CYSTS, FIBROIDS, CANCER?
IS YOUR WOOD OVERGROWN?

Growth… something we all strive for, and we're all very interested in, both on an inner and outer level. But when growth is either stifled or out of control, when it has a life of its own, distinct from the rest of our body/mind, it can create inner nodules, cysts, tumors, fibroids, warts, moles, or even cancer.

You might be wondering what a cyst, mole or wart has to do with cancer, but according to Chinese medical theory, every function in our body is regulated by a corresponding organ. And in the case of our growth—any growth at all—and the free flow of our creative energy, which promotes growth, the liver is the primary control mechanism. According to Chinese medicine, the liver function in the body is in charge of regulating all growth, whether wanted or unwanted.

In Chinese medicine, each organ has a corresponding season and element. The Five Element theory of Oriental medicine discusses correspondences between the elements, seasons and organs (see chart below).

Element	Organs	Season	Quality
Wood	Liver, Gall Bladder	Spring	Growth
Water	Bladder, Kidneys	Winter	Flow
Earth	Stomach, Spleen	Late Summer	Grounded
Metal	Lungs, Large Intestine	Fall	Letting Go
Fire	Heart, Small Intestine	Summer	Flourishing

As you can see, the Liver and Gall Bladder correspond to the Wood Element and growth or overgrowth in the body. The liver will actually create moles, warts and small cysts as a defense, or balancing mechanism, to keep itself in homeostasis. These small, unwanted growths, are what keep the liver from needing to create larger, more significant, unwanted growths, such as breast or ovarian cancer.

They are a sign of toxicity and imbalance in the body that is often genetically linked. If you cut them out, even a small wart or cyst, the body will first "try" to grow them back, to get your attention and bring you back to homeostasis. But if you keep cutting them out or freezing them off, the body will have no choice but to create larger, more serious, even life-threatening growths and tumors.

It may seem like an odd concept, but I'm talking here both about inner, spiritual/emotional growth and also the growths in our body, such as tumors, moles, cancers, etc. "What's the connection?" you might be asking. Well, if the energy of the liver becomes what we call in Chinese medicine "stagnant" or blocked, it creates an "overgrowth" or nodule, somewhere in the body. The area it "decides" to "place" this growth is dependent on where the blockage is occurring.

Polyps or tumors in the colon (large intestine), for instance, might arise if the primary issues you are dealing with are letting go, or boundary issues of separating what's worth keeping versus "getting rid" of. Uterine fibroids might have to do with issues of sexuality, reproduction and the ability to "re-create." Prostatitis or prostate cancer may have to do with a man's ability to "re-create" his masculine principle out into the world, just as fibrocystic breast disease or breast cancer may have to do with issues of the feminine principle of not feeling nurtured or not having the creative outlet in your life to nurture others.

The underlying theme in all growths in the body, whether they be moles and warts (early signs of blockage and stagnation in the liver) or tumors and cancer (advanced and progressed signs of blockage and stagnation), is commonly a lack of connection with one's inner creative, life-giving force. Lacking this connection on the spiritual and emotional levels, the body will be forced to manifest the imbalance in the form of physical "over-growth."

This said, what can we actually do to treat the liver to prevent these negative or pathological "growths" from occurring? The universe has fortunately provided us with many herbs and nutrients that we now know will keep the body detoxified and the energy of the liver flowing smoothly. The preventive treatment, and the treatment to begin with in all cases of any unwanted growth in your body, is to do a good detoxification, which should include the detoxification all your major body organs.

A Doctor of Chinese medicine can tell through traditional tongue and pulse diagnosis, coupled with blood tests, urine and hair analysis, which organs need to be detoxified.

A specific remedy for liver detoxification—one that was popularized by Edgar Cayce—is the castor oil pack. This should be done daily, or at least weekly. Don't worry, this isn't the castor oil your grandma made you drink when you were little! O.K., so we're first going to get castor oil from the health food store and spread it all over the abdomen, from your breast bone down to your pubic bone. Now, take a hot washcloth and place it over the castor oil. Then place a hot water bottle over the washcloth to keep it hot. Do this for about 20 minutes, ideally once per day, to get the energy of the liver and the other internal organs to start moving more freely. Another version of this is to make fresh ginger root tea and to soak your washcloth in the hot tea mixture before placing it on your abdomen. This has a stimulating effect on the organs.

Part of the detoxification process should also include a good colon cleanse. This is because you want to be sure that the toxins you're releasing from your liver, lungs and kidneys are leaving your body and not being re-absorbed by your colon. The detoxification formula and colon cleanse products I use are quite effective and have a proven track record among my many patients who have already gone through this program with great results! (Contact Dr. Martin for a list of available products.)

Strengthening the immune system is another vital component to your treatment regimen, and there are many herbs, vitamins and mineral supplements to help you.

I use a high potency vitamin E and antioxidant formula which has a lot of research supporting its effectiveness.

Additional immune-enhancing supplements include selenium, pycnogenols, CoQ$_{10}$, germanium, shark cartilage, proteolytic enzymes, apricot kernels, green tea extract, St. John's Wort, echinacea and astragalus.

If you're not a vegetarian, there are also some good animal-based products to stimulate immunity, including glandular extracts of thymus, spleen and liver. Aborigine cultures around the world have used glandular extracts and herbs as a part of their traditional treatments to prevent and treat serious illness. I use a product called Bio-Immunozyme Forte, which contains a well-rounded combination of immune-boosting products.

A specific Chinese herbal formula which has been used traditionally to shrink tumors and build immunity is Minor Bupluerum. My office sells a very high quality version of this traditional formula. Remember whenever you purchase herbs to buy from a reputable company, since the quality can vary significantly. More specific Chinese formulae need to be prescribed based specifically on where the growth is occurring, your particular body and personality type and metabolic imbalance.

When it comes to immunity, homeopathic medicine may be your number one best "ace-in-the-hole." And although for minor health problems it's great to use homeopathy to treat yourself, when it comes to more serious diseases, you need to consult your professional homeopath to get a constitutional remedy.

Research has found that most excess growths in the body correspond to an overly acidic body chemistry, so it's good to add herbs and foods to alkalinize your body. Alkalinizing herbs include garlic, comfrey, bladder wrack and Irish moss. Animal products tend to acidify your system, although in proper amounts can also be used to build your immune system if you are depleted. I have created a modified Zone Diet for my patients that is specifically geared to each individual's metabolic type. (See page 141)

A good drink to balance your body chemistry and help digestion is to boil a cup of water and then mix in one teaspoon of honey and one or two tablespoons of apple cider vinegar. Drink this with meals two to three times per day.

If you're trying to promote and strengthen immunity and get rid of a possible acid condition in your body, stay away from coffee, alcohol, red meat, sugar and all recreational drugs. Your primary diet should consist of complex carbohydrates such as beans, peas, soups, cooked vegetables and only low fat animal protein that is complementary with and necessary for your particular body-type.

For the pain associated with serious health problems such as tumors or cancers, there are a few herbs which are very helpful pain relievers including feverfew, white willow bark, valerian and hops.

If one needs to be treated with chemotherapy or radiation, there are also specific vitamins, herbs and homeopathics for reducing the side effects, but these need to be chosen based on the particular area being treated and the specific symptoms that arise. In general, you need to take very large doses of antioxidants before, during, and after any of these invasive types of treatments along with your homeopathic remedies. Acupuncture can also reduce the side-effects of a chemotherapy and radiation.

If you are on any medications prescribed by a physician, don't stop them without his or her advice. Many of the suggestions in this article can be used in conjunction with traditional medical treatments such as surgery, radiation or chemotherapy. So-called "alternative" medicine, is actually complementary, and can be used along with most of our traditional allopathic medical treatments.

> *One of these days the cancer research people ... will wake up to the fact that psychology has an influence on tissue cells, a proposition they have consistently regarded even until now as preposterous heresy.*
> —*Dr. Karl Menniger*

CANDIDA

Candida albicans is an opportunistic yeast that attacks the immune system and affects thousands of people each year. Candidiasis is a yeast infection that can cause poor digestion, vaginal yeast, headaches, migraines, allergies, ringing in the ears, skin rashes, diarrhea, constipation, mental fogginess or fuzziness, gas, bloating, and a host of other symptoms.

If you or someone you know has some of these symptoms, has a history of taking a lot of antibiotics, has been on the birth control pill for a long period of time, and has been unsuccessfully treated elsewhere, they should be checked for Candida.

The diagnosis of Candida is made in a variety of ways, including vaginal cultures, blood tests, stool samples, and throat cultures. The treatment for Candida is different for everyone. Some people prefer Chinese herbal formulas that kill off the Candida and boost the immune system. Others benefit from acupuncture and homeopathic treatments as well.

If you think that you have Candida, the most important thing is to realize that there is hope and you don't need to suffer any longer.

CANDIDA DIET

If you already know you suffer from Candida, this diet and supplement program will be a great help in getting it out of your system. If you are unsure, you may want to get a stool test and/or blood test to see for sure. If you are infected, make sure that anyone you are in intimate contact with is also on the program. Otherwise you can pass it back and forth, resulting in no improvement.

Symptoms of Candida include: headaches, bloating, gas, indigestion, tinnitis, sore throats, irritability, PMS, fungus on the nails or tongue, skin rashes, food allergies, cravings for fruit or for sweets or carbohydrates, frequent urinary infections, diarrhea or yeast infections, and a spiking fever after taking antibiotics.

FOODS TO AVOID:

- ✧ Chocolate
- ✧ Sugar
- ✧ Most sweets
- ✧ Wheat, gluten, rye, oats, barley (try amaranth, rice, buckwheat and quinoa instead)
- ✧ Fats and fried foods of all types
- ✧ Dairy products (except for yogurt, which is OK)
- ✧ Artificial sweeteners of all types
- ✧ Anything excessively sweet
- ✧ Summer fruits (moderate fruits are OK: sour apples, cherries, bananas, bosc and Asian pears)
- ✧ Excessive use of yeasty products (use non-yeast, non-wheat breads, or bake your own from rice flour)
- ✧ Coffee and caffeine
- ✧ Soy sauce
- ✧ Alcohol
- ✧ Excessively salty or excessively spicy foods

FOODS AND SUPPLEMENTS TO EMPHASIZE:

- ✧ Emphasize the use of cooked vegetables
- ✧ Tofu and soy products
- ✧ Goat cheese, sunflower seeds
- ✧ Eggs are also a good source of protein as are salmon, swordfish and shark
- ✧ Chlorophyll
- ✧ Saussarea and Cardamom (herbal formulas)
- ✧ Vitamin C, buffered
- ✧ Zinc
- ✧ Digestive enzymes with HCL and Enterogenic Capsules
- ✧ Aqua Flora Phase 1 and Phase 2
- ✧ Phellostatin Chinese Herbal Formula
- ✧ DAG Solution for mouth gargle and vaginal douche
- ✧ AVI Cream for Vaginal Yeast
- ✧ AC Formula for intestinal yeast or systemic yeast
- ✧ ADHS to kill the candida

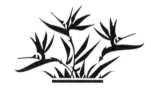

CHRONIC FATIGUE IMMUNE DEFICIENCY SYNDROME (CFIDS)

Introduction

Chronic Fatigue Immune Deficiency Syndrome, or CFIDS as it is called for short, is an opportunistic disease. As with all opportunists, it attacks the host when resistance is at its lowest. This includes resistance on any or all levels—spiritual, emotional, mental, or physical.

As a doctor of Oriental medicine and a classical homeopath, I have had the rather unique opportunity to see and assist others through their struggles and crises with CFIDS. I have been treating CFIDS since 1986 and am a member of the CFIDS national physician's honor role. I have also had the opportunity to guide many patients to partial and, in many cases, full recovery.

I perceive my role as healer and as a physician who treats CFIDS to be fourfold:

❁ To support my patients emotionally while they partake in the challenging task of working through any emotional blocks to getting well

❁ To strengthen their immune system through dietary counseling, therapeutic treatment with appropriate vitamin and mineral supplements, acupuncture, herbal remedies, and homeopathic medicine

❁ To monitor and give support to whatever lifestyle changes are necessary to bring them to a state of optimal health

❁ To integrate my treatment approach with that of the rest of their chosen treatment team, usually a psychotherapist or hypnotherapist, and sometimes a medical doctor or chiropractic doctor

History of CFIDS

Although the history of CFIDS can be traced back to the early 1800s, the most recent history is the most relevant. Names given to fatigue-causing diseases that affect large numbers of people have included chronic Epstein-Barr virus (EBV), Candida, environmental allergies, universal reactors, depression, hysteria, PMS, anxiety, and hypoglycemia. In Great Britain, the controversy has been raging since 1950, when nearly 200 staff members of the Royal Free Hospital of London become ill with what appeared to be the same illness.

In the U.S., the controversy began in 1984 with an outbreak in Incline Village, Nevada, which was originally blamed on EBV. The outbreak was subsequently dismissed as "yuppie flu" by the media, but the people in Nevada all had high blood test readings for both Epstein-Barr virus and another virus, which was not identified until later. Unfortunately, no definitive correlations could be made before research funding ran out.

The U.S. Center for Disease Control is now funding studies to determine the exact causes of CFIDS. Popular Western medical theory is that it is caused by a specific type of virus called a retrovirus, or it is perhaps linked to autoimmune diseases similar to Lupus or rheumatoid arthritis. Other doctors think it is simply clinical depression. It may be one, a combination, or all of these things and perhaps some others, depending on the individual case. The syndrome is broadly defined and not as specific as some might wish.

Definition of CFIDS

A working definition of CFIDS has three criteria:

1. The onset of severe fatigue in a previously healthy and energetic person

2. A typical pattern of symptoms (see list below)

3. Exclusion of other illnesses that cause fatigue (see chart of other illnesses and tests to consider)

Symptoms Typical of CFIDS Patients

✧ Mild or low grade fever, often persisting for long periods of time or recurring often

✧ Recurrent sore throat

✧ Painful lymph glands

✧ Muscle weakness

✧ Muscle pain

✧ Prolonged fatigue after exercise or even mild exertion

✧ Recurrent headache

✧ Migratory or constant joint pain

✧ Psychological problems such as anxiety or depression

✧ Sleep problems

✧ Sudden onset of any or all of these symptoms

✧ Onset following a bad cold or flu

Characteristics of CFIDS Patients

Here are some personality characteristics that might be found in someone suffering from CFIDS:

❂ Either having a lack of boundaries or too constricted, creating too many restrictions, keeping others' love and nurturing out. If they do not set boundaries, they take in too much of other people's problems and can't differentiate their problems from others' problems. This leads to a "burnout" condition.

❈ Lack of patience; wanting answers to problems now and solutions right away

❈ Black-and-white thinking; not accepting the nature of the universe and their reality as relative: "It is or it isn't." A setup for wanting simple, quick solutions. Unwilling to accept the complexity in things or in other people.

❈ Very critical and judgmental of themselves and others. This causes more constriction and difficulty in digestion. The body shuts down and "beats itself up."

❈ The type of person who cannot fit into the high-paced model of contemporary society—the "yin" type. This could be a woman with PMS who is told there is something wrong with her for feeling moody, or a person who is viewed as "sickly" because he does not conform to the fast pace of life. (In contrast, Native American cultures would allow the PMS-suffering woman time to do the creative work she needs to stay in balance.) Some people with CFIDS are simply very creative, introverted, intuitive types who—given another more congenial, slow-paced setting—would not be viewed as having a problem.

Lab Tests and Other Diseases to Consider in the Diagnosis

❈ Complete blood cell count (CBC)
❈ T-cell/B-cell ratio
❈ Chemistry Panel
❈ SED Rate
❈ Thyroid Panel
❈ EBV Panel
❈ Cytomegalo Virus (CMV) Panel
❈ Candida Panel
❈ Antinuclear Antibody
❈ Rheumatoid Factor
❈ Lyme Disease Antibody
❈ Hepatitis A and B Antibodies
❈ HIV Antibody
❈ HHV-6 Antibodies
❈ Coxacci Virus B Titer
❈ Natural Killer Cells

One must be careful in making a diagnosis of CFIDS because the disease has so many different possible presenting symptoms. It may appear to be many other diseases, which sometimes makes the diagnosis very difficult. In fact, a person suffering with CFIDS may also have a number of other immune problems.

There may often be slight anemia, a sluggish thyroid, a slightly low WBC (white blood cell count), slightly elevated enzymes, or other borderline abnormalities in the blood workup. An allopathically-trained physician may often find nothing wrong with a person, but when evaluated by someone trained in identifying CFIDS, the condition may become more apparent.

Causes of CFIDS

Hereditary factors are always said to play some role in all disease processes. If a person is not prone by heredity to a certain susceptibility, they will not contract this or any disease. Diet and lifestyle also play a role and will be discussed below. Emotions and attitude are also an important ingredient to examine in CFIDS. Finally, the environment and external factors must also be considered.

In terms of Oriental medical theory, each person is evaluated as an individual, but the most prevalent disease patterns are found in:

✧ A weakened water element and kidneys;
✧ Weakness in the immune system and the digestive organs, notably stomach and spleen;
✧ Toxic or stagnant energy in the liver and gallbladder; and/or
✧ Disturbed Shen and heart yin deficiency.

Psychological Considerations

One of the first tasks I have as a healer is to encourage all CFIDS clients to seek some type of help—counseling, hypnotherapy, or psychotherapy. CFIDS is opportunistic, and I notice that sufferers with this disease usually have emotional issues revolving around the setting of personal limits and boundaries.

A "typical" client, if there is such a person, may be overextending him/herself at work or in personal relationships. Usually the client comes from a dysfunctional family or is an adult child of an alcoholic (ACA) and has grown up accustomed to having his or her own boundaries severely compromised. As a result, in adult life these patients are usually unaware of others encroaching upon their boundaries—unaware, that is, until CFIDS stifles them physically.

CFIDS is a physical symbol or embodiment at the cellular level of an invasion or intrusion of personal boundaries on an emotional level. In other words, if the immune system is functioning well on the cellular level, CFIDS will not progress physically or emotionally.

Often the CFIDS patient needs in-depth work at setting limits on how much he can give of himself and at setting boundaries on how much he will let others into his emotional space. This may involve talking or cognitive therapy, or it may require more in-depth grief recovery work. The most effective type of therapy is often a type that integrates bodywork with cognitive work, such as Body-Mind Therapy, Radix or Reichian work, or Rebirthing. The relationship between the therapist and the patient is of critical importance, as this will be the model upon which the patient will learn to construct appropriate limits and boundaries.

Dealing with the deep-seated parental issues of invasiveness and abandonment is not an easy or simple process. Often patients have also been abused sexually, which further complicates their sense of personal boundaries.

Another psychological characteristic of the CFIDS patient, closely associated with the issues of setting boundaries and limits, is that the typical patient is one who has gone through life as a barometer for the thoughts and feelings of those around them. S/he is also often sensitive to the point of being psychic as well. These "human barometers," as I call them, carry a very heavy burden on their shoulders.

Depending on the context, this dynamic can manifest in several different yet similar ways. At work, she can be the employee who second-guesses her employer's needs and moods, and is constantly running on adrenaline to ensure that the boss is taken care of. In a family, he can be the person who is always there for everybody, and is everything to everybody else but himself. She can be the entrepreneur who sets no limits and is constantly running on overdrive, or the top performer at work after two or three years of concentrated performance and success.

Another dynamic that many people with CFIDS manifest is a severe contraction in several areas of life. Due to a difficulty in establishing realistic limits and boundaries, these individuals may have learned to "pull in" their boundaries and have turned uncompromising and inflexible. Obsessive-compulsive character styles and CFIDS often travel together.

In terms of Oriental medicine, we find that either of these behavior patterns involves excess. It is in the excess that the body gets out of harmony with itself and becomes diseased. Either an extreme of yang energy (overextending oneself) or an extreme of yin energy (contracting into oneself) will cause the kind of imbalance that makes one susceptible to CFIDS. In Oriental medicine, we strive to achieve an equilibrium, or balance, between yin and yang through the use of diet, herbs, and sometimes acupuncture.

Viewed from another holistic viewpoint, CFIDS patients often have many environmental sensitivities. These can manifest as allergies or sensitivities to carpet, filtered air in office buildings, detergents, deodorants, perfumes, smog, noise pollution, household cleaners, or any number of other smells or noises that others do not react to. They are often called "universal reactors."

On a cultural level, CFIDS patients can be seen as barometers of our global environmental health. In a way, they have become the global barometers of a culture off its track and out of touch with nature and its true resources.

I have treated some CFIDS patients who, in order to feel better, needed only a reduction in their work hours from 40 to 30 hours a week. Others needed more rest; some needed to stop watching TV news or reading the newspaper. The vast amount

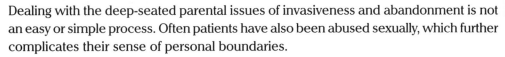

of data we are called upon to filter and integrate on a daily basis is escalating to an overwhelming level for increasingly greater numbers of people. CFIDS is just one of the many immune problems that people are experiencing as a result of our ever-faster pace of life.

It is also true that women tend to suffer from CFIDS more than men. In our culture, women tend to take on the role of caretaker, or a receptive role, more than men do. Women have been taught to subordinate their needs and attend to those around them more often than men have been taught to do so. In general, women also tend to have a more developed "receptive" mode when it comes to interpersonal communication skills.

It could be that these trained "receivers" and a small percentage of men who also have a strongly-developed sensitive or receptive sides are receiving a lot more than they, and our culture, have bargained for.

What is the nutritional approach for treating CFIDS?

My particular approach to diet and nutrition stems primarily from my background in Chinese medicine and its Law of the Five Elements. The first step is to diagnose the patient according to which of the five elements is the weakest, out of balance, or in need of nutritional support. Then I assess the patient in terms of the endocrine system and determine which of the endocrine glands is the weakest. Blood tests and hair analysis are sometimes used to get a more complete diagnosis.

Common weaknesses in CFIDS patients are found in the thyroid function, the adrenal glands, the spleen, stomach and digestive functions, and the liver and gallbladder complex. These organs and glands are assessed in terms of function from a Western and a Chinese medical viewpoint.

The thyroid function is weakened by foods such as sugar, sweets, and refined carbohydrates. The spleen is weakened by foods that are sweet or have a sweet taste, such as sugar, artificial sweeteners, honey, etc. The spleen is also weakened by foods that have qualities of cold or dampness. The Chinese often talk in metaphors. To this system of thinking, cold and damp include foods such as ice cream, frozen yogurt, iced drinks, dairy products in general, raw food diets, candy, and the like.

Foods that strengthen the spleen include cooked vegetables, whole grains, quality and easy to digest protein such as fish (but never shellfish), split peas, lentils, and tofu products. A moderate amount of naturally sweet unprocessed foods are also strengthening. These might include sweet brown rice, yam, sweet potato, carrot, beets, acorn squash, amasake beverage, barley, or kabocha pumpkin.

The liver is weakened and made toxic by simple carbohydrates such as sugar and white flour products as well as fats and deep fried foods. This also includes alcohol, recreational drugs, red fatty meats, and shellfish. An excess of any foods that are sour in flavor also weakens the liver. This includes vinegar, lemons, pickles, or sauerkraut. (A *moderate* amount of the sour flavor, such as a wedge of lemon in warm water after meals, actually helps the liver to heal and detoxify.)

Eating foods high in the amino acid lysine and low in arginine is also very important. Lysine is contained in all the legumes. Arginine foods include all grains and chocolate, to name a few. Lysine is known for strengthening immunity, and arginine is known to be an antagonist and a competitor to lysine.

Ultimately, each and every patient must be evaluated as to his or her own individual food needs. Special consideration must be given to food intolerance and allergies. In this regard, a good digestive enzyme or digestive tea following meals helps breakdown, assimilation, and uptake of food. Compulsive under-eaters and compulsive overeaters also have special food issues which must be taken into careful consideration and dealt with individually if a healthy meal plan and long-term behavioral changes are to be maintained.

Which vitamins and other supplements are best for CFIDS?

The subject of nutritional supplements is controversial and I try to be open to and incorporate all points of view as appropriate. If a patient does not have the time to eat an impeccable diet, then I use supplements to augment the protein, minerals, and vitamins missing from the diet. Also, the use of supplements usually will work well for those patients interested in faster progress.

The typical supplements that can be used are the following, always noting that each person must be evaluated individually: lysine, vitamin B, dry vitamin E, beta carotene, buffered, chelated, or esterfied vitamin C, CoQ_{10}, germanium, ginkgo, sea cucumber, and a host of other immune enhancers.

Herbs which can be used include golden seal, suma, astragalus, Pau D'arco, echinacea, and shiitake mushrooms. A full spectrum amino acid supplement is also helpful, but it is crucial to avoid any arginine in the supplement. Various Chinese herbal formulas are usually prescribed based on the patient's constitution and specific symptom picture.

How does acupuncture work to treat CFIDS?

Acupuncture therapy is aimed at treating the whole person as well as individual symptoms. In this regard, acupuncture points are chosen according to such general emotional symptoms as grief, depression, and anxiety, and also for such specific symptoms as insomnia, headaches, anemia, fatigue, flatulence, and bloating.

Acupuncture can be used very effectively for taking the "edge" off an anxious patient. It offers a natural approach to relaxation and a temporary stilling of the typical CFIDS overactive mind. It also works particularly well to energize the person, if the problem of fatigue is based on physical exhaustion or emotional depression.

Typical acupuncture points that I use are listed below, along with a listing of the symptoms which each is used to treat. There's also a Chinese translation of the point. Of course, each point in acupuncture is used for many more problems and symptoms than those listed. I am only giving a general idea for the reader's information. (See the reference section for a more in-depth source on this topic.)

- Stomach 36 (Foot Three Miles) for low energy or poor digestion. This acupuncture point strengthens and tones the spleen and stomach.

- Spleen 4 (Ancestor and Descendant) for flatulence, bloating, hypo-glycemia, and energy

- Heart 7 (Spirit's Gate) for insomnia, anxiety, desire for an excessive amount of cold drinks, and palpitations of the heart

- Liver 3 (Great Thoroughfare) for headaches, detox of the liver, for sore throat, and bloating

- Large Intestine 4 (Adjoining Valleys) is used for constipation or diarrhea, headaches over the eyes or in the sinus, abdominal pain, and sore throat.

- Urinary Bladder 23 (Kidney's Hollow) for weak adrenal glands, chronic fatigue, chronic back pain, memory loss, and sensation of heaviness in the head

- Yin Tang (Seal Hall) calms the emotions and also works on headaches, anxiety, insomnia, emotional insecurity, and a weak pituitary gland affecting the hormones.

- Conception Vessel 3 and 4 (Central Pole and Hinge at the Source) for low energy, lack of groundedness, feeling spacey, dizziness, and memory loss

- Conception Vessel 12 (Middle Stomach Cavity) strengthens and tones the spleen and stomach, works on flatulence, poor digestion, and low energy.

- Conception Vessel 17 (Central Altar) regulates the lungs and breathing, works on anxiety attacks, frequent colds and flu, worry, and asthma.

- Conception Vessel 22 (Heaven's Chimney) stimulates the thyroid gland, throat, low energy, difficulty in speaking one's truth and expressing oneself.

- Ear Acupuncture Points: Shen Men, Lung 1, Lung 2, Liver, and Adrenal

How does homeopathic medicine fit into your treatment program?

Homeopathic medicine can be applied on an emotional level for ongoing emotional themes in a person's life, or it can be used on the physical level to treat specific physical symptoms that are painful or causing the patient discomfort or limitation in other ways. Homeopathy does not cover up the patient's symptoms; it allows the body and emotions to come to terms with reality so that the patient becomes more grounded and centered in himself. Physically and emotionally, homeopathy allows the body to "shed another layer of the onion" of disease, metaphorically speaking. This could mean that a person who was never able to cry over the loss of a loved one many years ago may finally be able to experience the grief in a more authentic way. It could mean that a person who cannot stop crying over a recent loss would suddenly be able to gain a new sense of composure. Homeopathy never causes anything in and of itself; rather, it provides a catalyst for the body and mind to balance and achieve a more authentic equilibrium.

The homeopathic remedies are prescribed based on a wide array of the patient's physical and emotional symptoms. These symptoms are then "matched" to the closest or most similar homeopathic remedy "picture." One need not have all the typical indications of a remedy for the remedy to be effective. Some of the more typical remedy pictures for the CFIDS patient are listed below. (For more complete information on the homeopathic approach, see applicable sections in this book or purchase a homeopathic text.)

- ❀ *Natrum muriaticum* is for people whose symptoms began as a result of the death of a loved one, the trauma of a broken love affair, or death of a cherished pet. Grief, rejection, sadness, or loss are causal factors. The personality is closed off with fear of invasion or robbery. Insomnia with grief is common. They will be worse with consolation, may have migraine headaches at 10 A.M. or 3 P.M., suffer from hay fever, and possibly have fever blisters or suffer from herpes.

- ❀ *Sepia* treats those whose theme is fear or withdrawal, with indifference to those loved best. There may be weeping and irritability, especially before menses. They feel worse when alone, crave sweets and vinegar, have frequent headaches, and may experience hot flashes. They may be adverse to sex or it may cause them pain. All their symptoms are better when moving around, exercising, or dancing.

- ❀ *Arsenicum Album* paints the picture of perfectionism, constriction, obsessive compulsive behavior, insecurity, and anxiety about health. They may have insomnia and not be able to get to sleep until after midnight. They fear disease, cancer, poverty, and death. They can be fastidious, suicidal, restless, moving around all the time. Exhaustion is the keynote and all their symptoms surface and are worse from midnight to 2 A.M. They may have a burning or raw throat or diarrhea.

- ❀ *Nux Vomica* is for those who tend to be irritable, ambitious, hard-driving, impatient, jealous, and with a high sex drive. They fear commitment and marriage in particular, and need stimulants such as coffee, tea, alcohol, sweets, or pastries. Without these to stimulate a depleted system, they will feel exhausted. The system can shut down with toxicity and constipation. They may wake up from 3 to 4 A.M. thinking about business matters.

- ❀ *Pulsatilla* treats patients who lack physical boundaries and limits, so common in patients with CFIDS. They can be needy and clinging, with an unrealistic perception of relationship. They can also be soft, yielding, and mild. Their moods are changeable—they cry easily and feel better with a shoulder to cry on. Men may have a fear of women. Physical symptoms can include cystitis, PMS, chronic headaches, a craving for sweets, ice cream, and butter. They feel terrible after eating fats and rich foods.

- *Coffea cruda* is for people who are mentally and possibly physically hyperactive. They are very toxic. Thinking late at night keeps them awake. They have many neuralgic pains and are sensitive to noises and bright lights.

- *Aurum metallicum* treats those suffering from severe depression, even to the point of being suicidal. Many feel that life is not worth living due to their suffering; they may have financial worries and feel there is little or no possibility of recovery. Physically, they may suffer from joint pains, arthritis.

Which lifestyle changes are necessary for the CFIDS patient?

Although suggestions for lifestyle changes will normally arise in the process of a patient's counseling sessions, it is an important area to focus on from the point of view of the health practitioner as well. If the therapist is not too familiar with CFIDS, I may take the initiative and offer some suggestions.

Typical lifestyle issues that are well worth monitoring include the number of hours at work per day, sleep patterns, exercise levels, and the amount of time spent daily in entertainment, relaxation, meditation, or prayer. If the person is a smoker, takes drugs or alcohol or eats a lot of junk food, these are issues that will need to be seriously addressed as well.

One of the more difficult issues that have to be addressed is the existence of toxins in the home and workplace. Eliminating these impacts on the lifestyle of one's co-workers and those people with whom one lives and socializes. It can be a challenge to enlist their support in order to get one's own needs met. If the person is not in a primary relationship and is not receiving the emotional support they need from close friends, then it is important to establish a social and emotional support system as quickly as possible. Emotional support is a key ingredient to an effective wellness program.

Coordination of the Healing Team

Part of my role as a holistic health practitioner is to coordinate the entire healing process for the patient. This may take the form of serving as a clearinghouse for whatever team the person has assembled to help him through the healing process. Often this involves initiating telephone calls to others on the team, such as his medical doctor, chiropractor, or therapist. The main thing is to ensure that communication is open among all participants of the healing team. This will make certain that treatment goals and procedures are compatible and complementary.

What is health relative to CFIDS?

One important concept to keep in mind in treating CFIDS is that treatment involves the *process* of recovery, rather than the *product* of recovery. Emphasize is on the word *process* because CFIDS, even more than with nearly all other disease processes (emotional or physical), requires a process-oriented approach to achieve any real level of recovery.

Our Western cultural viewpoint on disease has been to dissect it into its constituent parts and then treat each individual part as an independent entity. The Western medical approach treats a headache as if it's a pain in the head, an ulcer as if the problem is with the stomach, constipation as if the bowel is at fault. After treating each separate part to get rid of the symptom, the Western doctor puts the patient back together again—stitches him up, so to speak, and expects health or healing to have occurred. But is this what real health is, and is this really the way the human body functions?

An increasing number of people are beginning to expect and demand more from our health care system. We are realizing a deeper connection and interrelatedness between the mind, the body, and all the various parts in the body. We are learning that if you affect with one part, it in turn affects other parts.

In reality, if our treatment is only to remove a symptom, then the symptom will keep recurring in another closely-related organ somewhere else. If an emotional symptom is "pushed down" by a drug, or suppressed and ignored, in many cases it will resurface in the physical body.

The human body is a complex interaction of various parts, inseparably connected to the mind, emotions, and spirit. A headache can be caused by indigestion, sun exposure, hypoglycemia, tension, structural problems, muscle spasms, emotional problems, etc. Constipation can be caused by emotional problems, poor diet, indigestion, allergy, or liver and gallbladder problems.

With CFIDS we have a tremendous opportunity, because the CFIDS patient displays such a wide array of symptoms and creates such a broad pattern of physiological and emotional symptoms. We have the unprecedented opportunity to approach CFIDS holistically—as a healing *process*.

To deal with the patient as a whole entity in an ongoing process, not just as a deficient immune system or an emotionally depressed person, offers an opportunity for self-discovery and integration in the midst of a health crisis.

Such a complex symptom picture will not be cured by one simple pill or surgical procedure. That's the wonderful perspective of CFIDS with this outlook—we are almost forced to see its cure as an ongoing process, rather than as a single event in time.

When fully understood, process healing work is much more palatable and easy to accept than the Band-Aid approach common in Western medicine. Process work allows us to accept the ups and downs so common with CFIDS. Not only that, it's the only thing that will truly work.

What does spirituality have to do with healing CFIDS?

Another important dimension of CFIDS is found in its potential for spiritual growth and newfound meaning to life. In other words, what *is* the ultimate meaning or purpose behind a patient "getting" or "allowing in" or "falling victim to" CFIDS? I do not mean to imply that the person suffering from CFIDS is responsible for getting the disease. This "wellness macho" philosophy isn't very helpful to the healing process; it only sets up a climate of guilt, blame, or shame. But there *is* an opportunity to obtain information on the meaning of one's life when one is suffering from this disease. Moreover, it has been my experience that unless one is ready to examine his life and make changes—attitudinal and behavioral—it is much harder to effect a long-term healing.

Although we do not cause illness or bring it on ourselves, often after careful examination we can discover underlying beliefs in our emotions, thoughts, and spirituality that can be changed in order to promote healing.

The following quote may help to create some clarity:

One woman described her cancer as "the gift for the person who has everything." By this she meant that all her life she had looked for a teacher, a way through the mental and emotional pain that so often accompanied her desires and resistance to life. But it was not until she got cancer that she started to focus on the greater work to be done, on the healing for which she took birth…

" When healing becomes our priority, when being fully alive becomes a necessity instead of a mild, dilettantish interest, then real healing can occur…we forget that our healing comes in a willingness to be healed, a readiness to go beyond the old to something absolutely new and enter into the present moment… All of this sounds good on paper, but it is often easier said than done… Yet what other choice do we have than to try to grow into our bodies?"*

The CFIDS patient may no longer have much of a choice. S/he is up against the wall. The only choice is the one to become present in the here and now with the pain and symptoms, to confront it head-on, and be open to whatever larger shifts in attitude and behavior may be required.

CFIDS offers us a powerful motivation to reevaluate our life's meaning, to slow down, to nurture our inner child, to reconnect with one's loved ones, to take up a hobby, and to begin or place added emphasis on a path to healthier relationships with ourselves, our life's work, and with other people in our lives.

Such an opportunity! An opportunity in the midst of crisis. And with the loving support of a healing team, this crisis can and is being turned into opportunity by many CFIDS sufferers.

---

* *Healers on Healing*, by Richard Carlson, Ph.D. and Benjamin Shield. Tarcher, Inc. 1989.

COMMON QUESTIONS ABOUT CFS

How common is chronic fatigue?

Most research has shown that it is about one percent of the population, or about 2.4 million people. Chronic fatigue usually affects people in their twenties and thirties, and twice as many women as men are likely to be affected.

Why are women more prone?

It may be that women are much more likely to go to doctors in the first place. It may also be that there is some hormonal involvement, and that imbalances of estrogen and progesterone make one more susceptible to chronic fatigue.

Why is Chronic Fatigue Syndrome (CFS) so hard to diagnose?

At first glance CFS looks a lot like PMS, hypothyroid, hypoglycemia, Candida albicans, Lyme disease, lupus, depression, anxiety, insomnia, and a host of other illnesses. Since it resembles so many other problems, a diagnosis becomes a process of ruling out all these other diseases.

Don't most doctors feel CFS is all in the head?

Yes! Many doctors just prescribe antidepressant medications. A survey of doctors showed that only ten percent would treat it with anything more than bed rest.

What are the symptoms of CFS?

Persistent flulike symptoms, aches and pain, fatigue, sore throat, mild fever, lymph gland swelling, headaches, joint pains, depression, forgetfulness, irritability, inability to concentrate and difficulty getting to sleep are the primary symptoms. But each patient is unique and may have very different symptoms. Also, different symptoms may surface over the course of the healing process than were present at the initial onset of the illness.

How does the illness usually start?

Most patients will develop more and more fatigue symptoms over a period of three to six months. It usually creeps up on you, rather than coming on suddenly, although it can sometimes begin after a cold or flu.

Is CFS contagious?

Opinions vary, and many people living in the same household as CFS patients never get the disease. It is probably contagious and only certain people, perhaps those with a weak immune system, are more susceptible than others.

Is it caused by a virus?

At first it was believe to be caused by the Epstein-Barr virus (a relative of mononucleosis). Although I routinely test for the EB virus in the blood, it is probably not the cause but rather an effect of the compromised immune system.

What about the scare that CFS may be some form of AIDS?

There is absolutely no connection between CFS and AIDS! CFS and AIDS are distinctly different illnesses with many different symptoms. A simple blood test can rule out AIDS, and also tell you whether you have any immune problems to be concerned about. .

Do doctors agree on the treatment for CFS?

There are basically five camps of doctors. 1) Those who don't even believe in the illness in the first place. 2) Those that believe it is a form of depression and give antidepression medications. 3) Those who believe it is a distinct illness but do not know how to treat it and just recommend bed rest. 4) Those who believe it is real but aren't exactly sure what to do to treat it. Many of these doctors confuse it with Candida and only use vitamins or recommend psychotherapy. 5) Those, like myself, who specialize in the treatment of CFS and utilize many different treatments including vitamin therapy, nutritional guidance, acupuncture, homeopathy and Chinese herbal remedies.

Does the illness ever run its course?

Most of my patients are better within three months after starting treatment. Some people recover faster and some take longer. It depends on how long they have had it and how many lifestyle changes they are willing to make to get rid of it.

How soon do you think there will be a cure for CFS?

There already is. It is only through ignorance and disbelief that many doctors claim there is no known treatment. I have wonderful success treating CFS.

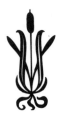

*Herpes simplex—An infectious virus which recurs in the same area of the skin, usually at a site where the mucous membrane joins the skin

Herpes Zoster—a type of herpes eruption (a painful blister type of eruption) which affects only certain parts of body, usually the face and upper body, and usually only occurs on one side

**Nosode—a type of homeopathic remedy made from human diseased tissue, such as tuberculinum or syphillinum.

THE HOLISTIC APPROACH TO THE TREATMENT OF CHICKENPOX

During the spring months chicken pox becomes more common than other times of the year. This is consistent with Oriental medical theory since chicken pox is a disease of Liver Wind. The liver is overactive during the spring months. For more information on the Five Element correlations, please see the section beginning on page 56.

The primary treatment for chicken pox according to Western medicine is to use antihistamines if the itching becomes unbearable. But with the use of herbs and homeopathic remedies, it is possible to lessen the effects of chicken pox substantially.

Chicken pox is a viral disease and is closely related to the virus of herpes zoster* (not herpes simplex*). The period of time between when you are exposed to it and when you actually begin to develop symptoms is from eleven to twenty-one days. The most common way to get it is to touch someone who has it already. You can give it to someone else (i.e. are "contagious") from a few days before you begin to break out yourself until the last pimple is crusted over.

To help the person (usually a child) heal faster, the following herbal formula is very effective: Take one tablespoon each of marigold flower, pennyroyal, and raspberry leaves. Steep them in a quart of boiled water, covered, for fifteen minutes, then strain. For a child age 4 and younger give two tablespoons, four times per day; for a child 5 years or older, give 4 tablespoons, four times per day.

If there is a fever, take two tablespoons elder flower and one tablespoon peppermint leaf; add to two cups boiled water and steep one-half hour; strain and give one-quarter cup to drink, four times per day.

For itching, add a couple handfuls of baking soda or cornstarch to a cool bath. Keep the body cool and away from drafts. Also, you can apply Rescue Remedy salve, Traumeel ointment, or Pau D'arco lotion directly to the blisters. Avena bath, available from most pharmacies, also makes a soothing bath.

Homeopathic remedies for chicken pox include the following:

- ✸ *Rhus tox:* for a restless or irritable child with itching and rashes;
- ✸ *Apis mel:* for extreme itching, with swelling, stinging pain or sudden puffing of large areas of the body;
- ✸ *Aconite:* in the first stages of fever, especially if the child is anxious, fearful and thirsty;
- ✸ *Belladonna:* for headache, flushing, sore throat and fever;
- ✸ *Pulsatilla:* as a preventative for other children or adults exposed to chickenpox;
- ✸ *Malandrinum:* as a preventative or as a nosode** for use concurrently with symptomatic remedies to lessen the amount of time the disease takes to heal.

DR. MARTIN'S SELF-HELP FOR
THE COMMON COLD AND FLU

Most of us sink into dread and depression at the thought of catching a cold or worse still, getting the flu. We fear it, we fight it, and we pump our bodies full of vitamin C to try to prevent it. Once we get a cold or the flu, our most common response is to pump our body full of over-the-counter drugs to dull the pain and discomfort we feel and to cover the symptoms enough to let us continue our normal work and social schedule.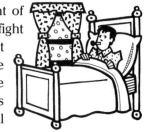

I would like to offer you another option in your outlook and treatment of a cold or flu. Briefly stated, it can actually be turned into a very positive experience. It can be interpreted as a sign that our body is releasing accumulated stress and toxins, that we are out of balance in some part of our life, or that we need to slow down a little, relax, unwind and take some time off.

What contributes to my getting a cold in the first place?

Anything that weakens the immune system can also lead you to get a cold or the flu. Common causal factors can be lack of sleep, emotional upset, undue stress in any part of your life, excess of any demanding physical activity, taking recreational drugs, undereating and/or not getting the proper nutrients into your system, overeating foods such as sugar, sweets, chocolate, greasy or fried foods, or overdoing beverages such as coffee, alcohol or black tea.

Overuse of space heaters during the winter months, or going back and forth between air conditioning and the warmth of outdoors during the spring or autumn months can also contribute.

Of course, to some extent, we are powerless over whether we get a cold or not. We all know some people who never catch colds. Others, have three or four per year. In other words, you must have a constitutional predisposition to getting colds in order to get one in the first place.

The seasonal changes also are beyond our control, and most colds begin during the fall or winter seasons. When houses and offices are sealed up to keep warmth in during the colder months, toxins can accumulate in the air and weaken our immune systems, sometimes called "Sick Building Syndrome."

What does Oriental medicine have to say about colds and the flu?

According to Oriental medicine, colds can be caused by at least three different factors:

Type 1 originates from excessive heat in the Stomach and Spleen Meridians. The primary symptoms might include sore throat, swollen glands, strep infection, fever, pain in the neck and shoulders and possible diarrhea or constipation with stomach upset. The cause is from excessive worry, anxiety, obsessive thinking or from an excess intake of fats, or hot, spicy foods and from overeating in general.

Type 2 originates from what is called Wind-Cold invading the Lung meridian. Symptoms may include runny nose, sneezing, soreness and aching all over the body, mucus, fever, chills and coughing. The cause is usually from not dressing warmly enough as the weather changes from warm to cold, from getting caught in a cold wind, from going back and forth between the warmth of indoors to the cold outdoors, or from the warmth outdoors to air-conditioning indoors. The emotions corresponding to the Lung type of cold include sadness, grief and hurt. If these emotions are held in and kept unconscious, especially during the fall season, one may be particularly susceptible to a Wind-Cold type of invasion.

Type 3 originates from a weakness in the Kidney meridian with a corresponding excessive quality in the Liver meridian. Typical symptoms of this are fever, red and itchy eyes, sore and tight muscles, sore throat, headaches, burning urination, pain in the right shoulder blade, low back pain and severe fatigue. The emotional factors contributing to this type of cold include excessive fear weakening the kidneys; or anger, resentment and pent-up feelings that have not been expressed causing the Liver meridian to stagnate and the liver to become toxic.

What is the treatment according to Oriental medicine?

Of course, the first treatment that we use in Oriental medicine is acupuncture and herbs. Each type of cold or flu, depending on the originating cause, has a specific type of treatment.

There are Chinese herbal formulas for all types of colds and flu. For example, *Yin Qiao Formula* is to be used during the first stages of the Wind-Cold or Wind-Heat type of cold with symptoms of congestion, fever, sore throat, swollen glands and aching shoulders and neck.

Zhong Gan Ling Formula is used when the fever and sore throat are the predominant symptoms. There may also be headaches and strep throat with a cough. *Minor Blue Dragon Formula* is used when a watery nasal discharge is the primary symptom. This formula is also useful in hay fever. *Minor Bupleurum Formula* is good for strengthening the immune system in general. It also helps to detoxify the liver in the case of Liver Heat. This formula can also be used for anxiety, poor appetite or poor sleep.

For treatment of fatigue, restlessness, lack of will power, low sex drive or dizziness, formulas for the kidney are used. *Quiet Contemplative Formula* is used to increase Kidney Yin and *Dynamic Warrior Formula* for weakness in Kidney Yang. Other formulas include *Gan Mao Ling* for strengthening the immune system, to reduce fever and reduce throat inflammation, and *Ping Chuan Pill* for asthma-like symptoms with cough, phlegm and difficulty breathing.

Pill Curing Formula is great for any type of digestive upset, especially if the cold began with some type of dietary indiscretion.

Herbal formulas are usually taken 2–3 tablets, three to four times per day. As soon as the symptoms lessen, the herbs should be stopped.

Acupuncture treatments are given at the onset of a cold and every two to three days until the cold has been resolved. Acupuncture works to strengthen the immune system and to resolve the blockage in whichever acupuncture meridians are involved in the cold.

Which common Western herbs can I use for a cold?

Garlic is probably the most well known cure-all. It has natural antibiotic properties, and can help to boost your resistance to infection, both bacterial and viral. You can add several mashed cloves to salads to help overcome the feeling of an oncoming cold and to cleanse the intestinal tract. You can also eat the cloves alone. Garlic capsules and tablets which have had the unpleasant smell removed are a good substitute for those who are taking homeopathic remedies (since raw garlic antidotes, i.e. negates, the effect of the remedies.)

Peppermint added to other teas has a cleansing effect on the whole body. With a pinch of yarrow and licorice root, peppermint will bring on the needed perspiration in case of a fever. It also has a settling effect on the stomach in case of nausea, poor appetite or vomiting. (*Note that mint in any form will also antidote homeopathic remedies.*)

Ginger Root is very good to bring on perspiration and to help in digestive problems. Many people know this herb for its healing properties during the morning sickness of pregnancy.

Cayenne Pepper is one of the great anti-cold herbs, especially useful if you have a lot of mucus, nasal and lung congestion. Either take one cayenne capsule three to four times per day or mix an eighth of a teaspoon into a cup of warm water and drink it down fast. This will clear out the lungs and nose. *Note that if you have ulcers or are prone to heartburn, do not take cayenne.*

Sage tea is good for a sore and red throat. Try gargling with sage tea and drinking eight ounces three to four times per day. Use ten ounces of boiled water to one teaspoon of sage leaves and let it steep for five to ten minutes.

What acupressure points can I use for a cold?

Massage the points indicated in "The Neck and Shoulder Release" (page 93) for a few minutes each. This will really help! These points relate primarily to the Lung and Gallbladder meridians.

What can I do for coughing?

The following acupressure points can be used for coughing. If the person is deficient, tired, lacks energy, has a weak cough and clear mucus, or is anemic, then use Lu 9 at the wrist crease. But if s/he has an excess condition with fever, red face, yellow mucus, or constipation, use Large Intestine 4 (LI 4 or *Hoku*, see page 94), Lung 5 and 6 (Lu 5 and Lu 6).

Which homeopathic remedies are good for colds?

(If you are new to homeopathy, you may want to try experimenting with a homeopathic formula from the health food store that is specifically for colds and the flu instead of trying to determine the correct single remedy for your particular set of symptoms.)

Remember that homeopathy is most effective when you can find the perfect match of one unique homeopathic remedy with your particular and unique set of symptoms. There are many different remedies for colds, and here are just a few of the most common ones.

Aconite 12X–30X is for the first stages of a cold, especially if it comes on after exposure to cold winds. You may awake at night, sometimes frightened, with a fever; no nasal discharge; hot dry skin; thirsty; dry cough; worse from 11–12 P.M.

Belladonna 12X–30X works well with sudden colds with high fever, burning hot skin, dreamy or spaced look, glassy eyes with wide pupils; red cheeks; sore throat; worse around midnight; worse from loud sounds or bright lights; better from rest and desires warmth.

Ferrum Phosphoricum 6X –30X is used when the onset is early in morning with slower and less dramatic symptoms, especially if you have tried other remedies for fever and sore throat and they have not cured the case; raw, scratchy throat; weakness; dull headache; pale face.

Arsenicum Album 12X–30X is for fever and chills; craves warmth; thin, watery nasal discharge that burns upper lip; watery, burning diarrhea; mental or physical restlessness at night, especially around midnight; anxiety; no desire for cold drinks; cough is better when sitting up and worse when lying down; insomnia.

Pulsatilla 12X–30X for an abundance of nasal discharge with thick, yellow-green mucus; no thirst; weepy and desiring company; cough with chest congestion; symptoms change readily and are worse in a warm, stuffy room and better in open air or with cool topical applications; craves affection.

Gelsemium 12X–30X for the aching muscles and chills that accompany colds; shivering up the spine with fever and weakness; trembling; no thirst; headache at the back of the head; watery runny nose which burns; sneezing; fatigue with droopy eyelids; preference for open air and quiet.

Eurpatorium Perf. 12X–30X when the predominant symptoms are aching bone pains; pain in the eye sockets; nausea; chills; feels bruised or sore in the low back.

How do I take the homeopathic remedies?

In general, take 4–6 tablets three to four times per day. If it is the correct remedy, a couple of doses should begin to bring relief so that you can cut down on the number of times you take the remedy. If the remedy does not work after a few doses, it is the wrong remedy. Wait three to four hours and try another remedy.

It is always best to begin with a low potency, such as 6X or 12X. If it begins to work and then suddenly stops, you may need the next higher potency. Try a 30X. It is best not to use any potency higher than a 30X unless you are experienced at using homeopathy.

Remember that sometimes homeopathy can cause a healing aggravation. If your symptoms get worse instead of better, remember that this is a good sign. It means that you have chosen the remedy well. But always be sure to stop the remedy immediately to let your body balance itself out *before* administering more remedies. When in doubt, wait! Don't give more medication if you are not sure what the current remedy is doing.

What else can I do to get rid of a cold?

Remember to slow down, stay at home, nurture yourself and use the time to let your creative, soft side emerge. Ask a friend for a massage (especially the upper back and neck area).

Should I keep covered up or is this an "old wives' tale"?

Yes, you should cover up. The acupressure points on the nape of the neck are called the Wind's Door and Lung's Hollow, and it is here that cold can enter the body easily. So to help prevent a cold or to keep a cold from getting worse, one should keep this part of the body covered and warm.

What do I have in my kitchen to take for a cold?

You can make a simple drink composed of five ½-inch slices of fresh ginger (with the skin left on), about three green onions (just the white part), and a little honey. Add 1 quart water, boil for about five minutes, turn the heat off, cover and steep for fifteen minutes. Sip on this throughout the day.

Another effective drink consists of grating a two-inch piece of fresh ginger root, adding two cups of boiling water and simmering for twenty minuets. Then add two tablespoons of lemon juice, one tablespoon of honey and a pinch of cayenne pepper.

What is the role of a fever?

A fever is the body's way of keeping a cold or flu virus from multiplying. It is a primary part of the body's natural arsenal to kill the virus by using your own natural immunity. It is best not to suppress a fever with drugs, since the use of even aspirin will be prolonging the life of the cold or flu and lessening your overall immune response.

Using homeopathic remedies for fever is the best approach since they will work with your body's immune system instead of against it. The properly selected homeopathic remedy is effective in lowering a fever not by suppressing it but by increasing your body's immune response.

A cool bath or cool towels placed on the forehead and feet may also be used. You may also want to take a warm bath with a strong dose of fresh brewed ginger tea added to the bath. After soaking for twenty minutes, wrap yourself up in blankets and try sweating out the fever and accumulated toxins.

What are some general supplements I can take for any type of cold or flu symptoms?

❋ *Zand Insure Herbal*—take three tablets, four times per day or two droppersful four times per day.

❋ *Oscillococcinum* or *Flu Solution*—this over-the-counter homeopathic remedy is great and will often stop a cold or flu before it gets started or stop it in its tracks.

❋ Vitamins C (buffered or esterfied), B (balanced), E (dry or emulsified), and beta carotene

❋ *Lysine*—an amino acid which works well for fighting viral infections

❋ *Suma* and *Astragalus Herbs*

❋ *Cyclone Cider*—available from health food stores. But if you are taking homeopathic remedies, don't take this since it has garlic in it.

What else should I do to get well fast?

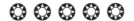

Be sure to keep your bowels open and moving. Constipation encourages the accumulation of toxins in the body. (On the other hand, diarrhea is just as bad because it depletes your body of yin and valuable minerals you need to get better.) Also be sure to get plenty of rest. Sleep as much as possible. Remember that if you have a fever, do not suppress it with over-the-counter drugs. A fever is a good sign that your body is fighting the infection.

Be considerate of others and stay at home if you are sneezing, coughing or have a lot of mucus. Although the reason for catching a cold is a lot more complex than the simple germ, it is a fact that without coming into contact with the cold or flu virus, you will not get it. Wash your hands frequently since research has shown that the way germs are most frequently passed is through the hands.

Eat very lightly, eating only easy-to-digest foods. You will want most of your energy going to fight the infection and not into digestion. Soups, broths, steamed vegetables and simple, well-cooked grains are best. For protein, try relying on vegetable sources such as tofu, split peas, lentils and beans. If you are having trouble with digestion, be sure to take digestive enzymes.

Most importantly, keep your emotions open. If you are uncertain as to whether you may have some emotional "constipation," try writing in a journal, talking to a good friend or opening an inner dialogue with your inner child. If you discover you have some long standing issues which are not being addressed, you may want to consider seeing a therapist for some deeper counseling work. Ask your health practitioner for a good referral.

❋ ❋ ❋ ❋ ❋

JOURNALING EXPERIENCE

Sit quietly with your journal beside you. Take a few deep breaths, let go of muscle tension, and try to relax. Give yourself permission to feel your whole body. Close your eyes and ask yourself which part is the most disturbed or in the most pain at this moment. Fully feel the sensation. Allow yourself to feel without judgment. If it is your throat, allow yourself to feel the pain. Swallow and feel the pain. If it is a congested nose and headache, feel this. No judgment.

Now ask this part of your body to speak. "If you could talk, what would you want to tell me?" Wait. Just wait for words to come up. If nothing comes up, try again. "If you could talk with a voice of your own, what would you tell me?" Now open your eyes and begin to write whatever comes.

The writing isn't necessarily supposed to make sense. Just be spontaneous and let your pen write whatever is coming up for you. If emotions occur, you may want to breathe deeply, or even let out some anger, tears, or moans. It's O.K. to feel. (Remember that it is not your fault that you got sick, but you may be able to use the experience to derive deeper meaning from what is going on in your life.)

Now that you have identified an inner voice that speaks for the part of you that is in pain, try opening a dialogue with this part. In your journal, allow yourself to write a question such as:

What do you want from me?

What did I do to you to make you feel so angry?

Don't you love me?

Why won't you let me go to work today?

I'm really angry with you; why did you do this to me?

Then write down the answer. Ask another question such as, "What would you like for me to do different in the future?" Ask again, and again write the answers as they come to you.

This type of journaling can be very effective in helping you to recover more quickly. If appropriate, it is always a good idea to share some or all of what you have written with a close friend, spiritual counselor, or therapist.

TREATING COLDS AND FLU WITH HERBS

The following are four of the most common herbs, with instructions for their use in the treatment of colds and the flu.

Garlic

This is probably the most well known "cure all" herb. It has natural antibiotic properties, and can help to boost your resistance to infection, both bacterial and viral. You can add several mashed cloves to salads to help overcome the feeling of an oncoming cold and to cleanse the intestinal tract. You can also eat the cloves alone, although most people find this a bit hard to stomach. Garlic capsules and Kyolic brand garlic are good substitutes for those who don't want to deal with the aroma of the raw cloves.

Another good formula is to crush a few cloves of garlic, add a dash of cayenne pepper and bring to boil. Then add the juice of one lemon and a tablespoon of honey, and sip. (If you are on homeopathic remedies, you must refrain from taking any kind of garlic.)

Peppermint

Peppermint added to other teas has a cleansing effect on the whole body. It helps with bad breath as well. With a pinch of yarrow and licorice and ginger root it will bring on the needed perspiration in the case of a fever. It also has a settling effect, as does ginger root, on the stomach in the case of nausea or vomiting. (Also do not use peppermint if you are using homeopathic remedies.)

Cayenne Pepper

This is one of the great anti-cold herbs, especially useful if you have a lot of mucus and congestion. Either take one cayenne capsule, or mix an eighth-teaspoon of the ground pepper into a cup of warm water and drink it down fast. This will clear out the lungs and nose. CAUTION: If you may have ulcers, do not take cayenne, as it will burn the stomach lining.

Sage

This common desert herb is great for a sore throat. Try making a concoction and gargling with sage tea and drinking the remainder. Use ten oz. boiling water to one teaspoon of the leaves and let it steep for five minutes. You can gather your own sage in the Western desert areas quite readily.

COLD & FLU FOLK REMEDY

(good for sore throat, cough, fever, aches and pains, headaches)

✧ ¼ cup of apple cider vinegar

✧ 1 to 2 cups of water

✧ 1–2 tablespoons honey

✧ ¼–1 teaspoon cayenne pepper (red pepper)

SIP THIS WHILE IT'S WARM

(for added benefit, sip while taking a hot bath)

SIMPLE MEASURES TO PREVENT FLU, COLDS, INFECTION & DISEASE

1. Never share your makeup, toothbrush, combs or hairbrush. Be careful when testing cosmetics in stores never to use products which others have touched. Shared makeup spreads bacteria, viruses and fungi, and possibly herpes.

2. Never sneeze or cough into your hands. Use a tissue and immediately discard it.

3. Wash your hands often, especially after coming into contact with others, and always before wiping your face or nose. Cold viruses are spread by shaking hands, touching doorknobs, etc.

4. Use a tissue when touching toilet seat handles or doorknobs in the public restrooms whenever possible.

5. Avoid contact with others who may be infected. Ask your co-workers to stay at home when they feel sick and are sneezing. Avoid plane travel if possible, since the air is recirculated. Eighty percent of illness enters through the membranes of the nose and eyes. Or purchase a personal ozone generator to protect you while flying.

6. Take plenty of buffered, esterified, or chelated Vitamin C, dry or emulsified vitamin E, and beta carotene and add the appropriate herbs and homeopathic remedies to your daily regimen.

7. Get plenty of quality rest, take naps when possible, don't "stuff" your feelings, and exercise daily.

FLU SHOTS: WHO NEEDS THEM?

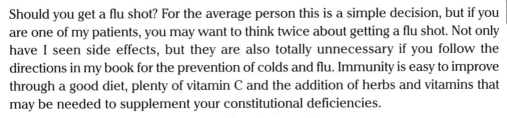

Should you get a flu shot? For the average person this is a simple decision, but if you are one of my patients, you may want to think twice about getting a flu shot. Not only have I seen side effects, but they are also totally unnecessary if you follow the directions in my book for the prevention of colds and flu. Immunity is easy to improve through a good diet, plenty of vitamin C and the addition of herbs and vitamins that may be needed to supplement your constitutional deficiencies.

If you are not being treated by classical homeopathy (which is by far the most effective way to strengthen your immune system), the next best thing is to follow the directions in my book and to take either homeopathic *influenzium* or *oscillococcinum*.

Over and over my patients tell me, "Everyone in my office is sick and I didn't get it," or "I got a cold and was back at work in one day, and everyone else was out for a week." The message: This holistic health thing really does work!!!

ON THE TREATMENT OF DIABETES USING HOMEOPATHY, ORIENTAL MEDICINE AND NUTRITIONAL COUNSELING

We often think of a disease like diabetes as a modern-day phenomenon, but ancient Chinese doctors were also battling with diabetes. They discovered an amazing detection method for detecting sugar in the urine. They had the patient pass urine on a wide, flat brick to see if ants gathered to collect the sugar in the urine. As far back as 752 A.D., pork pancreas was used as treatment for diabetes—an approach very similar to the use of modern-day insulin.

What is the cause of diabetes?

According to Western medicine, diabetes has a number of different causes and there are a number of different types of diabetes, but simply stated, most people who have diabetes have what is called diabetes mellitus. Technically, this is defined in the medical books as increased sugar in the blood.

There are two types of diabetes mellitus. Type 1, also known as juvenile onset diabetes, is a condition in which the body is unable to produce its own insulin. In Type 2, or adult onset diabetes, the body can usually produce insulin but is unable to make proper use of it. Type 1 is insulin-dependent and more difficult to treat and Type 2 can often be treated using less severe methods.

In healthy people, the amount of sugar, or glucose, in the blood is kept in balance by a mechanism in the body called blood sugar homeostasis. In other words, an organ called the pancreas secretes the proper amount of a chemical called insulin. Once the insulin is secreted and hits the bloodstream, the body knows how to utilize it properly.

But in diabetes mellitus, there is deficient insulin secreted by the pancreas, or it is not utilized properly by the body, and this causes the blood sugar to rise to excessive amounts. Typically, the diagnosis is made through taking a blood and urine sample and then noting elevated sugar in both.

Typical symptoms may include excessive urination, itching, excessive thirst, increased food intake or an abnormally strong desire for sweets. The cause of the pancreas dysfunction according to Western-trained medical doctors is uncertain, but it *is* known that such things as heredity, age and stress may be partial causes.

What is the treatment according to Western medicine?

As with most health problems, the Western approach to treating the problem is less concerned with finding and treating the cause than it is in trying to get rid of the symptoms of the problem. The basic Western treatment is to regulate the diet so that you never drive the blood sugar up to unacceptable levels. When the diet is adequate and excess glucose still appears in the blood and urine, then Western doctors prescribe insulin.

What is the treatment using homeopathic medicine?

According to homeopathic theory, we match the individual symptoms of the patient with the particular keynote symptoms of the homeopathic remedies. To do this, a thorough case history of the patient is taken along with a complete subjective description of symptoms in the patient's own words. In addition, all the other aspects of the patient's health are assessed and matched to a single, unique homeopathic remedy. For example, twenty diabetic patients may receive twenty **different** homeopathic remedies.

The emotional life of the patient may be very significant in determining the correct remedy. Other apparently unrelated physical factors such as digestion, sleep patterns, food likes and dislikes, skin problems, etc., may also be critical in determining the right remedy.

Note that there are many different approaches to prescribing homeopathic remedies. The approach I use is to prescribe single homeopathic remedies, one at a time. Although some other homeopaths may use multiple remedies, or give one remedy right after the other, I have found my approach, called Classical Homeopathy, to work best. Some Classical Homeopaths give **only** one remedy at a time, at intervals of three to six months. I usually give remedies more often than this. Depending on the patient and their particular problems and lifestyle, I sometimes will mix and match homeo-pathic approaches. I call this "eclectic homeopathy," but the Classical style of prescribing tends to work the best with most people.

A "typical" homeopathic remedy will be chosen based on the process of "repertorization." This is the process of matching the patient's symptoms with the keynotes of the homeopathic remedy. A "typical" patient's case follows, utilizing my computer program called MacRepertory. This program consists of more homeopathic data than any one person could possibly retain without the aid of a computer.

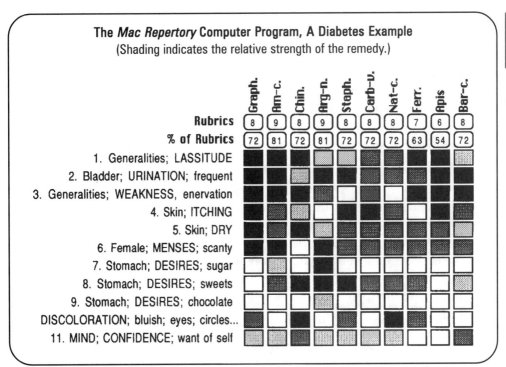

The *Mac Repertory* Computer Program, A Diabetes Example
(Shading indicates the relative strength of the remedy.)

	Graph.	Am-c.	Chin.	Arg-n.	Staph.	Carb-v.	Nat-c.	Ferr.	Apis	Bar-c.
Rubrics	8	9	8	9	8	8	8	7	6	8
% of Rubrics	72	81	72	81	72	72	72	63	54	72

1. Generalities; LASSITUDE
2. Bladder; URINATION; frequent
3. Generalities; WEAKNESS, enervation
4. Skin; ITCHING
5. Skin; DRY
6. Female; MENSES; scanty
7. Stomach; DESIRES; sugar
8. Stomach; DESIRES; sweets
9. Stomach; DESIRES; chocolate
10. DISCOLORATION; bluish; eyes; circles...
11. MIND; CONFIDENCE; want of self

As can be seen from the chart, across the top are listed the possible homeopathic remedies for this patient. Across the left side are listed the unique and individual symptoms I used for this particular patient. After assessing the patient and studying the individual remedies, one unique homeopathic remedy will be chosen to give this patient. After seeing the patient's progress and response to this remedy, the case will be taken again and a new homeopathic remedy then will be given. This process will be repeated over a period of four to twelve months, depending on the severity of the disease.

What is the treatment approach using Oriental medicine?

Similar to homeopathic medicine, the technique of Oriental medicine is more concerned with treating the cause of an illness than with only eradicating the symptoms. According to Oriental medicine, the cause of diabetes is a weakness of Yin. The Yin deficiency then causes excessive heat to invade and injure the various organs and acupuncture meridians.

Depending on the individual patient, the injury may occur primarily in the Lungs, Spleen or Kidneys. The first is characterized by excessive thirst, the second by excessive hunger, especially for sweets, and the third by frequent urination. Depending on the organ most affected by the Yin deficiency, and the individual symptoms of the patient, the treatment according to Oriental Medicine will be different for each patient.

Treatment is aimed at draining the excessive heat out of the body and strengthening the Yin. Treatment will include the use of Chinese herbal formulas and acupuncture. Treatment usually takes place once per week for a period of up to ten weeks.

Typical Chinese herbal formulas for the treatment of diabetes may include "Six Flavor Tea" or "Jade Spring Pills." The first is used primarily for nourishing the Kidney, Liver and Spleen Yin and in tonifying Kidney and Spleen Chi (energy). The primary indications and symptoms for the use of "Six Flavor Tea" are weakness or low back pain, restlessness, insomnia, night sweats, dizziness, sore throat, impotence and high blood pressure. The primary indications and symptoms for "Jade Spring Pills" are to regulate excessive appetite, relieve excessive thirst, and reduce the quantity of sugar in the urine. Another commonly used herbal formula is called "Quiet Contemplative." This formula is used to strengthen the Kidney Yin function.

Chinese medicine is often combined with assessment and additional treatment by a Western- trained physician, since it is common to utilize insulin at the same time Oriental medicine is used. There is **no conflict** in using the two together. But it is important to monitor the patient's blood sugar since the amount of insulin needed may be less with the introduction of acupuncture or herbs. Oriental medicine also has the potential to strengthen the body so that there will be less long-term side effects from the diabetes over the span of the patient's life.

What is the nutritional approach to treating diabetes?

Using a combined approach of Oriental medicine, nutrition and homeopathic medicine, it *is* possible to reverse the course of this disease. Often the amount of insulin that is needed can be reduced when these complementary treatments are used.

Nutritionally, the best diet must be geared to the individual and their particular diagnosis. Some of the general rules for everyone to follow will be follows: Reduce the intake of fats, fried foods, sugar and sweets, salt, refined carbohydrates, and most dairy products (milk and cheese); increase the intake of complex carbohydrates, low calorie foods, whole grains, whole fruits, and fermented dairy products (whole, live yogurt or kefir).

Fasting is not advisable for diabetics. Avoiding constipation and getting plenty of exercise are both very important. Specific supplements which are helpful include: Vitamin B complex, chromium, buffered, chelated or esterified vitamin C, dry or emulsified vitamin E, lecithin, blueberry leaf tea, garlic and kelp.

The most important thing to remember is to remain hopeful and to keep a positive outlook, reduce stress and stressful situations as much as possible and to begin at least one of the types of holistic treatment outlined in this short article along with your ongoing allopathic Western treatment.

ECZEMA TREATMENT

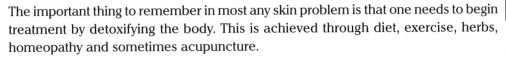

The important thing to remember in most any skin problem is that one needs to begin treatment by detoxifying the body. This is achieved through diet, exercise, herbs, homeopathy and sometimes acupuncture.

The herbal treatment involves the use of specific formulas designs to cleanse the blood and detoxify. I use combination WBC, which contains black walnut, burdock and cayenne, taking three capsules, three times per day. Jason Winters Tea may also be added, as well as a good colon and liver cleanser formula.

During stage one, a detox homeopathic may also be used, depending on the persons constitution. Common homeopathics may be *Sulphur*, *Kali sulph*, *Arsenicum alb*, or *Psorium*. It is important to remember that you may experience a flare up or healing aggravation when healing from the inside out, but that if this occurs it is a sign of progress and you must have patience.

Some of the specific acupuncture points for skin detox include Spleen 10 and Large Intestine 11. Other points are chosen based on the person's individual constitutional type.

The diet includes no eggs, red meat, chicken or fish. No stimulants, alcohol, wine, coffee, etc. No carbonated drinks, sugar or fats.

The diet should consist mainly of grains and vegetables and vegetable sources of protein. Warm water with lemon and fresh carrot juice is very good as well.

ACUTE URINARY TRACT INFECTIONS

Did you know that most acute urinary and bladder infections can be treated with either Chinese herbs, homeopathy, acupuncture or a combination of these three? Actually, most people run to get antibiotics for the first sign of urinary pain, but there is often no need. Here are some suggestions for self-treatment. (If you do not experience relief within twenty-four hours you had better come in to see your doctor as soon as possible. Usually the homeopathic approach will bring quick relief. If not, you are probably taking the wrong remedies.)

First, increase your intake of cranberry juice and other fluids. Also increase your intake of vitamin C, beta carotene and vitamin E in order to strengthen your immune system and ability to fight off whatever bug has attacked you.

The whole principle of this type of treatment is to strengthen your own system rather than needing to kill some bug. If your own system is strong enough, you will be fine in no time!!! Herbs to take include juniper berries, corn silk tea, sarsaparilla and equisetum.

Acupuncture is very effective in cases of infection, but obviously you can't do this on yourself. However, you *can* try a few homeopathic remedies. Some of the most common remedies are:

1. *Berberis vulg*: When the kidneys are also involved and shooting pains occur from the back to the groin.

2. *Cantharis*: This is the first remedy most people try. There is constant urging, burning, and rapid onset.

3. *Mercurius so*: You may also have a fever, pulsating in the urethra, bloody urine, with possible spasms or contractions in the urethra or rectum.

4. *Equisetum*: You may feel a full feeling in the bladder which not relieved by urination. Frequent urging to urinate with severe pain at the close of urination. Urine flows out drop by drop with sharp, burning or cutting pain in the urethra. There may be severe retention with deep pain in the kidney area. The right kidney area may be particularly painful.

A great Chinese formula is called Polyporus. This is useful when the symptoms include extreme thirst, insomnia, fever, decreased urine with pain, bloody urine and possible diarrhea.

Another good Chinese formula is Gentiana Formula. This useful when the cause is Liver-gallbladder damp-heat with headaches, skin heat such as herpes, candida, swelling and concentrated and painful urination.

There are many other homeopathic and herbal remedies, so by all means do not give up. Once you have cured your first infection without resorting to antibiotics your body begins to develop its own immunity and you find yourself less and less susceptible to future infections!!!!

INTERSTITIAL CYSTITIS TREATMENT
(a brief summary of treatment by Dr. Randy Martin)

As with any inflammatory process, we use herbal and homeopathic medications to reduce the inflammation and accompanying pain. We may also utilize acupuncture to relax the body and lower overall inflammation and to reinstate the healing process. Some of the specific suggestions that may be used include the following.

1. Antronex — a natural antihistamine complex by Standard Process

2. Inflavanoids — another natural antihistamine made up of antioxidants

3. Beta Carotene

4. Vitamin E

5. Ester C (an esterified Vitamin C)

6. Zinc Picolinate

7. Blueberry and Bilberry Herbal Extracts

8. Uva ursi tea

9. High potency antibiotics with other co-factors

10. A specific homeopathic remedy designed to aid in pain reduction and healing. This homeopathic remedy will be different for each individual, since every person has slightly different symptoms. Each person also has different stress factors in their life and based on these factors, we will tailor the program to the individual.

I usually will also perform a special urine test to check for enterococcus, which is the type of bacteria commonly involved in interstitial cystitis. This special culture may be positive even if previous urine tests have been negative. Based on the specific bacteria found, an herbal antibiotic may be used to counteract its effects and to strengthen the immune system.

We also perform blood lab tests to detect imbalances in your electrolytes. Based on these tests, we provide supplements to correct the blood deficiencies. This has the effect of healing the person by balancing the body chemistry and building immunity.

A HOLISTIC APPROACH TO ULCERATIVE COLITIS AND CROHN'S DISEASE

According to Chinese medicine, diseases are always an indication of an imbalance on a deeper level. Colitis and Crohn's both relate to other body functions and processes. It is when we have an understanding of the interconnectedness of all these body processes, that we have a better idea of how to treat ulcerative colitis and Crohn's from the holistic perspective.

This article is too short to go into specific diagnostic techniques, but I can share with you some of the general aspects of diagnosis from a holistic perspective. First I use Chinese tongue and pulse diagnosis. After this I perform a hair analysis, blood tests and diagnose according to "body type." I also take a complete history, consisting of about eight pages of information, from infancy to the present, and including your family. From all this information, I diagnose and treat your unique imbalances.

To treat the imbalances, I use acupuncture, Chinese herbs, constitutional homeopathic medicine, diet, and nutritional supplements. Some of the specific supplements and foods that have been shown to be effective for ulcerative colitis and Crohn's are listed below. Note that you should check with your doctor before trying anything new on your own.

Please be sure to **never** take yourself off any prescribed medications without your doctor's supervision. The quantities for supplements and herbs vary with each individual. Not all supplements work for everyone. Your doctor should individually prescribe the holistic program to meet your particular needs.

Sample Therapeutic Foods: potato broth, cooked carrots, okra, parsnips, squash, pumpkin, flax tea, papaya, rice porridge, miso soup, slippery elm gruel, cold water fish, evening primrose oil, black current seed oil, raw cabbage juice, celery juice.

Avoid the following: wheat-containing foods, corn, dairy products, peanuts, red meat, sugar-containing foods, coffee, caffeine, oranges, alcohol, spicy foods, fried foods, salty foods.

Supplements: beta carotene; zinc picolinate; magnesium; folic acid; omega-3 fatty acids; vitamins E, B, and C; lactobacillus acidophilus; liquid chlorophyll; alfalfa tablets; chlorella; quercetin.

THE NATURAL TREATMENT OF WARTS

Is there an alternative treatment for warts or moles?

Yes, most definitely! First, according to Oriental medicine warts are connected to the Liver and Gall Bladder, or the Wood element. So if you have warts or moles that keep growing back, they are most probably an indication of an imbalance or toxicity in your Liver or Gall Bladder meridians.

From the Western medical point of view,, the wart exists independently of any particular pathology. But this should not surprise you, since most problems, according to Western medicine, exist independently of any other body function or cause. Western medicine says that warts are caused by the HPV or the human papiloma virus. But Oriental medicine sees every symptom as connected to other parts of the body and meridian system.

What is the meaning of a wart?

First, it is important to remember that the wart represents an internal imbalance and toxicity and is actually a sign that your body is trying to rid itself of this toxicity. When the wart is burned off, it may drive the imbalance into a deeper part of the body (usually the liver), thus creating an even more difficult time of overall healing.

You must learn to respect your body's symptoms, no matter how benign in appearance or inconvenient they may be, and acknowledge the wisdom of the body to balance itself out by throwing toxicity to the surface where it will do less harm than if contained within the internal, more important organs.

What can I do to treat warts?

Here is what you can do. Nutritionally, you can take the following supplements, which have proven effective in removing warts:

1. Squeeze the contents of one vitamin E capsule on the wart and keep covered with a Band-Aid. Repeat daily for about one to two months.

2. Take vitamin E (in dry form) and beta carotene.

3. Topically apply homeopathic Thuja ointment.

4. Reduce your intake of fats, refined sugars, white flour and dairy products since all of these will cause further stagnation and toxicity in the liver and gall bladder meridians.

5. Consider doing a liver flush. The recipe is on page 179.

6. There are many homeopathic remedies that are very effective in treating warts and moles. Some of the most common are *Thuja*, *Antimonium cruda*, and *Causticum*. You may need the help of an experienced homeopath though since a wart is a symptom of a deeper imbalance and you will probably need to be treated constitutionally and over a longer period of time to permanently remove them.

What message do warts have to tell me on an emotional level?

The Liver and Gall Bladder meridians relate to the emotions of anger and resentment, so you should examine your mode of dealing with stress in your life. Establish coping mechanisms that allow you to release your stress patterns without harming yourself or others. Meditation, guided imagery, walking, swimming, or psychotherapy are some possibilities. You may have already noticed that more warts tend to "grow" during times of stress. This is because the constricted energy is creating further blockage in the liver.

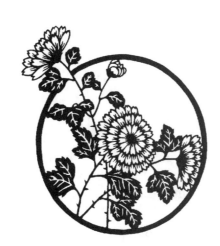

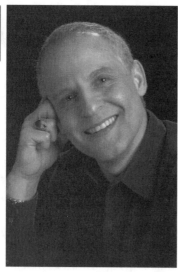

ABOUT THE AUTHOR

Dr. Randy W. Martin is an active member of his community. He serves on the Board of Directors for the local food co-op, volunteers at the local free clinic and donates to various environmental and citizen's rights groups. In addition to his health-related training, he has a B.A. in Psychology and a Master's degree in Urban Planning. Dr. Martin has worked as an environmental resource planner for more than eight years, both for government and as a representative of citizen activist groups, which has given him a unique awareness of how the environment affects our well-being.

Dr. Martin volunteers as a community leader for an AOL Classical Homeopathy chat group and has worked on the staff of many different holistic health clinics and organizations. He is a consultant to the entertainment industry and has appeared frequently on national radio and local television. He serves as an expert witness and has authored several articles for professional homeopathic and Chinese medical journals. He also has produced a series of video and audio tapes on a wide variety of health-related topics.

When not practicing medicine, Dr. Martin enjoys writing; studying kabala, metaphysics and meditation; various types of dance; hiking; and organic gardening.

CONTACT INFORMATION

All products mentioned in this book are available for purchase through Dr. Martin. If you would like more information on Dr. Martin's services, his lecture schedule, or would like a list of products, audio and video tapes that are available through his office, you may reach him at:

Dr. Randy Martin
17000 Ventura Blvd. #220
Encino, CA 91316
(818) 905-6171
e-mail: drrandymartin@optimalhealth4u.com

REFERENCES

Homeopathy

Bach, Edward, M.D. *The Bach Flower Remedies*. New Canaan, Conn.: Keats, 1979.

Coulter, Catherine R. *Portraits of Homeopathic Medicines*, Vol. 1–3. St. Louis: Quality Med. Pub., 1998.

Coulter, Harris L. *AIDS and Syphilis: The Hidden Link*. Berkeley, Calif.: North Atlantic Books, *1987.*

Cummings, Stephen, F.N.P., and Dana Ullman, M.P.H. *Everybody's Guide To Homeopathic Medicines*. New York: Putnam Pub. Group, 1984.

Herscu, Paul, N.D. *The Homeopathic Treatment of Children*. Berkeley, Calif.: North Atlantic Books, 1991.

IBIS Software from AMRITA, Portland, Oregon, 1999.

MacRepertory Software from Kent Homeopathic Associates, Fairfax, Calif., 1998.

Neustaedter, Randall, O.M.D., L.Ac. *The Immunization Decision: A Guide for Parents*. Berkeley, Calif.: North Atlantic Books, 1990.

Smith, Trevor. *The Homeopathic Treatment of Emotional Illness*. Rochester, Vermont: Inner Traditions International, 1998.

Ullman, Dana. *Homeopathy: Medicine for the 21st Century*. Berkeley, Calif.: North Atlantic Books, 1987.

Vitoulkas, George. *The Science of Homeopathy*. New York: Grove Press, distributed by Random House, 1980.

Whitmont, Edward C. *Psyche and Substance*. Richmond, Calif.: North Atlantic Books, 1983.

Herbal Medicine

Bensky, Dan and Andrew Gamble. *Chinese Herbal Medicine: Materia Medica*. Vista, Calif.: Eastland, 1990.

Fratkin, Jake. *Chinese Herbal Patent Formulas: A Practical Guide*. Portland, Oregon: ITM, 1986.

Fratkin, Jake Paul. *Chinese Classics: Popular Chinese Herbal Formulas*. Santa Fe, New Mexico: Shaya Pub., 1990.

Hsu, Hong-Yen, Ph.D., and Chau-Shin Hsu, Ph.D. *Commonly Used Chinese Herb Formulas with Illustrations*. Long Beach, Calif.: DHAI, 1993.

Lust, John. *The Herb Book*, New York: Bantam, 1983.

Treben, Maria. *Health Through God's Pharmacy*. New York: American Ed. Systems, 1995.

Nutrition and Healing

Abravanel, Elliot D., M.D. *Dr. Abravanel's Body Type Diet and Lifetime Nutrition Plan*. New York: Bantam Books, 1988.

Aihara, Herman. *Acid and Alkaline*. Oroville, Calif.: George Ohsawa Macrobiotic Found., 1980.

Airola, Paavo, Ph.D. *Hypoglycemia: A Better Approach*. Sherwood, Oregon: Health Plus Pub., 1977.

Barmakian, Richard, N.D. *Hypoglycemia: Your Bondage or Freedom*. Irvine, Calif.: Altura Health Pub., 1976.

Barnes, Broda O., M.D. *Hypothyroidism: The Unsuspected Illness*. New York: Crowell, 1976.

Bieler, Henry G. *Food Is Your Best Medicine*. New York: Vintage Books, 1973.

Bloomfield Frena, and Gary Butt. *Harmony Rules: The Chinese Way of Health through Food*. New Beach, Maine: Samuel Weiser, 1987.

Brodsky, Greg. *From Eden to Aquarius: The Book of Natural Healing*. New York: Bantam, 1972.

Buchman, Dian Dincin. *Herbal Medicine: The Natural Way to Get Well and Stay Well*. New York: Random House, 1988.

Chaitow, Leon, N.D., D.O. *The Healing Power of Amino Acids*. San Francisco: Thorsons, 1987.

Ferguson, James M., M.D. *Habits, Not Diets*. Menlo Park, Calif.: Bull Pub. Co., 1988.

Gagne, Steve. *Energetics of Food*. Santa Fe, New Mexico: Spiral Sciences, 1990.

Heller, Dr. Rachael F. and Dr. Richard F. *The Carbohydrate Addict's Diet*. New York: Dutton, 1993.

Kushi, Michio. *A Natural Approach to Allergies*. New York: Japan Pub., 1985.

Langer, Stephen E., M.D., and James F. Scheer. *Solved: The Riddle of Illness*. New Canaan, Conn.: Keats, 1995.

Lark, Susan M., M.D., *Premenstrual Syndrome Self-Help Book*. Berkeley, Calif.: Celestial Arts, 1995.

——*The Menopause Self-Help Book*. Berkeley, Calif.: Celestial Arts, 1995.

——*Making the Estrogen Deision*. Berkley, Calif.: Celestial Arts, 1996.

Marmorstein, Jerome, M.D. *The Psycho-Metabolic Blues*. Santa Barbara, Calif.: Woodbridge Press, 1979.

Pritikin, Nathan. *The Pritikin Promise*. New York: Pocket Books, 1991.

Reuben, Carolyn, C.A., and Joan Priestley, M.D. *Essential Supplements for Women*. New York: Perigee Books, 1988.

References

Roth, Geneen. *When Food Is Love*. New York: Dutton, 1992.

Tips, Jack, N.D., Ph.D. *Energy and Addictions*. Austin, Texas: Apple-A-Day, 1988.

Valentine, Tom and Carole. *Medicine's Missing Link: Metabolic Typing and Your Personal Food Plan*. Rochester, Vermont: Thorsons Pub., 1987.

Wilson, Denis, M.D. *Wilson's Syndrome*. Orlando, Florida: Cornerstone Pub Co., 1993.

Oriental Medicine

Beinfield, Harriet and Efrem Korngold. *Between Heaven and Earth: A Guide to Chinese Medicine*. New York: Ballantine, 1992.

Bensky, Dan and John O'Connor. *Acupuncture: A Comprehensive Text*. Vista, Calif.: Eastland, 1981.

Bin, Song Tian. *Atlas of the Tongue and Lingual Coatings in Chinese Medicine*. Beijing: People's Medical Publishing House, 1982.

Clogstoun-Willmott, Johathan. *Western Astrology and Chinese Medicine*. New York: Destiny Books, 1985.

Connelly, Dianne M. *Traditional Acupuncture: The Law of the Five Elements*. Columbia, MD, Centre for Traditional Acupuncture, Inc., 1979.

——*All Sickness is Home Sickness*. Columbia, Maryland: Centre for Traditional Acupuncture, Inc., 1982.

Hammer, Leon, M.D. *Dragon Rises and Red Bird Flies: Psychology and Chinese Medicine*. Barrytown, New York: Station Hill Press, 1980.

Kaptchuk, Ted J., O.M.D. *The Web That Has No Weaver*. Lincolnwood, Illinois: Cont. Pub. Co., 1984.

Kushi, Michio. *How To See Your Health: Book of Oriental Diagnosis*. New York: Japan Pub., 1980.

Requena, Yves. *Character and Health: The Relationship of Acupuncture and Psychology*. Brookline, Mass.: Paradigm Pub., 1995.

Personal Growth, Psychological and Spiritual Resources

Carlson, Richard, Ph.D., and Benjamin Shield. *Healers on Healing*. New York: Putnam, 1989.

Chia, Mantak. *Taoist Secrets of Love*. San Bruno, Calif.: Audio Literature, 1996.

Clow, Barbara Hand. *Liquid Light of Sex*. Santa Fe, New Mexico: Bear & Co., 1991.

Conger, John P. *Jung and Reich: The Body as Shadow*. Berkeley, Calif.: North Atlantic Books, 1988.

Cooper, David A. *Entering the Sacred Mountain*. New York: Random House, 1995.

Dossey, Larry, M.D. *Meaning and Medicine*. New York: Bantam Books, 1991.

Gendlin, Eugene T., Ph.D. *Focusing*. New York: Bantam, 1982.

Goldsmith, Joel S. *A Parenthesis in Eternity*. San Francisco, Calif.: Harper, 1986.

Hendricks, Gay, Ph.D., and Kathlyn Hendricks, Ph.D. *Breathing and the Art of Centering*. New York: Ingram Audio, 1989.

——*The Conscious Heart*. New York: Bantam, 1999.

Johnson, Robert A. *Owning Your Own Shadow: Understanding the Dark Side of the Psyche*. San Francisco, Calif.: Harper, 1993.

Merton, Thomas. *New Seeds of Contemplation*. New York: New Directions, 1972.

Miller, Alice. *The Drama of the Gifted Child*. New York: Basic Books, 1996.

Pollard, Dr. John K. III. *Self Parenting*. Deerfield Beach, Florida: Health Comm., 1992.

Rosenberg, Jack Lee, and Marjorie L. Rand. *Body, Self, and Soul*. Atlantic, Georgia: Humanics, 1985.

Upledger, John E. *Your Inner Physician and You: Craniosacral Therapy and Somatoemotional Release*. Berkeley: North Atlantic Books, 1997.

Bill, W. *As Bill Sees It*. New York: AA World Services, 1967.

Welwood, John, Ph.D. *Journey of the Heart*. New York: Harper Collins, 1996.

Weil, Andrew, M.D. *Health and Healing*. New York: Houghton Mifflin Co., 1995.

Whitmont, Edward C., M.D. *The Alchemy of Healing*. Berkeley, Calif.: North Atlantic Books, 1993.

Veterinary Medicine

Frazier, Anitra. *The New Natural Cat*. New York: Dutton, 1990.

A

B

C

Index

O

P

Q

R

S